Pathophysiology

made

Incredibly Easy!®

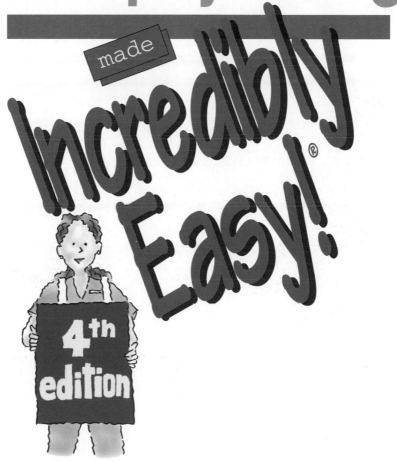

4th edition

Pathophysiology

made

Incredibly Easy! ®

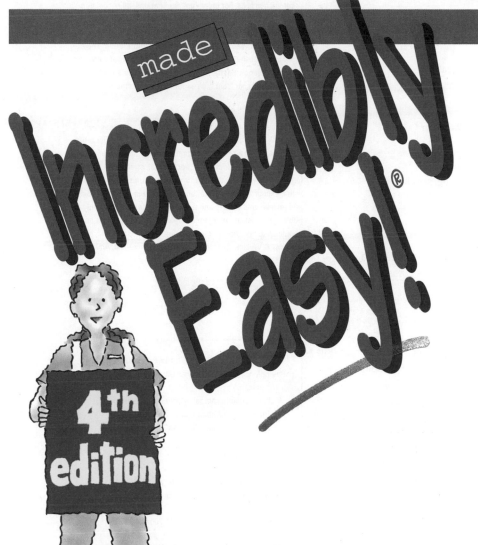

4th edition

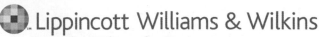

Lippincott Williams & Wilkins
a Wolters Kluwer business

Philadelphia · Baltimore · New York · London
Buenos Aires · Hong Kong · Sydney · Tokyo

Staff

Executive Publisher
Judith A. Schilling McCann, RN, MSN

Editorial Director
David Moreau

Clinical Director
Joan M. Robinson, RN, MSN

Art Director
Mary Ludwicki

Electronic Project Manager
John Macalino

Clinical Project Manager
Beverly Ann Tscheschlog, RN, BS

Editor
Elizabeth Rosto

Copy Editors
Rita Doyle, Amy Furman, Pamela Wingrod

Designer
Lynn Foulk

Illustrator
Bot Roda

Digital Composition Services
Diane Paluba (manager), Joyce Rossi Biletz,
Don Knauss, Donna Morris

Associate Manufacturing Manager
Beth J. Welsh

Editorial Assistants
Karen J. Kirk, Jeri O'Shea, Linda K. Ruhf

Design Assistant
Georg W. Purvis IV

Indexer
Barbara Hodgson

Library of Congress Cataloging-in-Publication Data
Pathophysiology made incredibly easy!—4th ed.
    p. ; cm.
    Includes bibliographical references and index.
    1. Physiology, Pathological. 2. Nursing.
    [DNLM: 1. Pathology—Nurses' Instruction. QZ 4
P3024 2008]
    RB113.P3636 2008
    616.07—dc22
    ISBN-13: 978-0-7817-7912-8 (alk. paper)
    ISBN-10: 0-7817-7912-X (alk. paper)

                                    2007040395

Contents

	Contributors and consultants	*vii*
	Not another boring foreword	*ix*
1	Pathophysiology basics	1
2	Cardiovascular system	17
3	Respiratory system	67
4	Neurologic system	119
5	Gastrointestinal system	167
6	Musculoskeletal system	213
7	Endocrine system	243
8	Renal system	279
9	Hematologic system	313
10	Immune system	339
11	Infection	367
12	Cancer	391
13	Genetics	435
	Practice makes perfect	*466*
	Less common disorders	*499*
	Glossary	*508*
	Selected references	*513*
	Credits	*514*
	Index	*515*

Contributors and consultants

Kim Cooper, RN, MSN
Nursing Department Chair
Ivy Tech Community College
Terre Haute, Ind.

Lillian Craig, RN, MSN, FNP-C
Adjunct Faculty
Oklahoma Panhandle State University
Goodwell

Ellen L. Cummings, RN, MSN, CNRN
Nursing Faculty
Maricopa Community College School District
GateWay Community College
Phoenix, Ariz.

Phyllis Magaletto, MSN, RN, BC
Instructor (Medical-Surgical)
Cochran School of Nursing
Yonkers, N.Y.

Pamela Moody, MSN, PhD, CRNP
Nurse Administrator, Area 3
Alabama Department of Public Health
Tuscaloosa

Theresa A. Petersen, RN, MSN, FNP
Assistant Professor
Montana State University – Northern
Havre

Catherine Shields, RN, BSN
Nurse Educator
Ocean County Vocational Technical School
Toms River, N.J.

Donna L. Van Houten, RN, MS
Nursing Faculty
GateWay Community College (Maricopa Community
    College District)
Phoenix, Ariz.

Sandra McSherry Waguespack, RN, MSN
Instructor
Health Sciences Center School of Nursing
Louisana State University
New Orleans

Colleen R. Walsh, RN, MSN, ONC, CS, ACNP-BC
Faculty, Graduate Nursing
University of Southern Indiana College of Nursing
Evansville

Sharon Wing, RN, MSN
Associate Professor
Cleveland State University

Not another boring foreword

If you're like me, you're too busy caring for your patients to have the time to wade through a foreword that uses pretentious terms and umpteen dull paragraphs to get to the point. So let's cut right to the chase! Here's why this book is so terrific:

 It will teach you all the important things you need to know about pathophysiology. (And it will leave out all the fluff that wastes your time.)

 It will help you remember what you've learned.

 It will make you smile as it enhances your knowledge and skills.

Don't believe me? Try these recurring logos on for size:

Now I get it! explains difficult concepts using illustrations and flowcharts.

Battling illness provides the latest treatments for diseases and disorders.

The genetic link connects genetics to many common disorders.

Memory joggers offer mnemonics and other aids to help you understand and remember difficult concepts.

See? I told you! And that's not all. Look for me and my friends in the margins throughout this book. We'll be there to explain key concepts, provide important care reminders, and offer reassurance. Oh, and if you don't mind, we'll be spicing up the pages with a bit of humor along the way, to teach and entertain in a way that no other resource can.

I hope you find this book helpful. Best of luck throughout your career!

Joy

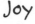

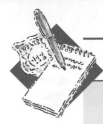

1

Pathophysiology basics

Just the facts

In this chapter, you'll learn:

♦ the structure of cells and how cells reproduce, age, and die

♦ the concept of homeostasis and how it affects the body

♦ the causes of disease

♦ the process of disease development.

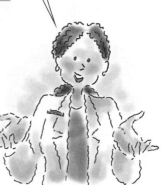

Understanding pathophysiology begins with understanding the body's basic building block: the cell.

Understanding cells

The cell is the body's basic building block. It's the smallest living component of an organism. Many organisms are made up of one independent, microscopically tiny cell. Other organisms, such as humans, consist of millions of cells grouped into highly specialized units that function together throughout the organism's life.

Large groups of individual cells form tissues, such as muscle, blood, and bone. Tissues form the organs (such as the brain, heart, and liver), which are integrated into body systems (such as the central nervous system [CNS], cardiovascular system, and digestive system).

Cell components

Cells are composed of various structures, or *organelles*, each with specific functions. (See *Just your average cell*, page 2.) The organelles are contained in the *cytoplasm*—an aqueous mass—that's surrounded by the cell membrane. The largest organelle, the *nucleus*, controls cell activity and stores deoxyribonucleic acid (DNA), which carries genetic material and is responsible for cellular reproduction or division.

Just your average cell

The illustration below shows cell components and structures. Each part has a function in maintaining the cell's life and homeostasis.

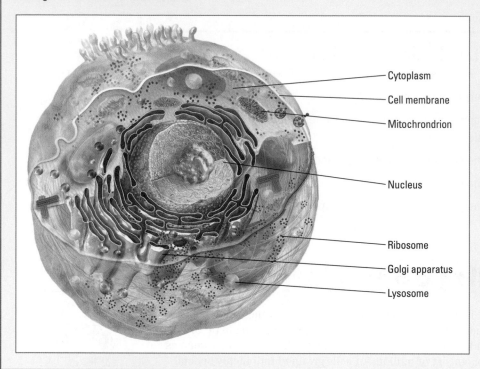

Cytoplasm

Cell membrane

Mitochrondrion

Nucleus

Ribosome

Golgi apparatus

Lysosome

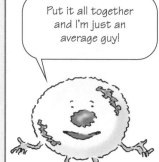

Put it all together and I'm just an average guy!

More components

The typical animal cell is characterized by several additional elements:

• Adenosine triphosphate, the energy that fuels cellular activity, is made by the mitochondria.

• Ribosomes and the endoplasmic reticulum synthesize proteins and metabolize fat within the cell.

• The Golgi apparatus holds enzyme systems that assist in completing the cell's metabolic functions.

• Lysosomes contain enzymes that allow cytoplasmic digestion to be completed.

Cell division and reproduction

Individual cells don't live as long as the organism they're a part of. They're subject to wear and tear and must reproduce and be replaced. Most cells reproduce as quickly as they die.

Cell reproduction occurs in two stages. In the first stage, called *mitosis*, the nucleus and genetic material divide. In the second stage, called *cytokinesis*, the cytoplasm divides, beginning during late anaphase or telophase. At the end of cytokinesis, the cell produces two daughter cells. (See *Replicate and divide.*)

The great divide

Before division, a cell must double its mass and content. This occurs during the growth phase, called *interphase*. Chromatin, the small, slender rods of the nucleus that give it its granular appearance, begins to form.

Replication and duplication of DNA occur during the four phases of mitosis:

 prophase

 metaphase

 anaphase

 telophase.

Replicate and divide

These illustrations show the different phases of cell reproduction, or *mitosis.*

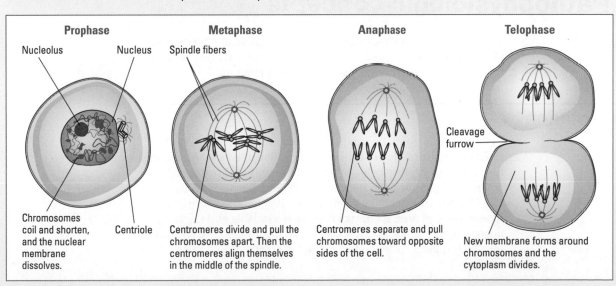

Prophase

Nucleolus   Nucleus

Chromosomes coil and shorten, and the nuclear membrane dissolves.

Centriole

Metaphase

Spindle fibers

Centromeres divide and pull the chromosomes apart. Then the centromeres align themselves in the middle of the spindle.

Anaphase

Centromeres separate and pull chromosomes toward opposite sides of the cell.

Telophase

Cleavage furrow

New membrane forms around chromosomes and the cytoplasm divides.

Prophase

During prophase, the chromosomes coil and shorten, and the nuclear membrane dissolves. Each chromosome is made up of a pair of strands called *chromatids*, which are connected by a spindle of fibers called a *centromere*.

Metaphase

During metaphase, the centromeres divide, pulling the chromosomes apart. The centromeres then align themselves in the middle of the spindle.

Anaphase

At the onset of anaphase, the centromeres begin to separate and pull the newly replicated chromosomes toward opposite sides of the cell. By the end of anaphase, 46 chromosomes are present on each side of the cell.

Telophase

In the final phase of mitosis—*telophase*—a new membrane forms around each set of 46 chromosomes. The spindle fibers disappear, cytokinesis occurs, and the cytoplasm divides, producing two identical new daughter cells.

Now that all the work is done, there's two of us where there once was one!

Pathophysiologic concepts

The cell faces a number of challenges through its life. Stressors, changes in the body's health, disease, and other extrinsic and intrinsic factors can alter the cells' normal functioning.

Adaptation

Cells generally continue functioning despite challenging conditions or stressors. However, severe or prolonged stress or changes may injure or destroy cells. When cell integrity is threatened, the cell reacts by drawing in its reserves to keep functioning, by adaptive changes or by cellular dysfunction. If cellular reserve is insufficient, the cell dies. If enough reserve is available and the body doesn't detect abnormalities, the cell adapts by atrophy, hypertrophy, hyperplasia, metaplasia, or dysplasia. (See *Adaptive cell changes*.)

Adaptive cell changes

When cells are stressed, they can undergo a number of changes.

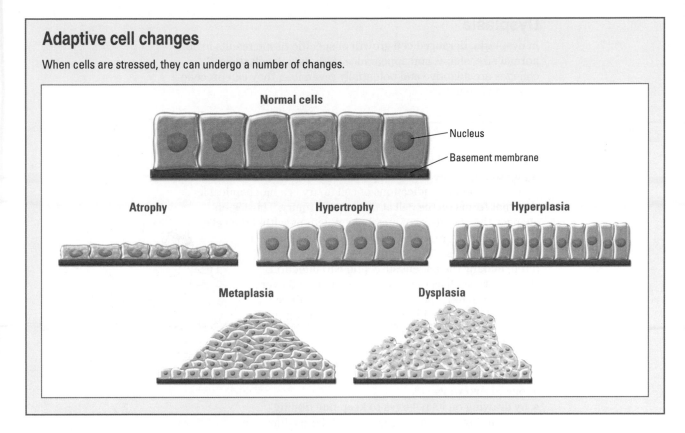

Normal cells

Nucleus

Basement membrane

Atrophy

Hypertrophy

Hyperplasia

Metaplasia

Dysplasia

Atrophy

Atrophy is a reversible reduction in the size of the cell. It results from disuse, insufficient blood flow, malnutrition, denervation, or reduced endocrine stimulation.

Hypertrophy

Hypertrophy is an increase in the size of a cell due to an increased workload. It can result from normal physiologic conditions or abnormal pathologic conditions.

Hyperplasia

Hyperplasia, an increase in the number of cells, is caused by increased workload, hormonal stimulation, or decreased tissue.

Metaplasia

Metaplasia is the replacement of one adult cell with another adult cell that can better endure the change or stress. It's usually a response to chronic inflammation or irritation.

Dysplasia

In dysplasia, deranged cell growth of specific tissue results in abnormal size, shape, and appearance. Although dysplastic cell changes are adaptive and potentially reversible, they can precede cancerous changes.

Cell injury

A person's state of wellness and disease is reflected in the cells. Injury to any of the cell's components can lead to illness.

One of the first indications of cell injury is a biochemical lesion that forms on the cell at the point of injury. This lesion changes the chemistry of metabolic reactions within the cell.

Consider, for example, a patient with chronic alcoholism. The cells of the immune system may be altered, making the patient susceptible to infection. Other cells, such as those of the pancreas and liver, are also affected. These cells can't be reproduced, which prevents a return to normal functioning.

> A cell can often adapt to injury by drawing on its reserves.

Draw on your reserves, adapt, or die

When cell integrity is threatened—for example, by toxins, infection, physical injury, or deficit injury—the cell reacts in one of two ways:
- by drawing on its reserves to keep functioning
- by adapting through changes or cellular dysfunction.

If enough cellular reserve is available and the body doesn't detect abnormalities, the cell adapts. If there isn't enough cellular reserve, cell death (*necrosis*) occurs. Necrosis is usually localized and easily identifiable.

Toxic injury

Toxic injuries may be caused by factors inside the body (called *endogenous factors*) or outside the body (called *exogenous factors*). Common endogenous factors include genetically determined metabolic errors, gross malformations, and hypersensitivity reactions. Exogenous factors include alcohol, lead, carbon monoxide, and drugs that alter cellular function. Examples of such drugs are chemotherapeutic agents used for cancer treatment and immunosuppressive drugs that prevent rejection in organ transplant recipients.

Infectious injury

Viral, fungal, protozoan, and bacterial agents can cause cell injury or death. These organisms affect cell integrity, usually by interfer-

Memory jogger

To remember the four causes of cell injury, think of how the injury tipped (or **TIPD**) the scale of homeostasis:

Toxin or other lethal (cytotoxic) substance

Infection

Physical insult or injury

Deficit, or lack of water, oxygen, or nutrients.

ing with cell synthesis, producing mutant cells. For example, human immunodeficiency virus alters the cell when the virus is replicated in the cell's ribonucleic acid.

Physical injury

Physical injury results from a disruption in the cell or in the relationships of the intracellular organelles. Two major types of physical injury are thermal (electrical or radiation) and mechanical (trauma or surgery). Causes of thermal injury include radiation therapy for cancer, X-rays, and ultraviolet radiation. Causes of mechanical injury include motor vehicle crashes, frostbite, and ischemia.

Deficit injury

When a deficit of water, oxygen, or nutrients occurs, or if constant temperature and adequate waste disposal aren't maintained, cellular synthesis can't take place. A lack of just one of these basic requirements can cause cell disruption or death.

> Without enough water, oxygen, and nutrients, I don't stand a chance!

Cell degeneration

A type of nonlethal cell damage known as *degeneration* generally occurs in the cytoplasm of the cell, while the nucleus remains unaffected. Degeneration usually affects organs with metabolically active cells, such as the liver, heart, and kidneys, and is caused by these problems:
- increased water in the cell or cellular swelling
- fatty infiltrates
- atrophy
- autophagocytosis, during which the cell absorbs some of its own parts
- pigmentation changes
- calcification
- hyaline infiltration
- hypertrophy
- dysplasia (related to chronic irritation)
- hyperplasia.

> Degeneration occurs in the cytoplasm of the cell; the nucleus remains unaffected.

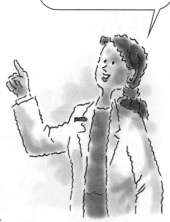

Talkin' 'bout degeneration

When changes within cells are identified, degeneration may be slowed or cell death prevented through prompt treatment. An electron microscope makes the identification of changes within cells easier. When a disease is diagnosed before the patient complains of any symptoms, it's termed *subclinical identifica-*

tion. Unfortunately, many cell changes remain unidentifiable even under a microscope, making early detection impossible.

Cell aging

During the normal process of cell aging, cells lose structure and function. Lost cell structure may cause a decrease in size or wasting away, a process called *atrophy.* Two characteristics of lost cell function are:

- hypertrophy, an abnormal thickening or increase in bulk
- hyperplasia, an increase in the number of cells.

Cell aging may slow down or speed up, depending on the number and extent of injuries and the amount of wear and tear on the cell.

Warning: This cell will self-destruct

Signs of aging occur in all body systems. Examples of the effects of cell aging include decreases in elasticity of blood vessels, bowel motility, muscle mass, and subcutaneous fat. The cell aging process limits the human life span. One theory says that cell aging is an inherent self-destructive mechanism that increases with a person's age.

Cell death may be caused by internal (intrinsic) factors that limit the cells' life span or external (extrinsic) factors that contribute to cell damage and aging. (See *In's and out's of cell aging.*)

Down with cell aging!

Homeostasis

The body is constantly striving to maintain a dynamic, steady state of internal balance called *homeostasis.* Every cell in the body is involved in maintaining homeostasis, both on the cellular level and as part of an organism.

Any change or damage at the cellular level can affect the entire body. When an external stressor disrupts homeostasis, illness may occur. A few examples of external stressors include injury, lack of nutrients, and invasion by parasites or other organisms. Throughout the course of a person's life, many external stressors affect the body's internal equilibrium.

In's and out's of cell aging

Factors that affect cell aging may be intrinsic or extrinsic, as outlined here.

Intrinsic factors
- Psychogenic
- Inherited
- Congenital
- Metabolic
- Degenerative
- Neoplastic
- Immunologic
- Nutritional

Extrinsic factors
Physical agents
- Force
- Temperature
- Humidity
- Radiation
- Electricity
- Chemicals

Infectious agents
- Viruses
- Bacteria
- Fungi
- Protozoa
- Insects
- Worms

Maintaining the balance

Three structures in the brain are responsible for maintaining homeostasis:

☞ the medulla oblongata, the part of the brain stem that's associated with vital functions, such as respiration and circulation

☞ the pituitary gland, which regulates the function of other glands and thereby a person's growth, maturation, and reproduction

☞ the reticular formation, a group of nerve cells or nuclei that form a large network of connected tissues that help control vital reflexes, such as cardiovascular function and respiration.

> Every cell in the body is involved in maintaining homeostasis, a dynamic, steady state of internal balance.

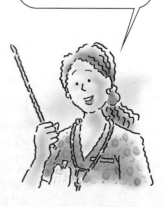

Feedback mechanisms

Homeostasis is maintained by self-regulating feedback mechanisms. These mechanisms have three components:

☞ a sensor mechanism that senses disruptions in homeostasis

☞ a control center that regulates the body's response to disruptions in homeostasis

☞ an effector mechanism that acts to restore homeostasis.

An endocrine (hormone-secreting) gland usually controls the sensor mechanism. A signal is sent to the control center in the CNS, which initiates the effector mechanism.

There are two types of feedback mechanisms:

☞ a negative feedback mechanism, which works to restore homeostasis by correcting a deficit within the system

☞ a positive feedback mechanism, which occurs when hormone secretion triggers additional hormone secretion. This indicates a trend away from homeostasis.

> Negative feedback cancels out the original response. Positive feedback exaggerates it.

Accentuate the negative

For negative feedback mechanisms to be effective, they must sense a change in the body—such as a high blood glucose level—and attempt to return body functions to normal. In the case of a high blood glucose level, the effector mechanism triggers increased insulin production by the pancreas, returning the blood glucose level to normal and restoring homeostasis. (See *Negative feedback, positive result,* page 10.)

Negative feedback, positive result

This flowchart shows how a negative feedback mechanism works to restore homeostasis in a patient with a high blood glucose level.

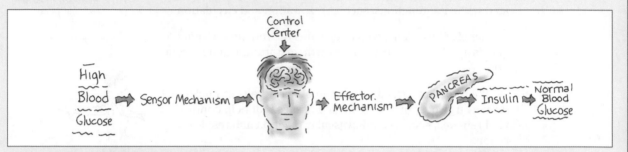

...and the positive

The positive feedback mechanism is far from positive. It takes the original response and exaggerates it. It's said to be positive because the change that occurs proceeds in the same direction as the initial disturbance, causing a further deviation from homeostasis. A positive feedback mechanism is responsible for intensifying labor contractions during childbirth.

Disease and illness

Although disease and illness aren't synonymous, they're commonly used interchangeably. Disease occurs when homeostasis isn't maintained. The patient has subjective complaints, a specific medical history, and signs, symptoms, and laboratory or radiologic findings characteristic of that disease. Illness occurs when a person is no longer in a state of normal health. It's highly individualized and personal.

For example, a person may have coronary artery disease, diabetes, or asthma but not be ill all the time because his body has adapted to the disease. In this situation, a person can perform necessary activities of daily living.

Genetic factors plus

Genetic factors (such as a tendency toward obesity), unhealthy behaviors (such as smoking), stress, and even the patient's perception of the disease (such as acceptance or denial) influence the course and outcome of a disease. Diseases are dynamic and may manifest in various ways, depending on the patient and his environment.

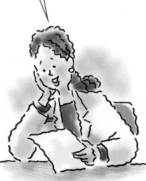

Genetic factors, plus unhealthy behaviors, plus personality type, plus attitude, plus perception may add up to disease.

Cause

One aspect of disease is its cause (the fancy term is *etiology*). The cause of disease may be intrinsic or extrinsic. Diseases with no known cause are called *idiopathic*.

Intrinsic or extrinsic

The cause of disease is intrinsic when the disease occurs because of a malfunction or change within the body. Intrinsic factors include inherited traits, the patient's age, and the patient's gender.

Extrinsic causes of disease come from outside the body. Examples of extrinsic causes include infectious agents, mechanical trauma, smoking, chemical exposure, nutritional problems, drug use, temperature extremes, radiation exposure, and psychological stress.

Development

A disease's development is called its *pathogenesis*. Unless identified and successfully treated, most diseases progress according to a typical pattern of symptoms. Some diseases are self-limiting or resolve quickly with limited or no intervention; others are chronic and never resolve. Patients with chronic diseases may undergo periods of remission and exacerbation. During remission, the patient's symptoms lessen in severity or disappear. During exacerbation, the patient experiences an aggravation of symptoms or an increase in the severity of the disease.

Telltale signs

Usually, a disease is uncovered because of an increase or decrease in metabolism or cell division. Signs and symptoms may include hypofunction, such as constipation; hyperfunction, such as increased mucus production; or increased mechanical function, such as a seizure.

How the cells respond to disease depends on the causative agent and the affected cells, tissues, and organs. Resolution of disease depends on many factors that occur over time.

Disease stages

Typically, diseases progress through these stages:
• *Exposure* or *injury*. Target tissue is exposed to a causative agent or is injured.
• *Latent* or *incubation period*. No signs or symptoms are evident.
• *Prodromal period*. Signs and symptoms are usually mild and nonspecific.

• *Acute phase.* The disease reaches its full intensity and complications commonly arise. If the patient can still function in a pre-illness fashion during this phase, it's called the *subclinical acute phase.*
• *Remission.* This second latent phase occurs in some diseases and is commonly followed by another acute phase.
• *Convalescence.* In this stage of rehabilitation, the patient progresses toward recovery after the termination of a disease.
• *Recovery.* In this stage, the patient regains health or normal functioning. No signs or symptoms of the disease occur.

> People with certain diseases never fully recover; periodic remission is their best outcome.

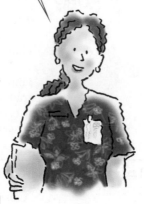

Stress and disease

When a stressor such as a life change occurs, a person can respond in one of two ways: by adapting successfully or by failing to adapt. A maladaptive response to stress may result in disease. The underlying stressor may be real or perceived.

When stress strikes

According to Hans Selye's General Adaptation Model, the body reacts to stress in the stages depicted below.

Physical or psychological stressor

⬇

Alarm reaction
• Arousal of the central nervous system begins.
• Epinephrine and norepinephrine, along with other hormones, are released, causing an increase in heart rate, increased force of heart contractions, increased oxygen intake, and increased mental activity.

> Also known as the *fight-or-flight response*

⬇

Resistance
• The body responds to the stressor and attempts to return to homeostasis.
• Coping mechanisms are used.

> If stress comes to an end, the body should be able to return to a normal state, leading to recovery.

> If the stress doesn't stop, the exhaustion stage begins.

⬇

Recovery

Exhaustion
• The body can no longer produce hormones as in the alarm stage.
• Organ damage begins.

> Exhaustion marks the onset of disease.

Stressful stages

Hans Selye, a pioneer in the study of stress and disease, described stages of adaptation to a stressful event: alarm, resistance, and exhaustion or recovery. (See *When stress strikes.*) In the alarm stage, the body senses stress, and the CNS is aroused. The body releases chemicals to mobilize the fight-or-flight response. This release is the adrenaline rush associated with panic or aggression. In the resistance stage, the body either adapts and achieves homeostasis or fails to adapt and enters the exhaustion stage, resulting in disease.

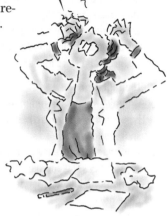

I have to find a way to adapt to all this stress!

Everything is under control

The stress response is controlled by actions taking place in the nervous and endocrine systems. These actions try to redirect energy to the organ—such as the heart, lungs, or brain—that's most affected by the stress.

Mind–body connection

Physiologic stressors may elicit a harmful response, leading to an identifiable illness or set of symptoms. Psychological stressors, such as the death of a loved one, may also cause a maladaptive response. Stressful events can exacerbate some chronic diseases, such as diabetes and multiple sclerosis. Effective coping strategies can prevent or reduce the harmful effects of stress.

That's a wrap!

Pathophysiology basics review

Understanding cell components
• Organelles—contained in the cytoplasm and surrounded by cell membrane
• Nucleus—responsible for cellular reproduction and division and stores DNA (genetic material)
• Other cell components:
  – Adenosine triphosphate
  – Ribosomes and endoplasmic reticulum
  – Golgi apparatus
  – Lysosomes

Cell reproduction
• Stage 1—mitosis (nucleus and genetic material divide)
• Stage 2—cytokinesis (cytoplasm divides)

Cell division phases
• Prophase—chromosomes coil and shorten, the nuclear membrane dissolves, and chromatids connect to a centromere
• Metaphase—centromeres divide, pulling the chromosomes apart, and align in the spindle

(continued)

Pathophysiology basics review *(continued)*

• Anaphase—centromeres separate and pull new replicated chromosomes to the opposite sides of the cell, resulting in 46 chromosomes on each side of the cell
• Telophase—final phase; new membrane forms around 46 chromosomes through cytokinesis, producing two identical new cells

Cell adaptation
• Atrophy—reversible reduction in size of cell
• Hypertrophy—increase in size of cell due to an increased workload
• Hyperplasia—increase in the number of cells
• Metaplasia—replacement of one adult cell with another adult cell that can better endure change or stress
• Dysplasia—deranged cell growth of specific tissue results in abnormal size, shape, and appearance—may precede cancerous changes.

Types of cell injury
• Toxic injury—endogenous (metabolic errors, gross malformations, hypersensitivity reactions), exogenous (alcohol, lead, carbon monoxide, drugs)
• Infectious injury—viruses, fungi, protozoa, bacteria
• Physical injury—thermal (electrical, radiation), mechanical (trauma, surgery)
• Deficit injury—lack of basic requirement

Maintaining homeostasis
• Medulla, pituitary gland, reticular formation are regulators.
• Two types of feedback mechanisms maintain homeostasis:
  – negative mechanism senses change and returns it to normal
  – positive mechanism exaggerates change.

Differentiating disease and illness
Disease
• Occurs when homeostasis isn't maintained.

• Influenced by genetic factors, unhealthy behaviors, personality type, and perception of the disease.
• Manifests in various ways depending on patient's environment.
Illness
• Occurs when a person is no longer in a state of "normal" health.
• Enables a person's body to adapt to the disease.

Causes of disease
• Intrinsic—hereditary traits, age, gender
• Extrinsic—infectious agents or behaviors, such as:
  – inactivity
  – smoking
  – drug use.
• Stressors, such as:
  – physiologic
  – psychological.

Disease development
Signs and symptoms
• Increase or decrease in metabolism or cell division
• Hypofunction such as constipation
• Hyperfunction such as increased mucus production
• Increased mechanical function such as a seizure

Disease stages
• Exposure or injury
• Latent or incubation period
• Prodromal period
• Acute phase
• Remission
• Convalescence
• Recovery

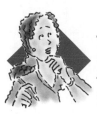

Quick quiz

Now that you've finished the first chapter, take our Quick quiz. We promise it will be low stress.

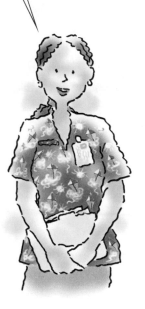

1. The organelle that contains the cell's DNA is the:
   A. mitochondria.
   B. Golgi apparatus.
   C. ribosome.
   D. nucleus.

Answer: D. The nucleus, the largest organelle, stores DNA and is responsible for cellular reproduction.

2. When a cell gets injured, the first sign is:
   A. a biochemical lesion.
   B. an area of hyperplasia.
   C. a chromatid.
   D. cellular necrosis.

Answer: A. Chemical reactions in the cell occur as a result of injury and form a biochemical lesion.

3. An extrinsic factor that can cause cell aging and death is:
   A. Down syndrome.
   B. sickle cell anemia.
   C. ultraviolet radiation.
   D. person's advanced age.

Answer: C. An extrinsic factor, such as ultraviolet radiation, comes from an outside source.

4. Homeostasis can be defined as:
   A. a steady, dynamic state.
   B. a state of flux.
   C. an unbalanced state.
   D. an exaggeration of an original response.

Answer: A. Homeostasis is a steady, dynamic state that may also be defined as a balancing act performed by the body to prevent illness.

Scoring

☆☆☆ If you answered all four items correctly, fantastic! Your intrinsic and extrinsic understanding of pathophysiology basics is excellent.

☆☆ If you answered three items correctly, wonderful! Your test-taking skills have achieved a nice homeostasis!

☆ If you answered fewer than three items correctly, no sweat! Twelve more Quick quizzes to go!

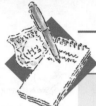

2

Cardiovascular system

Just the facts

In this chapter, you'll learn:

♦ the relationship between oxygen supply and demand

♦ risk factors for cardiovascular disease

♦ causes, pathophysiology, diagnostic tests, and treatments for several common cardiovascular disorders.

Understanding the cardiovascular system

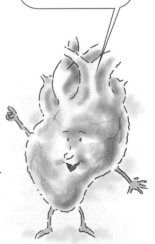

My function is so vital that it defines the very presence of life.

The cardiovascular system begins its activity when the fetus is barely 1 month old, and it's the last system to cease activity at the end of life.

The heart, arteries, veins, and lymphatics make up the cardiovascular system. These structures transport life-supporting oxygen and nutrients to cells, remove metabolic waste products, and carry hormones from one part of the body to another. Circulation requires normal heart function, which propels blood through the system by continuous rhythmic contractions.

Still the leading cause of death

Despite advances in disease detection and treatment, cardiovascular disease remains the leading cause of death in the United States. Heart attack, or myocardial infarction (MI), is the primary cause of cardiovascular-related deaths. MI typically occurs with little or no warning.

Oxygen balancing act

A critical balance exists between myocardial oxygen supply and demand. A decrease in oxygen supply or an increase in oxygen demand can disturb this balance and threaten myocardial function.

The four major determinants of myocardial oxygen demand are:

 heart rate

 contractile force

 muscle mass

 ventricular wall tension.

Cardiac workload and oxygen demand increase if the heart rate speeds up or if the force of contractions becomes stronger. This can occur in hypertension, ventricular dilation, or heart muscle hypertrophy.

The heart's law of supply and demand

If myocardial oxygen demand increases, so must oxygen supply. To effectively increase oxygen supply, coronary perfusion must also increase. Tissue hypoxia—the most potent stimulus—causes coronary arteries to dilate and increases coronary blood flow. Normal coronary vessels can dilate and increase blood flow five to six times above resting levels. However, stenotic, diseased vessels can't dilate, so oxygen deficit may result.

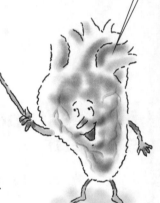

If myocardial oxygen demand increases, so must oxygen supply.

One-way ticket

Normally, blood flows unimpeded across the valves in one direction. The valves open and close in response to a pressure gradient. When the pressure in the chamber proximal to the valve exceeds the pressure in the chamber beyond the valve, the valves open. When the pressure beyond the valve exceeds the pressure in the proximal chamber, the valves close. The valve leaflets, or cusps, are so responsive that even a pressure difference of less than 1 mm Hg between chambers will open and close them.

How low can you flow?

Valvular disease is the major cause of low blood flow. A diseased valve allows blood to flow backward across leaflets that haven't closed securely. This phenomenon is called *regurgitation*. The backflow of blood through the valves forces the heart to pump more blood, increasing cardiac workload. The valve opening may also become restricted and impede the forward flow of blood. This is referred to as *stenosis*.

The heart may fail to meet the tissues' metabolic requirements for blood and fail to function as a pump. Eventually, the circulatory system may fail to perfuse body tissues, and blood volume and vascular tone may be altered.

Inner awareness

The body closely monitors both blood volume and vascular tone. Blood flow to each tissue is monitored by microvessels, which measure how much blood each tissue needs and control the local blood flow. The nerves that control circulation also help direct blood flow to tissues.

How the heart responds

The heart pays attention to the tissues' demands. It responds to the return of blood through the veins and to nerve signals that make it pump the required amounts of blood.

Under pressure

Arterial pressure is carefully regulated by the body: If it falls below or rises above its normal mean level, immediate circulatory changes occur.

If arterial pressure falls below normal, then an increase occurs in:
• heart rate
• force of contraction
• constriction of arterioles.

If arterial pressure rises above normal, these changes occur:
• reflex slowing of heart rate
• decreased force of contraction
• vasodilation.

Risk factors

Risk factors for cardiovascular disease fall into two categories: those that are modifiable and those that are nonmodifiable.

Modifiable risk factors

Some risk factors can be avoided or altered, potentially slowing the disease process or even reversing it. These factors include:
• elevated serum lipid levels
• hypertension
• cigarette smoking
• diabetes mellitus
• sedentary lifestyle
• stress
• obesity—especially abdominal (waist measurement greater than 40″ [101.6 cm] in men and greater than 35″ [88.9 cm] in women)
• excessive intake of saturated fats, carbohydrates, and salt.

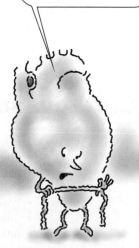

Oh no! If my waist measurement increases, I may be at increased risk for heart disease!

Nonmodifiable risk factors

Four nonmodifiable factors increase a person's risk of cardiovascular disease:

 age

 male gender

 family history

 race.

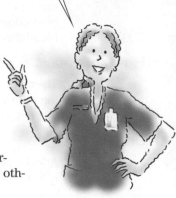

Most risk factors for heart disease are modifiable.

Better to be young at heart

Susceptibility to cardiovascular disease increases with age; disease before age 40 is unusual. However, the age-disease correlation may simply reflect the longer duration of exposure to other risk factors.

An estrogen effect?

Women are less susceptible than men to heart disease until after menopause; then they become as susceptible as men. One theory proposes that estrogen has a protective effect.

Nature vs. nurture

A positive family history also increases a person's chances of developing premature cardiovascular disease. For example, genetic factors can cause some pronounced, accelerated forms of atherosclerosis such as lipid disease. However, family history of cardiovascular disease may reflect a strong environmental component. Risk factors—such as obesity or a lifestyle that causes tension—may recur in families.

Color blind (for the most part)

Although it affects all races, blacks are most susceptible to cardiovascular disease.

Cardiovascular disorders

The disorders discussed in this section include:
- abdominal aortic aneurysm
- cardiac tamponade
- cardiogenic shock
- coronary artery disease (CAD)
- dilated cardiomyopathy
- heart failure
- hypertension

- hypertrophic cardiomyopathy
- MI
- pericarditis
- rheumatic fever and rheumatic heart disease.

Abdominal aortic aneurysm

In abdominal aortic aneurysm, an abnormal dilation in the arterial wall occurs in the aorta between the renal arteries and the iliac branches. In a saccular aneurysm, the outpouching occurs in the arterial wall. In a fusiform aneursym, the outpouching appears spindle-shaped and encompasses the entire aortic circumference. In a false aneurysm, the outpouching occurs when the entire vessel wall is injured and leads to a sac formation affecting the artery or heart. (See *Types of aortic aneurysms.*)

Aneurysms are four times more common in men than in women and are most prevalent in whites ages 50 to 80. An aneurysm that measures 6 cm has a 20% chance of rupturing within a year.

How it happens

About 95% of abdominal aortic aneurysms result from arteriosclerosis; the rest from cystic medial necrosis, trauma, syphilis, and other infections. These aneurysms develop slowly over time.

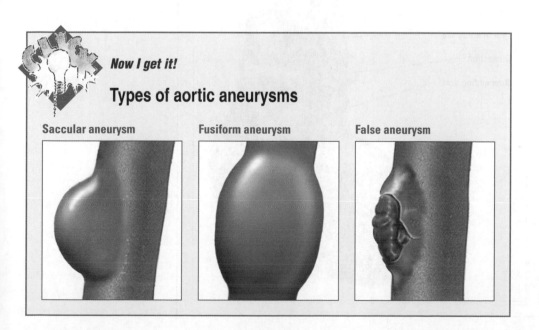

Now I get it!

Types of aortic aneurysms

Saccular aneurysm   **Fusiform aneurysm**   **False aneurysm**

It begins locally

First, a local weakness in the muscular layer of the aorta (tunica media), due to degenerative changes, allows the inner layer (tunica intima) and outer layer (tunica adventitia) to stretch outward. Blood pressure within the aorta progressively weakens the vessel walls and enlarges the aneurysm. Aneurysms can dissect or rip when bleeding into the weakened artery causes the artery wall to split (see *Dissecting aneurysm*).

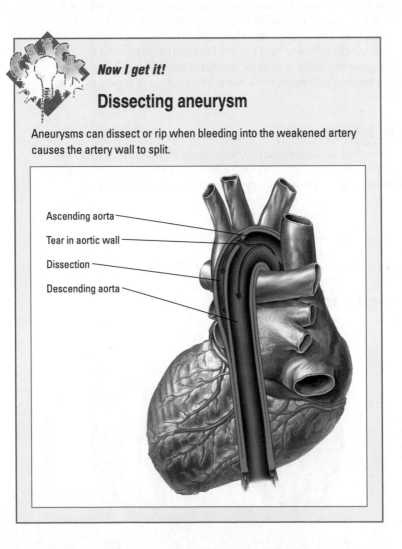

Now I get it!

Dissecting aneurysm

Aneurysms can dissect or rip when bleeding into the weakened artery causes the artery wall to split.

Ascending aorta

Tear in aortic wall

Dissection

Descending aorta

What to look for

Although abdominal aortic aneurysms usually don't produce symptoms, larger aneurysms may be evident (unless the patient is obese) as a pulsating mass in the periumbilical area, accompanied by a systolic bruit over the aorta.

Reaching the breaking point

A large aneurysm may continue to enlarge and eventually rupture. Lumbar pain that radiates to the flank and groin from pressure on lumbar nerves may signify enlargement and imminent rupture. If the aneurysm ruptures into the peritoneal cavity, it causes severe, persistent abdominal and back pain.

Other signs and symptoms of enlargement and rupture include:
• weakness
• sweating
• tachycardia
• hypotension (may be subtle if rupture into the retroperitoneal space produces a tamponade effect that prevents continued hemorrhage).

Patients with such rupture may remain stable for hours before shock and death occur, although 20% die immediately. (See *Treating abdominal aortic aneurysm.*)

What tests tell you

Because an abdominal aortic aneurysm rarely produces symptoms, in many cases it's detected accidentally as the result of an X-ray or a routine physical examination. Several tests can confirm suspected abdominal aortic aneurysm:

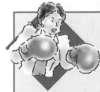

Battling illness

Treating abdominal aortic aneurysm

Treatments for abdominal aortic aneurysm are few. They include invasive interventions and drug therapy.

Invasive interventions

Usually, an abdominal aortic aneurysm requires resection of the aneurysm and replacement of the damaged aortic section with a Dacron or polytetrafluroethylene graft. Surgery is advised when the aneurysm is 5 to 6 cm in diameter.

Another invasive treatment option is a procedure known as endoluminal stent grafting. In this procedure, the doctor inserts a catheter through the femoral artery. Guided by angiography, he advances the catheter to the aneurysm. A balloon within the catheter is then inflated, pushing the stent open. The stent attaches with tiny hooks above and below the aneurysm. This creates a path for blood flow that bypasses the aneurysm.

Drug options

If the patient's aneurysm is small and produces no symptoms, surgery may be delayed. Beta-adrenergic blockers may be administered to decrease the rate of growth of the aneurysm.

• Serial ultrasonography allows accurate determination of aneurysm size, shape, and location.
• Anteroposterior and lateral X-rays of the abdomen can detect aortic calcification, which outlines the mass at least 75% of the time.
• Computed tomography can visualize the aneurysm's effect on nearby organs, particularly the position of the renal arteries in relation to the aneurysm.
• Aortography shows the condition of vessels proximal and distal to the aneurysm and the extent of the aneurysm but may underestimate the aneurysm's diameter because it visualizes only the flow channel and not the surrounding clot.

Cardiac tamponade

In cardiac tamponade, a rapid rise in intrapericardial pressure impairs diastolic filling of the heart. The rise in pressure usually results from blood or fluid accumulation in the pericardial sac. As little as 200 ml of fluid can create an emergency if it accumulates rapidly. If the condition is left untreated, cardiogenic shock and death can occur.

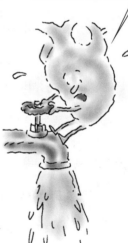

As little as 200 ml of fluid can cause cardiac tamponade.

Stretching it out

If fluid accumulates slowly and pressure rises—such as in pericardial effusion caused by cancer—signs and symptoms may not be evident immediately. This is because the fibrous wall of the pericardial sac can stretch to accommodate up to 2 L of fluid. (See *Understanding cardiac tamponade.*)

How it happens

Cardiac tamponade may result from:
• effusion, such as in cancer, bacterial infections, tuberculosis and, rarely, acute rheumatic fever
• hemorrhage caused by trauma, such as a gunshot or stab wound in the chest, cardiac surgery, or perforation by a catheter during cardiac or central venous catheterization and pacemaker insertion
• hemorrhage from nontraumatic causes, such as rupture of the heart or great vessels and anticoagulant therapy in a patient with pericarditis
• viral, postirradiation, or idiopathic pericarditis
• acute MI
• chronic renal failure during dialysis
• drug reaction from procainamide, hydralazine, minoxidil, isoniazid, penicillin, methysergide, or daunorubicin
• connective tissue disorders, such as rheumatoid arthritis, systemic lupus erythematosus, rheumatic fever, vasculitis, and scleroderma.

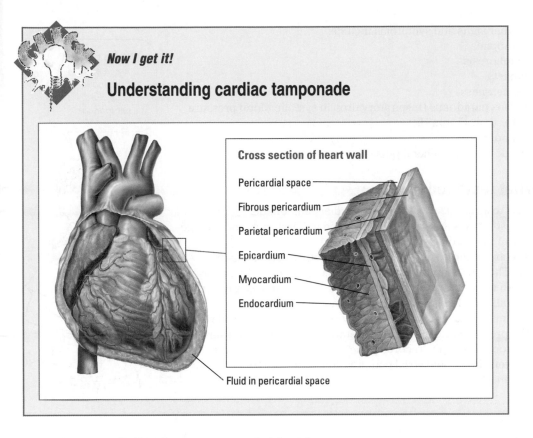

Now I get it!

Understanding cardiac tamponade

Cross section of heart wall

Pericardial space

Fibrous pericardium

Parietal pericardium

Epicardium

Myocardium

Endocardium

Fluid in pericardial space

Too much fluid, not enough blood

In cardiac tamponade, the progressive accumulation of fluid in the pericardium causes compression of the heart chambers. This obstructs blood flow into the ventricles and reduces the amount of blood that can be pumped out of the heart with each contraction. Reduced cardiac output may be fatal without prompt treatment.

The amount of fluid necessary to cause cardiac tamponade varies greatly. It may be as small as 200 ml when the fluid accumulates rapidly or more than 2,000 ml if the fluid accumulates slowly and the pericardium stretches to adapt.

What to look for

Cardiac tamponade has three classic features known as *Beck's triad:*
- hypotension with narrowing pulse pressure
- elevated central venous pressure (CVP) with neck vein distention
- muffled heart sounds.

Other signs and symptoms include:
* orthopnea
* diaphoresis
* anxiety
* restlessness
* pulsus paradoxus (inspiratory drop in systolic blood pressure greater than 15 mm Hg)
* cyanosis
* weak, rapid peripheral pulse.

These tests are used to diagnose cardiac tamponade.

What tests tell you

These tests are used to diagnose cardiac tamponade:
* Chest X-ray shows a slightly widened mediastinum and enlargement of the cardiac silhouette.
* Electrocardiography (ECG) rules out other cardiac disorders. The QRS amplitude may be reduced, and electrical alternans of the P wave, QRS complex, and T wave may be present. Generalized ST-segment elevation is noted in all leads.
* Pulmonary artery pressure monitoring reveals increased right atrial pressure or CVP and right ventricular diastolic pressure.
* Echocardiography records pericardial effusion with signs of right ventricular and atrial compression. (See *Treating cardiac tamponade.*)

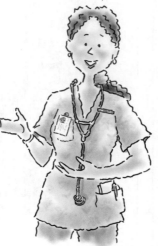

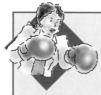

Battling illness

Treating cardiac tamponade

The goal of treatment for cardiac tamponade is to relieve intrapericardial pressure and cardiac compression by removing the accumulated blood or fluid. This can be done three different ways:

pericardiocentesis, or needle aspiration of the pericardial cavity

surgical creation of an opening, commonly called a *pericardial window*

insertion of a drain into the pericardial sac to drain the effusion.

Hypotensive patients

In the hypotensive patient, cardiac output is maintained through trial volume loading with I.V. normal saline solution, albumin and, perhaps, an inotropic drug such as dopamine, or a vasopressor such as phenylephrine.

Additional treatment

Depending on the cause of tamponade, additional treatment may be required, for example:
* in traumatic injury, blood transfusion or a thoracotomy to drain reaccumulating fluid or to repair bleeding sites
* in heparin-induced tamponade, the heparin antagonist protamine
* in warfarin-induced tamponade, vitamin K, and infusion of fresh-frozen plasma, if necessary.

Cardiogenic shock

Sometimes called *pump failure*, cardiogenic shock is a condition of diminished cardiac output that severely impairs tissue perfusion as well as oxygen delivery to the tissues. It reflects severe left-sided heart failure and occurs as a serious complication in some patients hospitalized with acute MI.

Cardiogenic shock typically affects patients whose area of infarction exceeds 40% of the heart's muscle mass. In these patients, mortality may exceed 85%. Most patients with cardiogenic shock die within 24 hours of onset. The prognosis for those who survive is extremely poor.

How it happens

Regardless of the underlying cause, left ventricular dysfunction triggers a series of compensatory mechanisms that attempt to increase cardiac output and, in turn, maintain vital organ function.

As cardiac output falls, baroreceptors in the aorta and carotid arteries initiate responses in the sympathetic nervous system. These responses, in turn, increase heart rate, left ventricular filling pressure, and peripheral resistance to flow to enhance venous return to the heart.

A vicious cycle

These compensatory responses initially stabilize the patient but later cause the patient to deteriorate as the oxygen demands of the already compromised heart rise. These events comprise a vicious cycle of low cardiac output, sympathetic compensation, myocardial ischemia, and even lower cardiac output. (See *Cycle of decompensation*, page 28.)

What to look for

Cardiogenic shock produces signs of poor tissue perfusion, such as:
- cold, pale, clammy skin
- drop in systolic blood pressure to 30 mm Hg below baseline or a sustained reading below 80 mm Hg that isn't attributable to medication
- weak peripheral pulses
- tachycardia
- rapid, shallow respirations
- oliguria (urine output less than 20 ml/hour)
- restlessness
- confusion
- narrowing pulse pressure

Now I get it!

Cycle of decompensation

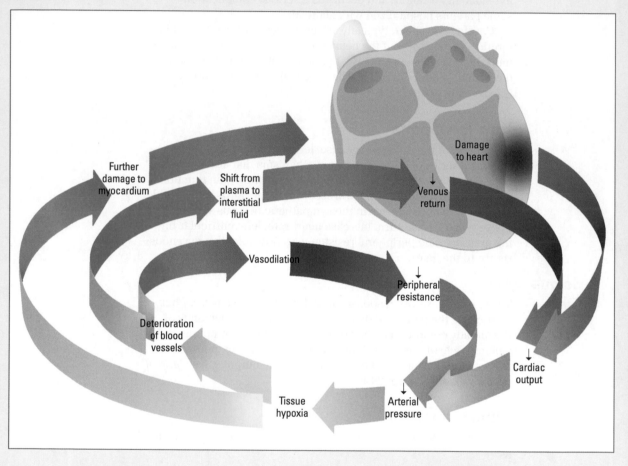

Damage
to heart

↓
Venous
return

Further
damage to
myocardium

Shift from
plasma to
interstitial
fluid

Vasodilation

↓
Peripheral
resistance

Deterioration
of blood
vessels

↓
Cardiac
output

Tissue
hypoxia

↓
Arterial
pressure

- cyanosis
- S_3 and S_4 heart sounds.

What tests tell you

These tests help diagnose cardiogenic shock:
- Pulmonary artery pressure (PAP) monitoring shows increased
PAP and increased pulmonary artery wedge pressure (PAWP),
which reflects a rise in left ventricular end-diastolic pressure (preload) and increased resistance to left ventricular emptying (after-

Battling illness

Treating cardiogenic shock

The aim of treatment is to enhance cardiovascular status by increasing cardiac output, improving myocardial perfusion, and decreasing cardiac workload. Treatment combines various cardiovascular drugs and mechanical-assist techniques.

Cardiovascular drugs

Drug therapy may include I.V. dopamine, a vasopressor that increases blood pressure and blood flow to the kidneys, and I.V. inamrinone, milrinone, or dobutamine, inotropic agents that increase myocardial contractility and cardiac output. Norepinephrine or phenylephrine may be used when a potent vasoconstrictor is needed.

I.V. nitroprusside, a vasodilator, may be used with a vasopressor to further improve cardiac output by decreasing afterload and reducing preload. However, the patient's blood pressure must be adequate to support nitroprusside therapy and must be monitored closely.

Mechanical-assist techniques

The intra-aortic balloon pump (IABP) is a mechanical-assist device that attempts to improve coronary artery perfusion and decrease cardiac workload. The inflatable balloon pump is surgically inserted through the femoral artery into the descending thoracic aorta.

After it's in place, the balloon inflates during diastole to increase coronary artery perfusion pressure and deflates before systole (before the aortic valve opens) to reduce resistance to ejection (afterload) and therefore lessen cardiac workload and improve cardiac output.

The line of last assistance

When drug therapy and IABP insertion fail, treatment may require a ventricular-assist device until transplantation is possible.

---

load). Cardiac output measured by thermodilution reveals a diminished cardiac output.
- Invasive arterial pressure monitoring shows hypotension.
- Arterial blood gas analysis reveals metabolic acidosis and hypoxia.
- ECG may reveal evidence of an acute MI, myocardial ischemia, or ventricular aneurysm.
- Cardiac enzymes and troponin levels are elevated.
- Echocardiography shows left ventricular dysfunction, valvular disease, dilation caused by an aneurysm, and ventricular septal defects. (See *Treating cardiogenic shock.*)

Coronary artery disease

CAD causes the loss of oxygen and nutrients to myocardial tissue because of poor coronary blood flow. This disease is nearly epidemic in the Western world. About 250,000 people a year die in the United States of CAD without being hospitalized—about one-half of all the deaths caused by CAD. It's most prevalent in white, middle-age men and in elderly people, with more than 50% of men age 60 or older showing signs of CAD on autopsy.

How it happens

Atherosclerosis is the most common cause of CAD. In this condition, fatty, fibrous plaques, possibly including calcium deposits, progressively narrow the coronary artery lumens, which reduces the volume of blood that can flow through them. This can lead to myocardial ischemia (a temporary deficiency of blood flow to the heart) and eventually necrosis (heart tissue death).

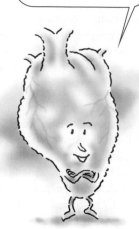

Quitting smoking, reducing stress, and lowering blood pressure can help prevent CAD.

What you can and can't control

Many risk factors are associated with atherosclerosis and CAD. Some are modifiable and some are nonmodifiable.

Nonmodifiable risk factors include being older than age 40, being male, being white, and having a family history of CAD. (See *Genes implicated in CAD*.)

Modifiable risk factors include:
• systolic blood pressure greater than 140 mm Hg or diastolic blood pressure greater than 95 mm Hg
• increased low-density and decreased high-density lipoprotein levels
• elevated homocysteine levels
• smoking (risk dramatically drops within 1 year of quitting)
• stress

The genetic link

Genes implicated in CAD

Overwhelming evidence confirms a genetic link to coronary artery disease (CAD). Researchers have identified more than 250 genes that may play a role in CAD. CAD commonly results from combined effects of multiple genes. These effects make the genetics of CAD very complicated because many genes can influence a person's risk.

Some of the best understood genes linked to CAD include:
• low-density lipoprotein (LDL) receptor—a protein that removes LDL from the bloodstream; a mutation in this gene is responsible for familial hypercholesterolemia
• apolipoprotein E—mutations in this gene, commonly called *apo E,* also affect blood levels of LDL

• apolipoprotein B-100—commonly called *apo B-11,* it's a component of LDL; mutations of this gene cause LDL to stay in the blood longer than normal, leading to very high LDL levels
• apolipoprotein A—a glycoprotein that combines with LDL to form a particle called *Lp(a).* Lp(a) appears as part of plaque on blood vessels.
• MTHFR—one of the enzymes that clears homocysteine from the blood; mutations in MTHFR genes may cause higher homocysteine levels
• cystathionine B-synthase—also known as *CBS,* it's another enzyme involved in homocysteine metabolism; CBS mutations cause a condition known as *homocystinuria* (homocysteine levels are so high that homocysteine can be detected in the urine).

- obesity, which increases the risk of diabetes mellitus, hypertension, and high cholesterol
- inactivity
- diabetes mellitus, especially in women.

Other risk factors that can be modified include increased levels of serum fibrinogen and uric acid, elevated hematocrit, reduced vital capacity, high resting heart rate, thyrotoxicosis, and the use of hormonal contraceptives.

More blood-flow blockers

Other factors that can reduce blood flow include:
- dissecting aneurysm
- infectious vasculitis
- syphilis
- congenital defects in the coronary vascular system.

Coronary artery spasms can also impede blood flow. These spontaneous, sustained contractions of one or more coronary arteries occlude the vessel, reduce blood flow to the myocardium, and cause angina pectoris (chest pain). Without treatment, ischemia and, eventually, MI result.

A precarious balance

As atherosclerosis progresses, luminal narrowing is accompanied by vascular changes that impair the diseased vessel's ability to dilate. This causes an imbalance between myocardial oxygen supply and demand, threatening the myocardium beyond the lesion. When oxygen demand exceeds what the diseased vessels can supply, localized myocardial ischemia results.

From aerobic to anaerobic

Transient ischemia causes reversible changes at the cellular and tissue levels, depressing myocardial function. Untreated, it can lead to tissue injury or necrosis. Oxygen deprivation forces the myocardium to shift from aerobic to anaerobic metabolism. As a result, lactic acid (the end product of anaerobic metabolism) accumulates. This reduces cellular pH.

With each contraction, less blood

The combination of hypoxia, reduced energy availability, and acidosis rapidly impairs left ventricular function. The strength of contractions in the affected myocardial region is reduced as the fibers shorten inadequately with less force and velocity. In addition, the ischemic section's wall motion is abnormal. This generally results in less blood being ejected from the heart with each contraction.

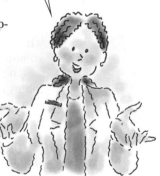

As atherosclerosis progresses, vascular changes occur that cause an imbalance between myocardial oxygen supply and demand.

Haphazard hemodynamics

Because of reduced contractility and impaired wall motion, the hemodynamic response becomes variable. It depends on the ischemic segment's size and the degree of reflex compensatory response by the autonomic nervous system.

Depression of left ventricular function may reduce stroke volume and thereby lower cardiac output. Reduction in systolic emptying increases ventricular volumes. As a result, left-sided heart pressures and pulmonary wedge pressure increase.

Compliance counts

These increases in left-sided heart pressures and PAWP are magnified by changes in wall compliance induced by ischemia. Compliance is reduced, magnifying the elevation in pressure.

A sympathetic response

During ischemia, sympathetic nervous system response leads to slight elevations in blood pressure and heart rate before the onset of pain. With the onset of pain, further sympathetic activation occurs.

What to look for

Angina is the classic sign of CAD. The patient may describe a burning, squeezing, or crushing tightness in the substernal or precordial area that radiates to the left arm, neck, jaw, or shoulder blade. He may clench his fist over his chest or rub his left arm when describing it. Pain is commonly accompanied by nausea, vomiting, fainting, sweating, and cool extremities.

Angina commonly occurs after physical exertion but may also follow emotional excitement, exposure to cold, or the consumption of a large meal. Sometimes, it develops during sleep and awakens the patient.

When to label it stable or unstable

If the pain is predictable and relieved by rest or nitrates, it's called *stable angina*. If it increases in frequency and duration and is more easily induced, it's called *unstable* or *unpredictable angina*. Unstable angina is classified as an acute coronary syndrome and is much more likely to progress to an MI. Unstable angina is thought to result from unstable plaque rupture that can lead to thrombus with an MI. (See *Treating CAD*.)

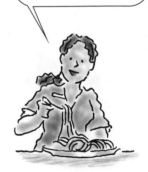

Angina is the classic sign of CAD. It usually occurs after physical exertion but can also follow emotional excitement, exposure to cold, or the consumption of a large meal.

What tests tell you

These diagnostic tests confirm CAD:
• ECG during an episode of angina shows ischemia, as demonstrated by T-wave inversion, ST-segment depression and, possibly,

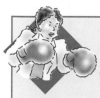

Battling illness

Treating CAD

Because coronary artery disease (CAD) is so widespread, controlling risk factors is important. Other treatment may focus on one of two goals: reducing myocardial oxygen demand or increasing the oxygen supply and alleviating pain. Interventions may be noninvasive or invasive.

Controlling risk

Because CAD is so widespread, patients should limit calories and their intake of salt, fats, and cholesterol as well as stop smoking. Regular exercise is important, although it may need to be done more slowly to prevent pain. If stress is a known pain trigger, patients should learn stress reduction techniques.

Other preventive actions include controlling hypertension with diuretics, beta-adrenergic blockers, or angiotensin-converting enzyme inhibitors; controlling elevated serum cholesterol or triglyceride levels with antilipemics; and minimizing platelet aggregation and blood clot formation with aspirin.

Noninvasive measures

Drug therapy also consists of nitrates, such as nitroglycerin, isosorbide dinitrate, or beta-adrenergic blockers that dilate vessels.

Invasive measures

Three invasive treatments are commonly used: coronary artery bypass graft (CABG) surgery, percutaneous transluminal coronary angioplasty (PTCA), and laser angioplasty.

CABG

Critically narrowed or blocked arteries may need CABG surgery to alleviate uncontrollable angina and prevent myocardial infarction (MI). In this procedure, a part of the saphenous vein in the leg or the internal mammary artery in the chest are grafted between the aorta and the affected artery beyond the obstruction.

Minimally invasive CABG requires a shorter recovery period and has fewer complications postoperatively. Instead of sawing open the patient's sternum and spreading the ribs apart, several small cuts are made in the torso through which small surgical instruments and fiber-optic cameras are inserted. This procedure was designed to correct blockages in one or two easily reached arteries and may not be appropriate for more complicated cases.

PTCA

PTCA may be performed during cardiac catheterization to compress fatty deposits and relieve occlusion. In patients with calcification, this procedure may reduce the obstruction by fracturing the plaque.

PTCA causes fewer complications than surgery, but it does have risks, which include:
- circulatory insufficiency
- MI
- restenosis of the vessels
- retroperitoneal bleeding
- sudden coronary reocclusions
- vasovagal response and arrhythmias
- death (in rare instances).

PTCA is a good alternative to grafting in elderly patients and others who can't tolerate cardiac surgery. However, patients with left main coronary artery occlusions or lesions in extremely tortuous vessels aren't candidates for PTCA.

Stenting may also be done in conjunction with PTCA. A stent is introduced into the artery and placed in the area where the vessel has narrowed to keep the artery open. Drug-eluding stents may help prevent restenosis.

Laser angioplasty

Laser angioplasty corrects occlusion by vaporizing fatty deposits with a hot-tip laser device. Percutaneous myocardial revascularization (PMR) is a procedure that uses a laser to create channels in the heart muscle to improve perfusion to the myocardium. A carbon dioxide laser is used to create transmural channels from the epicardial layer to the myocardium, extending into the left ventricle. This technique is also known as transmyocardial revascularization and appears to be up to 90% effective.

Rotational ablation, or rotational atherectomy, removes plaque with a high-speed, rotating burr covered with diamond crystals.

arrhythmias such as premature ventricular contractions. Results may be normal during pain-free periods. Arrhythmias may occur without infarction, secondary to ischemia.

• Treadmill or bicycle exercise stress test may provoke chest pain and ECG signs of myocardial ischemia. Monitoring of electrical rhythm may demonstrate T-wave inversion or ST-segment depression in the ischemic areas.

• Coronary angiography reveals the location and extent of coronary artery stenosis or obstruction, collateral circulation, and the arteries' condition beyond the narrowing.

• Myocardial perfusion imaging with thallium-201 during treadmill exercise detects ischemic areas of the myocardium, visualized as "cold spots."

Dilated cardiomyopathy

Also called *congestive cardiomyopathy*, dilated cardiomyopathy results from extensively damaged myocardial muscle fibers. This disorder interferes with myocardial metabolism and grossly dilates every heart chamber, giving the heart a globular shape.

This disorder usually affects middle-age men but can occur in any age-group. Because it usually isn't diagnosed until the advanced stages, the prognosis is generally poor. Most patients, especially those older than age 55, die within 2 years of symptom onset.

How it happens

Cardiomyopathy involves the ventricular myocardium, as opposed to other heart structures, such as the valves or coronary arteries. Dilated cardiomyopathy is characterized by a grossly dilated, hypodynamic ventricle that contracts poorly and, to a lesser degree, myocardial hypertrophy. All four chambers become dilated as a result of increased volumes and pressures. Thrombi commonly develop within these chambers due to blood pooling and stasis, which may lead to embolization.

If hypertrophy coexists, the heart ejects blood less efficiently. A large volume remains in the left ventricle after systole, causing heart failure.

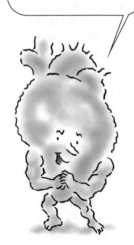

I'm in good shape now, but damage to my muscle fibers will leave me rounded and weak.

The onset of the disease is usually insidious. It may progress to end-stage refractory heart failure. If so, the patient's prognosis is poor. He may need heart transplantation.

Dilated cardiomyopathy can lead to intractable heart failure, arrhythmias, and emboli. Ventricular arrhythmias may lead to syncope and sudden death. (See *Understanding dilated cardiomyopathy.*)

Now I get it!

Understanding dilated cardiomyopathy

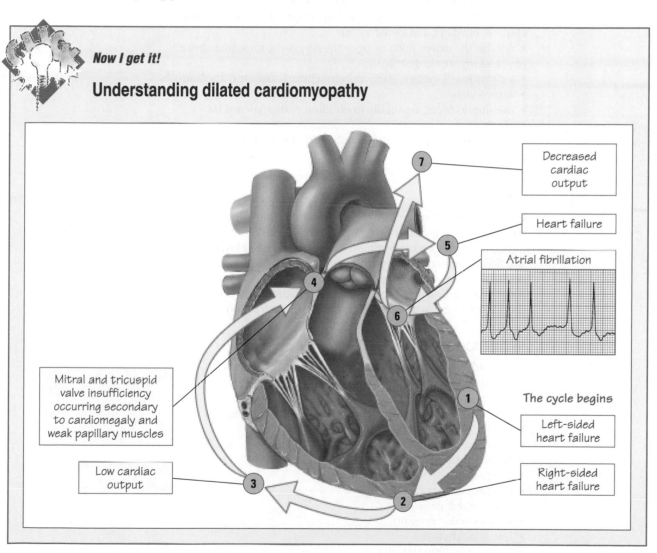

7 → Decreased cardiac output

5 → Heart failure

Atrial fibrillation

6

4

Mitral and tricuspid valve insufficiency occurring secondary to cardiomegaly and weak papillary muscles

1 — The cycle begins

Left-sided heart failure

Low cardiac output — 3

2 — Right-sided heart failure

Seeds of destruction

The exact cause of dilated cardiomyopathy is unknown. It may be linked to myocardial destruction caused by:

• infectious agents, as in viral myocarditis (especially after infection with coxsackievirus B, poliovirus, or influenza virus) and acquired immunodeficiency syndrome
• metabolic agents that cause endocrine and electrolyte disorders and nutritional deficiencies, as in hyperthyroidism, pheochromocytoma, beriberi, and kwashiorkor
• muscle disorders, such as myasthenia gravis, muscular dystrophy, and myotonic dystrophy
• infiltrative disorders, such as hemochromatosis and amyloidosis
• sarcoidosis
• rheumatic fever, especially in children with myocarditis
• alcoholism
• use of doxorubicin, cyclophosphamide, cocaine, and fluorouracil
• X-linked inheritance patterns.

Taking a pregnant pause

In addition, dilated cardiomyopathy may develop during the last trimester of pregnancy or a few months after delivery. Its cause is unknown, but it's most common in multiparous women older than age 30, particularly those with malnutrition or preeclampsia. In some patients, cardiomegaly and heart failure reverse with treatment, allowing a subsequent normal pregnancy. However, if cardiomegaly persists despite treatment, prognosis is poor.

What to look for

Signs and symptoms of dilated cardiomyopathy include:

• shortness of breath
• orthopnea
• dyspnea on exertion and paroxysmal nocturnal dyspnea
• fatigue
• dry cough at night
• palpitations
• nausea
• peripheral edema
• vague chest pain
• narrow pulse pressure
• irregular rhythms
• S_3 and S_4 gallop rhythms
• pansystolic murmur.

What tests tell you

No single test confirms dilated cardiomyopathy. Diagnosis requires elimination of other possible causes of heart failure and arrhythmias. These tests are used:
• ECG and angiography rule out ischemic heart disease. ECG may also show biventricular hypertrophy, sinus tachycardia, atrial enlargement, ST-segment and T-wave abnormalities and, in 20% of patients, atrial fibrillation or left bundle-branch block. QRS complexes are decreased in amplitude.
• Chest X-ray demonstrates moderate to marked cardiomegaly, usually affecting all heart chambers, along with pulmonary congestion, pulmonary venous hypertension, and pleural effusion. Pericardial effusion may give the heart a globular shape.
• Echocardiography may identify ventricular thrombi, global hypokinesis, and the degrees of left ventricular dilation and dysfunction.
• Cardiac catheterization can show left ventricular dilation and dysfunction, elevated left ventricular and right ventricular filling pressures, and diminished cardiac output.
• Gallium scans may identify patients with dilated cardiomyopathy and myocarditis.
• Transvenous endomyocardial biopsy may be useful in some patients to determine the underlying disorder, such as amyloidosis or myocarditis. (See *Treating dilated cardiomyopathy.*)

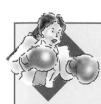

Battling illness

Treating dilated cardiomyopathy

The goals of treatment for dilated cardiomyopathy are to correct the underlying causes and to improve the heart's pumping ability. The second goal is achieved with cardiac glycosides, diuretics, oxygen, anticoagulants, vasodilators, and a low-sodium diet supplemented by vitamin therapy. Antiarrhythmics may be used to treat arrhythmias.

Therapy may also include prolonged bed rest and selective use of corticosteroids, particularly when myocardial inflammation is present. Vasodilators reduce preload and afterload, decreasing congestion and increasing cardiac output.

Acute and long-term therapy
Acute heart failure necessitates vasodilation with I.V. nitroprusside or nitroglycerin. Long-term treatment may include prazosin, hydralazine, isosorbide dinitrate, and anticoagulants if the patient is on bed rest. Dopamine, dobutamine, milrinone, and inamrinone may be useful during the acute stage.

Final option
When these treatments fail, heart transplantation may be the only option for carefully selected patients.

Heart failure

When the myocardium can't pump effectively enough to meet the body's metabolic needs, heart failure occurs. Pump failure usually occurs in a damaged left ventricle, but it may also happen in the right ventricle. Usually, left-sided heart failure develops first.

Heart failure is classified as:
• high-output or low-output
• acute or chronic
• left-sided or right-sided (see *Understanding left-sided and right-sided heart failure*)
• forward or backward. (See *Classifying heart failure*, page 41.)

Heart failure affects approximately 5 million people in the United States. Symptoms of heart failure may restrict a person's ability to perform activities of daily living and severely affect quality of life.

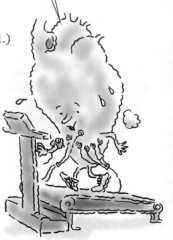

I could fail... gasp... if my myocardium can't pump enough to meet the body's metabolic needs.

But the good news is...

Advances in diagnostic and therapeutic techniques have greatly improved the outlook for these patients. However, the prognosis still depends on the underlying cause and its response to treatment.

How it happens

Heart failure may result from a primary abnormality of the heart muscle—for example, an infarction—that impairs ventricular function and prevents the heart from pumping enough blood.

Heart failure may also be caused by problems unrelated to MI:
• Mechanical disturbances in ventricular filling during diastole, due to blood volume that's too low for the ventricle to pump, occur in mitral stenosis secondary to rheumatic heart disease or constrictive pericarditis and in atrial fibrillation.
• Systolic hemodynamic disturbances—such as excessive cardiac workload caused by volume overload or pressure overload—limit the heart's pumping ability. This problem can result from mitral or aortic insufficiency, which leads to volume overload. It can also result from aortic stenosis or systemic hypertension, which causes increased resistance to ventricular emptying and decreased cardiac output.

Factors favorable to failure

Certain conditions can predispose a patient to heart failure, especially if he has underlying heart disease. These include:
• arrhythmias, such as tachyarrhythmias, which can reduce ventricular filling time; arrhythmias that disrupt the normal atrial and

Now I get it!

Understanding left-sided and right-sided heart failure

These illustrations show how myocardial damage leads to heart failure.

Left-sided heart failure

1. Increased workload and end-diastolic volume enlarge the left ventricle (see illustration below). Because of lack of oxygen, the ventricle en-larges with stretched tissue rather than func-tional tissue. The patient may experi-ence increased

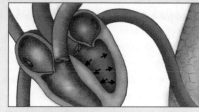

heart rate, pale and cool skin, tingling in the extremities, de-creased cardiac output, and arrhythmias.

2. Diminished left ventricular function allows blood to pool in the ventricle and the atrium and eventually back up into the pul-monary veins and capillaries, as shown below. At this stage, the patient may ex-perience dyspnea on exertion, confu-sion, dizziness, or-thostatic hypoten-sion, decreased pe-ripheral pulses and

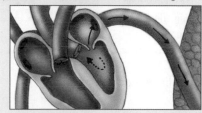

pulse pressure, cyanosis, and an S_3 gallop.

3. As the pulmonary circulation becomes engorged, rising capillary pressure pushes sodium and water into the interstitial space (as shown below), causing pulmonary edema. You'll note coughing, subcla-vian retractions, crackles, tachyp-nea, elevated pul-monary artery pres-sure, diminished pulmonary compli-

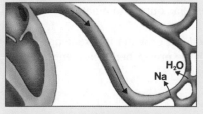

ance, and increased partial pressure of carbon dioxide.

4. When the patient lies down, fluid in the extremities moves into the systemic circulation (see illustration below). Because the left ventricle can't handle the in-creased venous re-turn, fluid pools in the pulmonary cir-culation, worsening pulmonary edema.

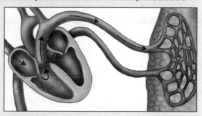

You may note decreased breath sounds, dullness on percus-sion, crackles, and orthopnea.

5. The right ventricle may now become stressed because it's pumping against greater pulmonary vascular resistance and left ventricular pressure (see illustration below). When this oc-curs, the patient's symptoms worsen.

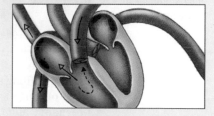

(continued)

Understanding left-sided and right-sided heart failure *(continued)*

Right-sided heart failure

6. The stressed right ventricle enlarges with the formation of stretched tissue (see illustration below). Increasing conduction time and deviation of the heart from its normal axis can cause arrhythmias. If the patient doesn't already have left-sided heart failure,

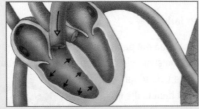

he may experience increased heart rate, cool skin, cyanosis, decreased cardiac output, palpitations, and dyspnea.

7. Blood pools in the right ventricle and right atrium. The backed-up blood causes pressure and congestion in the vena cava and systemic circulation (see illustration below). The patient will have elevated central venous pressure, jugular vein distention, and hepatojugular reflux.

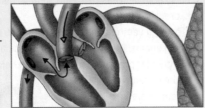

8. Backed-up blood also distends the visceral veins, especially the hepatic vein. As the liver and spleen become engorged (see illustration below), their function is impaired. The patient may develop anorexia, nausea, abdominal pain, palpable liver and spleen, weakness, and dyspnea secondary to abdominal distention.

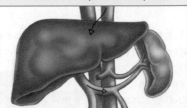

9. Rising capillary pressure forces excess fluid from the capillaries into the interstitial space (see illustration below). This causes tissue edema, especially in the lower extremities and abdomen. The patient may experience weight gain, pitting edema, and nocturia.

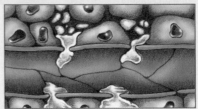

ventricular filling synchrony; and bradycardia, which can reduce cardiac output
- pregnancy and thyrotoxicosis, which increase cardiac output
- pulmonary embolism, which elevates PAP, causing right-sided heart failure
- infections, which increase metabolic demands and further burden the heart
- anemia, which leads to increased cardiac output to meet the oxygen needs of the tissues
- increased physical activity, increased salt or water intake, emotional stress, or failure to comply with the prescribed treatment regimen for the underlying heart disease.

Getting complicated

Eventually, sodium and water may enter the lungs, causing pulmonary edema, a life-threatening condition. Decreased perfusion to the brain, kidneys, and other major organs can cause them to fail. MI can occur because the oxygen demands of the overworked heart can't be met.

Classifying heart failure

Heart failure may be classified different ways according to its pathophysiology.

Right-sided or left-sided

Right-sided heart failure is a result of ineffective right ventricular contractile function. It may be caused by an acute right ventricular infarction or pulmonary embolus. However, the most common cause is profound backward flow due to left-sided heart failure.

Left-sided heart failure is the result of ineffective left ventricular contractile function. It may lead to pulmonary congestion or pulmonary edema and decreased cardiac output. Left ventricular myocardial infarction (MI), hypertension, and aortic and mitral valve stenosis or insufficiency are common causes.

As the decreased pumping ability of the left ventricle persists, fluid accumulates, backing up into the left atrium and then into the lungs. If this worsens, pulmonary edema and right-sided heart failure may also result.

Systolic or diastolic

In systolic heart failure, the left ventricle can't pump enough blood out to the systemic circulation during systole and the ejection fraction falls. Consequently, blood backs up into the pulmonary circulation, pressure rises in the pulmonary venous system, and cardiac output falls.

In diastolic heart failure, the left ventricle can't relax and fill properly during diastole and the stroke volume falls. Therefore, larger ventricular volumes are needed to maintain cardiac output.

Acute or chronic

"Acute" refers to the timing of the onset of symptoms and whether compensatory mechanisms kick in. Typically, fluid status is normal or low, and sodium and water retention don't occur.

In chronic heart failure, signs and symptoms have been present for some time, compensatory mechanisms have taken effect, and fluid volume overload persists. Drugs, diet changes, and activity restrictions usually control symptoms.

Acute or insidious

The patient's underlying condition determines whether heart failure is acute or insidious.

Heart failure is commonly associated with systolic or diastolic overloading and myocardial weakness. As stress on the heart muscle reaches a critical level, the muscle's contractility is reduced and cardiac output declines. Venous input to the ventricle remains the same, however.

The body's responses to decreased cardiac output include:
- reflex increase in sympathetic activity
- release of renin from the juxtaglomerular cells of the kidney
- anaerobic metabolism by affected cells
- increased extraction of oxygen by the peripheral cells.

The long and short of it

When blood in the ventricles increases, the heart compensates, or adapts. Adaptations may be short term or long term:
- *Short-term adaptations*—As the end-diastolic fiber length increases, the ventricular muscle responds by dilating and increasing the force of contraction. (This is called the *Frank-Starling curve*.)

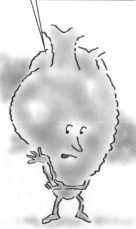

I'm an incredibly adaptable organ, if I do say so myself.

• *Long-term adaptations*—Ventricular hypertrophy increases the heart muscle's ability to contract and push its volume of blood into the circulation.

Compensation may occur for long periods before signs and symptoms develop.

What to look for

The early signs and symptoms of heart failure include:
• fatigue
• exertional, paroxysmal, and nocturnal dyspnea
• neck vein engorgement
• hepatomegaly.
    Later signs and symptoms include:
• tachypnea
• palpitations
• dependent edema
• unexplained, steady weight gain
• nausea
• chest tightness
• slowed mental response
• anorexia
• hypotension
• diaphoresis
• narrow pulse pressure
• pallor
• oliguria
• gallop rhythm
• inspiratory crackles on auscultation
• dullness over the lung bases
• hemoptysis
• cyanosis
• marked hepatomegaly
• pitting ankle enema
• sacral edema in bedridden patients.

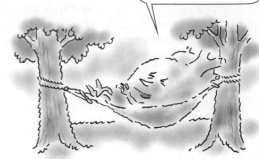

Geez, look what happens if I'm laid up and can't do my job!

What tests tell you

These tests help diagnose heart failure:
• ECG reveals ischemia, tachycardia, and extrasystole.
• Echocardiogram identifies the underlying cause as well as the type and severity of the heart failure.
• Laboratory studies, such as B-type natriuretic peptide, confirm the presence of heart failure.
• Chest X-ray shows increased pulmonary vascular markings, interstitial edema, or pleural effusion and cardiomegaly.
• PAP monitoring shows elevated PAP, PAWP, and left ventricular end-diastolic pressure in left-sided heart failure and elevated right

Battling illness

Treating heart failure

The goal of treatment for heart failure is to improve pump function, thereby reversing the compensatory mechanisms that produce or intensify the clinical effects.

Heart failure can usually be controlled quickly with treatment, including:
• administration of diuretics (such as furosemide, hydrochlorothiazide, ethacrynic acid, bumetanide, spironolactone, or triamterene) to reduce total blood volume and circulatory congestion
• bed rest
• oxygen administration to increase oxygen delivery to the myocardium and other vital organs
• administration of inotropic drugs (such as digoxin) to strengthen myocardial contractility; sympathomimetics (such as dopamine and dobutamine) in acute situations; or inamrinone or milrinone to increase contractility and cause arterial vasodilation
• administration of vasodilators to increase cardiac output or angiotensin-converting enzyme inhibitors to decrease afterload
• antiembolism stockings to prevent venostasis and thromboembolism formation.

Acute pulmonary edema

As a result of decreased contractility and elevated fluid volume and pressure, fluid may be driven from the pulmonary capillary beds into the alveoli, causing pulmonary edema. Treatment for acute pulmonary edema includes:

• administration of morphine
• administration of nitroglycerin or nitroprusside to diminish blood return to the heart
• administration of dobutamine, dopamine, inamrinone, or milrinone to increase myocardial contractility and cardiac output
• administration of diuretics to reduce fluid volume
• administration of supplemental oxygen
• placement of the patient in high Fowler's position.

Continued care

After recovery, the patient must continue medical care and usually must continue taking digoxin, angiotensin-converting enzyme inhibitors, beta-adrenergic blockers, diuretics, and potassium supplements. The patient with valve dysfunction who has recurrent, acute heart failure may need surgical valve replacement.

What's left?

Left ventricular remodeling surgery may also be performed. This surgical procedure involves cutting a wedge about the size of a small slice of pie out of the left ventricle of an enlarged heart. The left ventricle is repaired. The result is a smaller ventricle that can pump blood more efficiently. The only option for some patients is heart transplantation. A left ventricular assist device may be necessary until a heart is available for transplantation.

atrial pressure or CVP in right-sided heart failure. (See *Treating heart failure.*)

Hypertension

Hypertension is an intermittent or sustained elevation of diastolic or systolic blood pressure. Generally, a sustained systolic blood pressure of 139 mm Hg or higher or a diastolic blood pressure of 89 mm Hg or higher indicates hypertension.

Hypertension affects about 50 million adults in the United States. Blacks are more likely than Whites to be affected.

Listen up—this is essential

The two major types of hypertension are essential (also called *primary* or *idiopathic*) and secondary. The etiology of essential hypertension, the most common type, is complex. It involves several interacting homeostatic mechanisms. Hypertension is classified as secondary if it's related to a systemic disease that raises peripheral vascular resistance or cardiac output. Malignant hypertension is a severe, fulminant form of the disorder that may arise from either type.

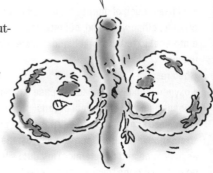

Stop pushing so hard! I don't need all this pressure.

How it happens

Hypertension may be caused by increases in cardiac output, total peripheral resistance, or both. Cardiac output is increased by conditions that increase heart rate or stroke volume. Peripheral resistance is increased by factors that increase blood viscosity or reduce the lumen size of vessels, especially the arterioles.

Family history, race, stress, obesity, a diet high in fat or sodium, use of tobacco or hormonal contraceptives, a sedentary lifestyle, and aging may all play a role. Their effects continue to be studied.

Sly as a fox

Essential hypertension usually begins insidiously as a benign disease. If left untreated, even mild cases can cause major complications and death. Carefully managed treatment, which may include lifestyle modifications and drug therapy, improves prognosis.

Why? Why? Why?

Several theories help to explain the development of hypertension. For example, it's thought to arise from:
• changes in the arteriolar bed, causing increased resistance
• abnormally increased tone in the sensory nervous system that originates in the vasomotor system centers, causing increased peripheral vascular resistance
• increased blood volume resulting from renal or hormonal dysfunction
• an increase in arteriolar thickening caused by genetic factors, leading to increased peripheral vascular resistance
• abnormal renin release resulting in the formation of angiotensin II, which constricts the arterioles and increases blood volume. (See *Understanding hypertension.*)

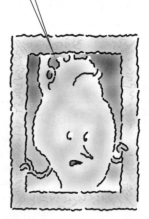

Do you get the picture? Essential hypertension is sneaky. It may begin benign, but it will slowly get nasty.

Now I get it!

Understanding hypertension

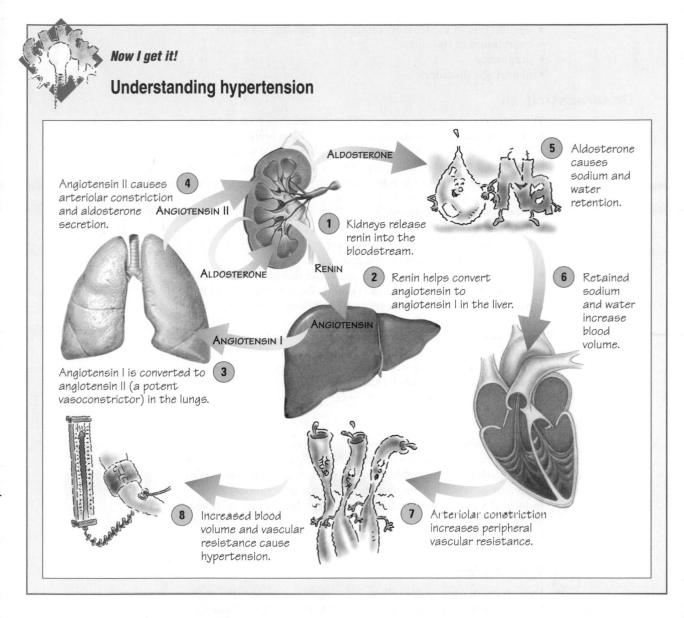

Angiotensin II causes arteriolar constriction and aldosterone secretion. **4**

ANGIOTENSIN II

ALDOSTERONE

ALDOSTERONE

RENIN

ANGIOTENSIN I

Angiotensin I is converted to angiotensin II (a potent vasoconstrictor) in the lungs. **3**

ANGIOTENSIN

1 Kidneys release renin into the bloodstream.

2 Renin helps convert angiotensin to angiotensin I in the liver.

5 Aldosterone causes sodium and water retention.

6 Retained sodium and water increase blood volume.

8 Increased blood volume and vascular resistance cause hypertension.

7 Arteriolar constriction increases peripheral vascular resistance.

Secondary hypertension

Secondary hypertension may be caused by:
- renovascular disease
- renal parenchymal disease
- pheochromocytoma
- primary hyperaldosteronism
- Cushing's syndrome
- diabetes mellitus

- dysfunction of the thyroid, pituitary, or parathyroid gland
- coarctation of the aorta
- pregnancy
- neurologic disorders.

Underneath it all

The pathophysiology of secondary hypertension is related to the underlying disease. For example, consider these points:

- The most common cause of secondary hypertension is chronic renal disease. Insult to the kidney from chronic glomerulonephritis or renal artery stenosis interferes with sodium excretion, the renin-angiotensin-aldosterone system, or renal perfusion. This causes blood pressure to rise.
- In Cushing's syndrome, increased cortisol levels raise blood pressure by increasing renal sodium retention, angiotensin II levels, and vascular response to norepinephrine.
- In primary aldosteronism, increased intravascular volume, altered sodium concentrations in vessel walls, or very high aldosterone levels cause vasoconstriction (increased resistance).
- Pheochromocytoma is a secreting tumor of chromaffin cells, usually of the adrenal medulla. It causes hypertension due to increased secretion of epinephrine and norepinephrine. Epinephrine functions mainly to increase cardiac contractility and rate. Norepinephrine functions mainly to increase peripheral vascular resistance.

Late complications

Complications occur late in the disease and can attack any organ system. Cardiac complications include CAD, angina, MI, heart failure, arrhythmias, and sudden death. Neurologic complications include stroke and hypertensive encephalopathy. Hypertensive retinopathy can cause blindness. Renovascular hypertension can lead to renal failure. (See *A close look at blood vessel damage in hypertension*.)

What to look for

Hypertension usually doesn't produce signs and symptoms until vascular changes in the heart, brain, or kidneys occur. Severely elevated blood pressure damages the intima of small vessels, resulting in fibrin accumulation in the vessels, local edema and, possibly, intravascular clotting.

Location, location, location

Symptoms depend on the location of the damaged vessels, for example:
- *brain*—stroke, transient ischemic attacks

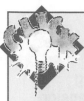

Now I get it!

A close look at blood vessel damage in hypertension

Sustained hypertension damages blood vessels. Vascular injury begins with alternating areas of dilation and constriction in the arterioles. The illustrations below show how damage occurs.

Increased intra-arterial pressure damages the endothelium. Angiotensin induces endothelial wall contraction, allowing plasma to leak through interendothelial spaces. Plasma constituents deposited in the vessel wall cause medial necrosis.

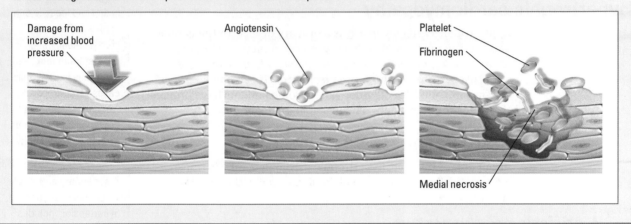

- *retina*—blindness
- *heart*—MI
- *kidneys*—proteinuria, edema and, eventually, renal failure.

A heavy heart workload

Hypertension increases the heart's workload. This causes left ventricular hypertrophy and, later, left-sided heart failure, pulmonary edema, and right-sided heart failure.

What tests tell you

The following tests may reveal predisposing factors and help identify the cause of hypertension:

- Urinalysis may show protein, red blood cells, or white blood cells (WBCs), suggesting renal disease; or glucose, suggesting diabetes mellitus.
- Excretory urography may reveal renal atrophy, indicating chronic renal disease. One kidney that's more than ⅝″ (1.6 cm) shorter than the other suggests unilateral renal disease.
- Serum potassium levels less than 3.5 mEq/L may indicate adrenal dysfunction (primary hyperaldosteronism).

- Blood urea nitrogen (BUN) levels that are elevated to more than 20 mg/dl and serum creatinine levels that are elevated to more than 1.5 mg/dl suggest renal disease.

These tests may help detect cardiovascular damage and other complications:
- ECG may show left ventricular hypertrophy or ischemia.
- Chest X-ray may demonstrate cardiomegaly. (See *Treating hypertension.*)

Hypertrophic cardiomyopathy

Hypertrophic cardiomyopathy is a primary disease of the cardiac muscle. You may hear it called several other names, including *idiopathic hypertrophic subaortic stenosis, hypertrophic obstructive cardiomyopathy,* or *muscular aortic stenosis.*

The course of this disorder varies. Some patients have progressive deterioration; others remain stable for years.

How it happens

About 50% of the time, hypertrophic cardiomyopathy is transmitted genetically as an autosomal dominant trait. Other causes aren't known.

A stiffening of the septum

Hypertrophic cardiomyopathy is characterized by left ventricular hypertrophy and an unusual cellular hypertrophy of the upper ventricular septum. These changes may result in an outflow tract pressure gradient, a pressure difference that results in an obstruction of blood outflow. The obstruction may change between examinations and even from beat to beat.

Hypertrophy of the intraventricular septum can pull the papillary muscle out of its usual alignment. This causes altered function of the anterior leaflet of the mitral valve and mitral insufficiency. The myocardial wall may stiffen over time, causing increased resistance to blood entering the right ventricle and an increase in diastolic filling pressures.

Inevitable pump failure

Cardiac output may be low, normal, or high, depending on whether the stenosis is obstructive or nonobstructive. Eventually, left ventricular dysfunction—a result of rigidity and decreased compliance—causes pump failure.

Getting complicated

Pulmonary hypertension and heart failure may occur secondary to left ventricular stiffness. Sudden death is also possible and usually

Battling illness

Treating hypertension

Although essential hypertension has no cure, drugs and modifications in diet and lifestyle can control it. Generally, lifestyle modification is the first treatment used, especially in early, mild cases. If this doesn't work, the doctor may prescribe diuretics and various types of antihypertensives.

A secondary approach
Treatment of secondary hypertension includes correcting the underlying cause and controlling hypertensive effects. Hypertensive crisis, or severely elevated blood pressure, may not respond to drugs and may be fatal.

results from ventricular arrhythmias, such as ventricular tachycardia and ventricular fibrillation. (See *Looking at hypertrophic cardiomyopathy.*)

Now I get it!

Looking at hypertrophic cardiomyopathy

1. The left ventricle and interventricular septum hypertrophy and become stiff, noncompliant, and unable to relax during ventricular filling.

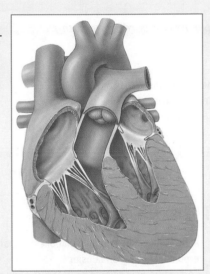

3. The left ventricle forcefully contracts but can't sufficiently relax.

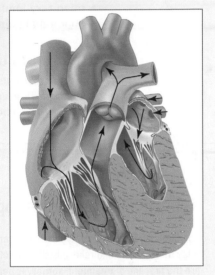

2. As the ventricle's ability to fill decreases, the pressure increases and left atrial and pulmonary venous pressures rise.

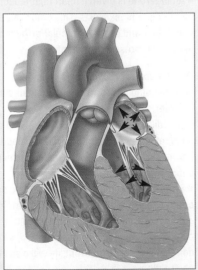

4. The anterior leaflet of the mitral valve is drawn toward the interventricular septum as the blood is forcefully ejected. Early closure of the outflow tract results because of the decreasing ejection fraction.

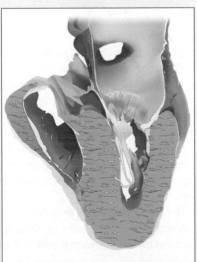

What to look for

Signs and symptoms of hypertrophic cardiomyopathy include:
- atrial fibrillation
- orthopnea
- dyspnea on exertion
- syncope
- angina
- fatigue
- edema
- tachypnea
- migratory joint pain
- abdominal pain. (See *Treating hypertrophic cardiomyopathy.*)

What tests tell you

These tests are used to diagnose hypertrophic cardiomyopathy:
- Echocardiography shows left ventricular hypertrophy and a thick, asymmetrical intraventricular septum in obstructive dis-

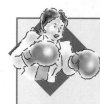

Battling illness

Treating hypertrophic cardiomyopathy

The goals of treatment for hypertrophic cardiomyopathy are to relax the ventricle and relieve outflow tract obstruction. Drugs are the first line of treatment; surgery is performed rarely and only when all else fails.

Drug therapy
These drugs are used to treat the disorder:
- Either propranolol or metoprolol, both beta-adrenergic blocking agents, is used to slow the heart rate and increase ventricular filling by relaxing the obstructing muscle, thereby reducing angina, syncope, dyspnea, and arrhythmias.
- Calcium channel blockers may reduce elevated diastolic pressures, decrease the severity of outflow tract gradients, and increase exercise tolerance. Disopyramide can be used to reduce left ventricular hypercontractility and the outflow gradient.
- Heparin is given during episodes of atrial fibrillation. When accompanying hypertrophic cardiomyopathy, atrial fibrillation is a medical emergency that calls for cardioversion. Because

of the high risk of systemic embolism, heparin must be administered until fibrillation subsides.
- Amiodarone is given if heart failure occurs, unless an atrioventricular block exists. This drug is also effective in reducing ventricular and supraventricular arrhythmias and improving left ventricular pressure gradients.

Don't reach for these drugs
The following drugs are contraindicated in treatment of this disorder:
- Vasodilators, such as nitroglycerin and diuretics, reduce venous return by permitting pooling of blood in the periphery. This decreases ventricular volume and chamber size and may cause further obstruction.
- Sympathetic stimulators and inotropic drugs increase cardiac contractility. If the septum is asymmetrically enlarged, it may obstruct left ventricular outflow, resulting in decreased cardiac output. Under these circumstances, any condition or medication that increases contractility will also increase the degree of obstruction.

ease. In nonobstructive disease, ventricular areas are hypertrophied and the septum may have a ground-glass appearance. Poor septal contraction, abnormal motion of the anterior mitral leaflet during systole, and narrowing or occlusion of the left ventricular outflow tract in obstructive disease may also be seen. The left ventricular cavity looks small, with vigorous posterior wall motion but reduced septal excursion.

• Cardiac catheterization reveals elevated left ventricular end-diastolic pressure and, possibly, mitral insufficiency.

• ECG usually shows left ventricular hypertrophy; ST-segment and T-wave abnormalities; Q waves in leads II, III, aV_F, and in V_4 to V_6 (due to hypertrophy, not infarction); left anterior hemiblock; left axis deviation; and ventricular and atrial arrhythmias.

• Chest X-ray may show a mild to moderate increase in heart size.

• Thallium scan usually reveals myocardial perfusion defects.

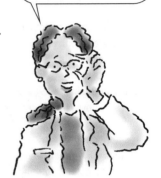

In MI, one of the heart's arteries fails to deliver enough blood to the part of the heart muscle it serves.

Myocardial infarction

MI, an acute coronary syndrome, results from reduced blood flow through one of the coronary arteries. This causes myocardial ischemia, injury, and necrosis. (See *What is an acute coronary syndrome?* and *Understanding MI*, pages 52 and 53.)

What is an acute coronary syndrome?

Acute coronary syndrome (ACS) is an umbrella term that covers a range of thrombotic coronary artery diseases, including unstable angina, ST-elevation myocardial infarction (STEMI or Q-wave MI), and non-ST elevation myocardial infarction (NSTEMI or non-Q wave MI). Patients with ACS have some degree of coronary artery occlusion. The term is useful because the initial symptoms and management of these three diseases are similar. Diagnosis requires a focused history, a physical examination, electrocardiogram, and serial serum cardiac marker studies. Differentiating acute coronary syndrome from noncardiac chest pain is the primary challenge.

Development begins with a rupture or erosion of plaque—an unstable and lipid-rich substance. The rupture results in adhesions, fibrin clots, and activation of thrombin. A thrombus progresses and occludes blood flow, although an early throm-

bus doesn't necessarily totally block blood flow. Depending on the degree of occlusion, the effect is an imbalance in myocardial oxygen supply and demand.

• If the patient has unstable angina, a thrombus partially occludes a coronary vessel. This thrombus is full of platelets. The partially occluded vessel may have distal microthrombi that cause necrosis in some myocytes.

• If smaller vessels infarct, the patient is at higher risk for MI, which may progress to a non-ST elevation MI. Usually, only the innermost layer of the heart is damaged.

• If reduced blood flow through one of the coronary arteries causes myocardial ischemia, injury, and necrosis, ST-segment elevation MI results. The damage extends through all myocardial layers.

Leading the way

In North America and Western Europe, MI is one of the leading causes of death. Death usually results from cardiac damage or complications. Mortality is about 25% in men and 38% in women within 1 year of experiencing an MI. However, more than 50% of

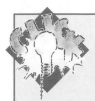

Now I get it!

Understanding MI

In myocardial infarction (MI), blood supply to the myocardium is interrupted. Here's what happens:

1. Injury to the endothelial lining of the coronary arteries causes platelets, white blood cells, fibrin, and lipids to converge at the injured site, as shown to the right. Foam cells, or resident macro-

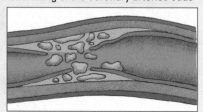

phages, congregate under the damaged lining and absorb oxidized cholesterol, forming a fatty streak that narrows the arterial lumen.

2. Because the arterial lumen narrows gradually, collateral circulation develops and helps maintain myocardial perfusion distal to the obstruction. The illustration to the right shows collateral circulation.

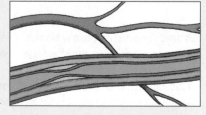

3. When myocardial demand for oxygen is more than the collateral circulation can supply, myocardial metabolism shifts from aerobic to anaerobic, producing lactic acid (represented by

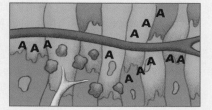

"A"), which stimulates nerve endings, as shown above.

4. Lacking oxygen, the myocardial cells die (as shown below). This decreases contractility, stroke volume, and blood pressure.

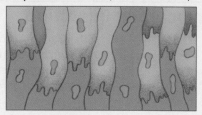

5. Hypoperfusion stimulates baroreceptors, which, in turn, stimulate the adrenal glands to release epinephrine and norepinephrine. This cycle is shown to the right. These catecholamines (C) increase heart rate and cause peripheral vasoconstriction, further increasing myocardial oxygen demand.

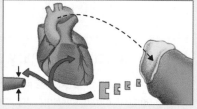

6. Damaged cell membranes in the infarcted area allow intracellular contents into the vascular circulation, as shown to the right. Ventricular arrhythmias then develop with elevated serum levels of potassium (■), CK-MB (▲), cardiac troponin (●), and lactate dehydrogenase (○).

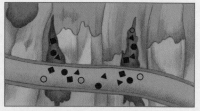

Understanding MI *(continued)*

7. All myocardial cells are capable of spontaneous depolarization, so the electrical conduction system may be affected by infarct, injury, and ischemia. The illustration to the right shows an injury site.

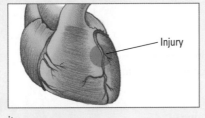

Injury

8. Extensive damage to the left ventricle may impair its ability to pump, allowing blood to back up into the left atrium and, eventually, into the pulmonary veins and capillaries, as shown in the illustration to the right. Crackles may be heard in the lungs on auscultation. Pulmonary artery and capillary wedge pressures are increased.

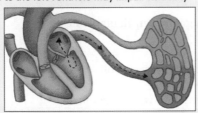

9. As back pressure rises, fluid crosses the alveolocapillary membrane, impeding diffusion of oxygen (O_2) and carbon dioxide (CO_2) (as shown to the right). Arterial blood gas measurements may show decreased partial pressure of arterial oxygen and arterial pH and increased partial pressure of arterial carbon dioxide.

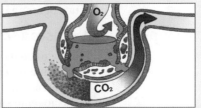

sudden deaths occur within 1 hour after the onset of symptoms, before the patient reaches the hospital.

Men are more susceptible to MI than premenopausal women, although the incidence is increasing in women who smoke and take hormonal contraceptives. The incidence in postmenopausal women is similar to that in men.

How it happens

MI results from occlusion of one or more of the coronary arteries. Occlusion can stem from atherosclerosis, thrombosis, platelet aggregation, or coronary artery stenosis or spasm. Predisposing factors include:
- aging
- diabetes mellitus
- elevated serum triglyceride, low-density lipoprotein, cholesterol, and homocysteine levels and decreased serum high-density lipoprotein levels
- excessive intake of saturated fats, carbohydrates, or salt
- hypertension
- obesity

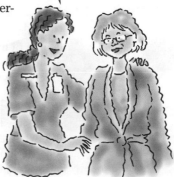

After menopause, women are as susceptible to MI as men.

- positive family history of CAD
- sedentary lifestyle
- smoking
- stress
- use of amphetamines or cocaine.

Susceptibility increases with age

Elderly patients are more prone to complications and death. The most common complications after an acute MI include:
- arrhythmias
- cardiogenic shock
- heart failure causing pulmonary edema
- pericarditis.
    Other complications include:
- rupture of the atrial or ventricular septum, ventricular wall, or valves
- ventricular aneurysms
- mural thrombi causing cerebral or pulmonary emboli
- extensions of the original infarction
- post-MI pericarditis (Dressler's syndrome), which occurs days to weeks after an MI and causes residual pain, malaise, and fever
- psychological problems caused by fear of another MI or organic brain disorder from tissue hypoxia
- personality changes.

Heavy reductions

MI results from prolonged ischemia to the myocardium with irreversible cell damage and muscle death. Functionally, MI causes:
- reduced contractility with abnormal wall motion
- altered left ventricular compliance
- reduced stroke volume
- reduced ejection fraction
- elevated left ventricular end-diastolic pressure. (See *Treating MI.*)

Insult...that is...ischemia added to injury

All MIs have a central area of necrosis or infarction surrounded by an area of injury. The area of injury is surrounded by a ring of ischemia. Tissue regeneration doesn't occur after an MI because the affected myocardial muscle is dead.

A compensatory kick

Scar tissue that forms on the necrotic area may inhibit contractility. When this occurs, the compensatory mechanisms (vascular constriction, increased heart rate, and renal retention of sodium and water) kick in to try to maintain cardiac output. Ventricular dilation also may occur. If a lot of scar tissue forms, contractility

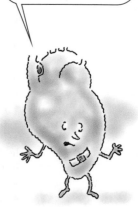

When scar tissue inhibits contractility, compensatory mechanisms kick in.

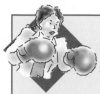

Battling illness

Treating MI

Arrhythmias, the most common problem during the first 48 hours after myocardial infarction (MI), require antiarrhythmics, a pacemaker (possibly), and cardioversion (rarely). Treatment for MI has three goals:
• to relieve chest pain
• to stabilize heart rhythm
• to reduce cardiac workload.

Drug therapy

Drugs are the mainstay of therapy. Typical drugs include:
• thrombolytic agents (such as tissue plasminogen activator [tPA] and streptokinase) to revascularize myocardial tissue
• procainamide or another antiarrhythmic (such as lidocaine or amiodarone) or disopyramide for ventricular arrhythmias
• glycoprotein IIb/IIIa inhibitor or aspirin to minimize platelet aggregation
• I.V. atropine for heart block or bradycardia
• sublingual, topical, transdermal, or I.V. nitroglycerin and calcium channel blockers (such as diltiazem), given by mouth or I.V. to relieve angina
• I.V. morphine (drug of choice) for pain and sedation
• drugs that increase myocardial contractility (such as dobutamine, inamrinone, and milrinone)
• beta-adrenergic blockers (such as propranolol, metoprolol, and timolol) after acute MI to help prevent reinfarction by decreasing myocardial workload and oxygen demand
• antilipemic to reduce elevated serum cholesterol or triglyceride levels

• angiotensin-converting enzyme (ACE) inhibitor to reduce afterload and preload and prevent remodeling.

Other therapies

Other therapies include:
• temporary pacemaker for heart block or bradycardia
• oxygen administered by face mask or nasal cannula at a modest flow rate for 24 to 48 hours, or at a lower concentration if the patient has chronic obstructive pulmonary disease
• bed rest with bedside commode to decrease cardiac workload
• pulmonary artery catheterization to detect left-sided or right-sided heart failure and to monitor the patient's response to treatment (not routinely done)
• intra-aortic balloon pump for cardiogenic shock
• cardiac catheterization, percutaneous transluminal coronary angioplasty, stent placement, and coronary artery bypass grafting.

Revascularization therapy

Revascularization therapy may be performed on patients who don't have a history of stroke, bleeding, GI ulcers, marked hypertension, recent surgery, or chest pain lasting longer than 6 hours. It must begin within 6 hours after the onset of symptoms, using I.V. intracoronary or systemic streptokinase or tPA. The best response occurs when treatment begins within 1 hour after symptoms first appear.

may be greatly reduced. The patient may develop heart failure or cardiogenic shock.

Siting the infarctions

The infarction site depends on the vessels involved:
• Occlusion of the circumflex coronary artery causes lateral wall infarctions.
• Occlusion of the left anterior coronary artery causes anterior wall infarctions.

• Occlusion of the right coronary artery or one of its branches causes posterior and inferior wall infarctions and right ventricular infarctions. Right ventricular infarctions can also accompany inferior infarctions and may cause right-sided heart failure.

What to look for

The cardinal symptom of MI is persistent, crushing substernal pain that may radiate to the left arm, jaw, neck, or shoulder blades. The pain is commonly described as heavy, squeezing, or crushing and may persist for 12 hours or more. However, in some patients—particularly elderly or diabetic patients—pain may not occur at all. In others, it may be mild and confused with indigestion.

An infarction on the horizon?

In patients with CAD, angina of increasing frequency, severity, or duration (especially if not provoked by exertion, a heavy meal, or cold and wind) may signal an impending infarction.

Other clinical effects include:
• a feeling of impending doom
• fatigue
• nausea
• vomiting
• shortness of breath
• cool extremities
• diaphoresis
• anxiety
• restlessness.

Fever is unusual at the onset of an MI, but a low-grade temperature may develop during the next few days. Blood pressure varies. Hypotension or hypertension may occur.

What tests tell you

These tests help diagnose MI:
• Serial 12-lead ECG may be normal or inconclusive during the first few hours after an MI. Abnormalities include serial ST-segment depression in NSTEMI and ST-segment elevation and Q waves, representing scarring and necrosis, in STEMI.
• Serum creatine kinase (CK) levels are elevated, especially the CK-MB isoenzyme, the cardiac muscle fraction of CK.
• Troponin I, a structural protein found in cardiac muscle, is elevated. Troponin levels increase within 4 to 6 hours of myocardial injury.
• Myoglobin is released with cardiac muscle damage and elevated levels may be detected as soon as 2 hours after an MI.

• Echocardiography shows ventricular wall dyskinesia with a STEMI and is used to evaluate the ejection fraction.
• Nuclear ventriculography (multiple gated acquisition scanning or radionuclide ventriculography) can show acutely damaged muscle by picking up accumulations of radionuclide, which appear as a "hot spot" on the film. Myocardial perfusion imaging with thallium-201 or cardiolite reveals a "cold spot" in most patients during the first few hours after a STEMI.

Pericarditis

The pericardium is the fibroserous sac that envelops, supports, and protects the heart. Inflammation of this sac is called *pericarditis*.

This condition occurs in acute and chronic forms. The acute form can be fibrinous or effusive, with serous, purulent, or hemorrhagic exudate. The chronic form, called *constrictive pericarditis*, is characterized by dense, fibrous pericardial thickening. The prognosis depends on the underlying cause but is typically good in acute pericarditis, unless constriction occurs.

How it happens

Common causes of pericarditis include:
• bacterial, fungal, or viral infection (infectious pericarditis)
• neoplasms (primary or metastatic from lungs, breasts, or other organs)
• high-dose radiation to the chest
• uremia
• hypersensitivity or autoimmune disease, such as systemic lupus erythematosus, rheumatoid arthritis, or acute rheumatic fever (most common cause of pericarditis in children)
• drugs, such as hydralazine or procainamide
• idiopathic factors (most common in acute pericarditis)
• postcardiac injury, such as MI (which later causes an autoimmune reaction in the pericardium), trauma, and surgery that leaves the pericardium intact but allows blood to leak into the pericardial cavity
• aortic aneurysm with pericardial leakage (less common)
• myxedema with cholesterol deposits in the pericardium (less common).

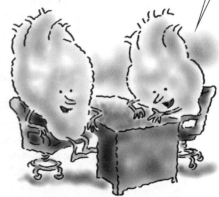

My pericardium and I have a great relationship—it envelops, supports, and protects me.

But what about the bad times, the times it became inflamed? Let's talk about pericarditis.

The effusion conclusion

Pericardial effusion is the major complication of acute pericarditis. If fluid accumulates rapidly, cardiac tamponade may occur. This may lead to shock, cardiovascular collapse and, eventually, death.

A scarred heart

As the pericardium becomes inflamed, it may become thickened and fibrotic. If it doesn't heal completely after an acute episode, it may calcify over a long period and form a firm scar around the heart. This scarring interferes with diastolic filling of the ventricles. (See *Understanding pericarditis.*)

What to look for

In acute pericarditis, a sharp, sudden pain usually starts over the sternum and radiates to the neck, shoulders, back, and arms. However, unlike the pain of MI, this pain is commonly pleuritic, increasing with deep inspiration and decreasing when the patient sits up and leans forward, pulling the heart away from the diaphragmatic pleurae of the lungs. A friction rub (a distinct sound heard when two dry surfaces rub together) is audible on auscultation.

Pericardial effusion, the major complication of acute pericarditis, may produce effects of heart failure, such as dyspnea, orthopnea, and tachycardia. It may also produce ill-defined substernal chest pain and a feeling of chest fullness.

If the fluid accumulates rapidly, cardiac tamponade may occur, causing pallor, clammy skin, hypotension, pulsus paradoxus, neck vein distention and, eventually, cardiovascular collapse and death.

Close to chronic right-sided heart failure

Chronic constrictive pericarditis causes a gradual increase in systemic venous pressure and produces symptoms similar to those of chronic right-sided heart failure, including fluid retention, ascites, and hepatomegaly. (See *Treating pericarditis,* page 60.)

What tests tell you

These laboratory test results reflect inflammation and may identify the disorder's cause:
• WBC count may be normal or elevated, especially in infectious pericarditis.
• Erythrocyte sedimentation rate (ESR) is elevated.

Now I get it!

Understanding pericarditis

Pericarditis occurs when a pathogen or other substance attacks the pericardium, leading to the events described below.

1. Inflammation

Pericardial tissue damaged by bacteria or other substances releases chemical mediators of inflammation (such as prostaglandins, histamines, bradykinins, and serotonins) into the surrounding tissue, starting the inflammatory process. Friction occurs as the inflamed pericardial layers rub against each other.

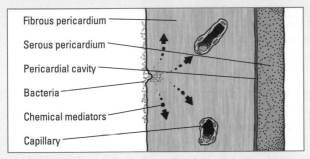

Fibrous pericardium
Serous pericardium
Pericardial cavity
Bacteria
Chemical mediators
Capillary

2. Vasodilation and clotting

Histamines and other chemical mediators cause vasodilation and increased vessel permeability. Local blood flow (hyperemia) increases. Vessel walls leak fluids and proteins (including fibrinogen) into tissues, causing extracellular edema. Clots of fibrinogen and tissue fluid form a wall, blocking tissue spaces and lymph vessels in the injured area. This wall prevents the spread of bacteria and toxins to adjoining healthy tissues.

3. Initial phagocytosis

Macrophages already present in the tissues begin to phagocytose the invading bacteria but usually fail to stop the infection.

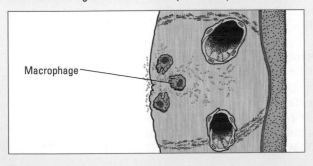

Macrophage

4. Enhanced phagocytosis

Substances released by the injured tissue stimulate neutrophil production in the bone marrow. Neutrophils then travel to the injury site through the bloodstream and join macrophages in destroying pathogens. Meanwhile, additional macrophages and monocytes migrate to the injured area and continue phagocytosis.

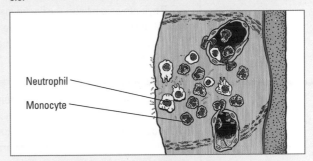

Neutrophil
Monocyte

5. Exudation

After several days, the infected area fills with an exudate composed of necrotic tissue, dead and dying bacteria, neutrophils, and macrophages. Thinner than pus, this exudate forms until all infection ceases, creating a cavity that remains until tissue destruction stops. The contents of the cavity autolyze and are gradually reabsorbed into healthy tissue.

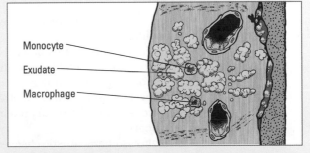

Monocyte
Exudate
Macrophage

6. Fibrosis and scarring

As the end products of the infection slowly disappear, fibrosis and scar tissue may form. Scarring, which can be extensive, may ultimately cause heart failure if it restricts movement.

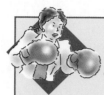

Battling illness

Treating pericarditis

Treatment for pericarditis strives to relieve symptoms, prevent or treat pericardial effusion and cardiac tamponade, and manage the underlying disease.

Bed rest and drug therapy
In idiopathic pericarditis, postmyocardial infarction pericarditis, and postthoracotomy pericarditis, treatment is twofold: bed rest as long as fever and pain persist and nonsteroidal antiinflammatory drugs, such as aspirin and indomethacin, to relieve pain and reduce inflammation.

If symptoms continue, the doctor may prescribe corticosteroids. Although they provide rapid and effective relief, corticosteroids must be used cautiously because pericarditis may recur when drug therapy stops.

More involved treatment
When infectious pericarditis results from disease of the left pleural space, mediastinal abscesses, or septicemia, the patient requires antibiotics, surgical drainage, or both. If cardiac tamponade develops, the doctor may perform emergency pericardiocentesis and may inject antibiotics directly into the pericardial sac.

Heavy-duty treatment
Recurrent pericarditis may require partial pericardectomy, which creates a window that allows fluid to drain into the pleural space. In constrictive pericarditis, total pericardectomy may be necessary to permit the heart to fill and contract adequately.

• Serum CK-MB levels are slightly elevated with associated myocarditis.
• Pericardial fluid culture obtained by open surgical drainage or pericardiocentesis sometimes identifies a causative organism in bacterial or fungal pericarditis.
• BUN levels detect uremia, antistreptolysin-O titers detect rheumatic fever, and purified protein derivative skin test detects tuberculosis.
• ECG shows characteristic changes in acute pericarditis. They include elevated ST segments in the limb leads and most precordial leads. The QRS segments may be diminished when pericardial effusion is present. Rhythm changes may also occur, including

atrial ectopic rhythms, such as atrial fibrillation and sinus arrhythmias.

• Echocardiography diagnoses pericardial effusion when it shows an echo-free space between the ventricular wall and the pericardium.

Rheumatic fever and rheumatic heart disease

A systemic inflammatory disease of childhood, acute rheumatic fever develops after infection of the upper respiratory tract with group A beta-hemolytic streptococci. It mainly involves the heart, joints, central nervous system, skin, and subcutaneous tissues and commonly recurs. If rheumatic fever isn't treated, scarring deformity of the cardiac structures results in rheumatic heart disease.

Worldwide, 12 million new cases of rheumatic fever are reported each year. The disease strikes most often during cool, damp weather in the winter and early spring. In the United States, it's most common in the north.

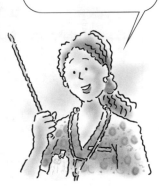

Rheumatic heart disease refers to the cardiac effects of rheumatic fever.

All in the family?

Rheumatic fever tends to run in families, lending support to the existence of genetic predisposition. Environmental factors also seem to be significant in development of the disorder. For example, in lower socioeconomic groups, the incidence is highest in children between ages 5 and 15, probably due to malnutrition and crowded living conditions.

How it happens

Rheumatic fever appears to be a hypersensitivity reaction. For some reason, antibodies produced to combat streptococci react and produce characteristic lesions at specific tissue sites. Because only about 0.3% of people infected with *Streptococcus* bacteria contract rheumatic fever, altered immune response probably is involved in its development or recurrence.

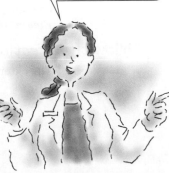

Carditis is the most destructive effect of rheumatic fever.

Getting complicated

The mitral and aortic valves are commonly destroyed by rheumatic fever's long-term effects. Their malfunction leads to severe heart inflammation (called *carditis*) and, occasionally, produces pericardial effusion and fatal heart failure. Of the patients who survive this complication, about 20% die within 10 years.

Carditis develops in up to 50% of patients with rheumatic fever and may affect the endocardium, myocardium, or peri-

Now I get it!

Sequelae of rheumatic heart disease

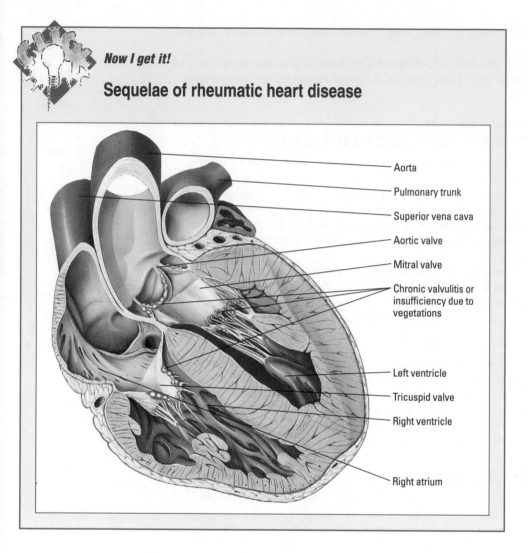

Aorta

Pulmonary trunk

Superior vena cava

Aortic valve

Mitral valve

Chronic valvulitis or insufficiency due to vegetations

Left ventricle

Tricuspid valve

Right ventricle

Right atrium

cardium during the early acute phase. Later, the heart valves may be damaged, causing chronic valvular disease. (See *Sequelae of rheumatic heart disease.*)

Follow the infection

The extent of heart damage depends on where the infection strikes:

• Myocarditis produces characteristic lesions called *Aschoff bodies* in the interstitial tissue of the heart as well as cellular swelling and fragmentation of interstitial collagen. These lesions lead to formation of progressively fibrotic nodules and interstitial scars.

• Endocarditis causes valve leaflet swelling, erosion along the lines of leaflet closure, and blood, platelet, and fibrin deposits, which form beadlike vegetation. Endocarditis strikes the mitral valve most commonly in females and the aortic valve in males. It affects the tricuspid valves in both sexes and, rarely, affects the pulmonic valve.

What to look for

In 95% of patients, rheumatic fever follows a streptococcal infection that appeared a few days to 6 weeks earlier. A temperature of at least 100.4° F (38° C) occurs.

Most patients complain of migratory joint pain or polyarthritis. Swelling, redness, and signs of effusion usually accompany such pain, which most commonly affects the knees, ankles, elbows, and hips.

Rash talk

About 5% of patients (usually those with carditis) develop a nonpruritic, macular, transient rash called *erythema marginatum*. This rash gives rise to red lesions with blanched centers. These same patients may also develop firm, movable, nontender subcutaneous nodules about 3 mm to 2 cm in diameter, usually near tendons or bony prominences of joints. These nodules persist for a few days to several weeks.

What tests tell you

No specific laboratory tests can determine the presence of rheumatic fever, but these test results support the diagnosis:

• WBC count and ESR may be elevated during the acute phase; blood studies show slight anemia caused by suppressed erythropoiesis during inflammation.

• C-reactive protein is positive, especially during the acute phase.

• Cardiac enzyme levels may be increased in severe myocarditis.

• Antistreptolysin-O titer is elevated in 95% of patients within 2 months of onset.

Battling illness

Treating rheumatic fever and rheumatic heart disease

Effective treatment for rheumatic fever and rheumatic heart disease aims to eradicate the streptococcal infection, relieve symptoms, and prevent recurrence, thus reducing the chance of permanent cardiac damage.

Acute phase

During the acute phase, treatment includes penicillin or erythromycin for patients with penicillin hypersensitivity. Salicylates, such as aspirin, relieve fever and minimize joint swelling and pain. If the patient has carditis, or if salicylates fail to relieve pain and inflammation, the doctor may prescribe corticosteroids.

Patients with active carditis require strict bed rest for about 5 weeks during the acute phase, followed by a progressive increase in physical activity. The increase depends on clinical and laboratory findings and the patient's response to treatment.

Long-term treatment

After the acute phase subsides, a monthly I.M. injection of penicillin G benzathine or daily doses of oral sulfadiazine or penicillin G may be used to prevent recurrence. This treatment usually continues for at least 5 years or until age 25.

Complications

Heart failure requires continued bed rest and diuretics. Severe mitral or aortic valvular dysfunction that causes persistent heart failure will require corrective surgery, such as commissurotomy (separation of the adherent, thickened leaflets of the mitral valve), valvuloplasty (inflation of a balloon within a valve), or valve replacement (with a prosthetic valve). However, this surgery is seldom necessary before late adolescence.

• Throat cultures may continue to show group A beta-hemolytic streptococci; however, they usually occur in small numbers and isolating them is difficult.
• ECG reveals no diagnostic changes, but 20% of patients show a prolonged PR interval.
• Chest X-ray shows normal heart size, except with myocarditis, heart failure, and pericardial effusion.
• Echocardiography helps evaluate valvular damage, chamber size, ventricular function, and the presence of a pericardial effusion.
• Cardiac catheterization evaluates valvular damage and left ventricular function in severe cardiac dysfunction. (See *Treating rheumatic fever and rheumatic heart disease.*)

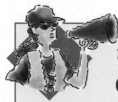

That's a wrap!

Cardiovascular system review

Understanding the cardiovascular system
The cardiovascular system is made up of the heart, arteries, veins, and lymphatics.
• Organs transport life-supporting oxygen and nutrients to cells, remove metabolic waste products, and carry hormones from one part of the body to another.

Myocardial function
• Increase in oxygen demand must be met by increase in oxygen supply.
• Blood normally flows in one direction across heart valves.
• Pressure gradient causes the valves to open and close.

Response to blood pressure drop
• Heart rate increases.
• Force of contraction increases.
• Arterioles constrict.

Response to blood pressure increase
• Heart rate decreases.
• Force of contraction decreases.
• Vasodilation occurs.

Cardiovascular disorders
• *Abdominal aortic aneurysm*—abnormal dilation in the arterial wall that occurs in the aorta between the renal arteries and the iliac branches
• *Cardiogenic shock*—condition of diminished cardiac output that severely impairs tissue perfusion as well as oxygen delivery to the tissues

• *Cardiac tamponade*—condition caused by blood or fluid accumulation in the pericardium, which leads to compressed heart chambers and decreased cardiac output
• *Coronary artery disease*—occurs when oxygen demand exceeds the supply from diseased vessels, leading to myocardial ischemia
• *Dilated cardiomyopathy*—disorder that's caused by extensive damage to the heart's muscle fibers, which results in dilated heart chambers
• *Heart failure*—impaired ventricular function due to a heart muscle abnormality that prevents the heart from pumping enough blood
• *Hypertension*—intermittent or sustained elevation of diastolic or systolic blood pressure
• *Hypertrophic cardiomyopathy*—primary disease of the myocardium that's characterized by a thickened, inflexible heart muscle
• *MI*—caused by blockage of one or more coronary arteries, which leads to prolonged myocardial ischemia, resulting in irreversible cell damage and muscle death
• *Pericarditis*—acute or chronic condition that's caused by an attack of bacteria or other substances that results in fibrosis and scar tissue after the infection ceases
• *Rheumatic fever and heart disease*—systemic inflammatory disease of childhood that develops after infection of the upper respiratory tract with group A beta-hemolytic streptococci

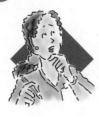

Quick quiz

1. Which factor is a major modifiable risk factor for CAD?
A. High cholesterol
B. Genetic predisposition
C. Age
D. Family history

Answer: A. High cholesterol is a risk factor that can be modified.

2. Which cause accounts for 50% of all cases of hypertrophic cardiomyopathy?
A. Autoimmune disease
B. Malnutrition
C. Genetic predisposition
D. MI

Answer: C. Genetic predisposition accounts for 50% of all cases of hypertrophic cardiomyopathy. The other 50% have unknown causes.

3. Which of the following is the major pathophysiologic effect of cardiac tamponade?
A. Atelectasis
B. Hypertension
C. Compressed heart
D. Distended pericardium

Answer: C. Cardiac tamponade is the progressive accumulation of fluid in the pericardium and causes compression of the heart chambers.

4. Which liver enzyme stimulates the adrenal cortex to secrete aldosterone?
A. Angiotensin I
B. Angiotensin II
C. Renin
D. Antidiuretic hormone

Answer: B. Angiotensin II works to increase preload and afterload by stimulating the adrenal cortex to secrete aldosterone.

Scoring

⭐⭐⭐ If you answered all four items correctly, hats off! There's only one way to say it: You're all heart!

⭐⭐ If you answered three items correctly, great job! Your heart is in the right place and so is your nose (your nose is in this book).

⭐ If you answered fewer than three items correctly, don't fret! You have shown a lot of heart.

3

Respiratory system

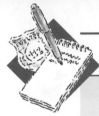

Just the facts

In this chapter, you'll learn:

♦ structures of the respiratory system

♦ how the respiratory system functions

♦ pathophysiology, diagnostic tests, and treatments for several respiratory diseases.

Understanding the respiratory system

The respiratory system consists of two lungs, conducting airways, and associated blood vessels.

The major function of the respiratory system is gas exchange. During ventilation, air is taken into the body on inhalation (inspiration) and travels through respiratory passages to the lungs. Oxygen (O_2) in the lungs replaces carbon dioxide (CO_2) in the blood (at the alveoli) during perfusion, and then CO_2 is expelled from the body on exhalation (expiration).

Disease or trauma may interfere with the respiratory system's vital work, affecting any of the following structures and functions:
- conducting airways
- lungs
- breathing mechanics
- neurochemical control of ventilation.

Conducting airways

The conducting airways allow air into and out of structures within the lung that perform gas exchange. The conducting airways include the upper airway and the lower airway.

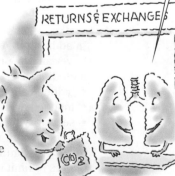

Gas exchange, that's the name of the game.

RETURNS & EXCHANGES

Upper airway

The upper airway consists of the:
- nose
- mouth
- pharynx
- larynx.

Going up

The upper airway allows air flow into and out of the lungs. It warms, humidifies, and filters inspired air and protects the lower airway from foreign matter.

Blocked!

Upper airway obstruction occurs when the nose, mouth, pharynx, or larynx becomes partially or totally blocked, cutting off the O_2 supply. Several conditions can cause upper airway obstruction, including trauma, tumors, and foreign objects.

If not treated promptly, upper airway obstruction can lead to hypoxemia (insufficient O_2 in the blood) and then progress quickly to severe hypoxia (lack of O_2 available to body tissues), loss of consciousness, and death. (See *The upper and lower airways*.)

Lower airway

The lower airway consists of:
- trachea
- right and left mainstem bronchi
- five secondary bronchi
- bronchioles.

The lower airways facilitate gas exchange. Each bronchiole descends from a lobule and contains terminal bronchioles, alveolar ducts, and alveoli. Terminal bronchioles are "anatomic dead spaces" because they don't participate in gas exchange. The alveoli are the chief units of gas exchange. (See *A close look at a pulmonary airway*, page 70.)

On the defense

In addition to warming, humidifying, and filtering inspired air, the lower airway provides the lungs with defense mechanisms, including:
- irritant reflex
- mucociliary system
- secretory immunity.

The irritant reflex is triggered when inhaled particles, cold air, or toxins stimulate irritant receptors. Reflex bronchospasm then occurs to limit the exposure, followed by coughing, which expels the irritant.

The upper and lower airways

The structures of the respiratory system (the airways, lungs, bony thorax, respiratory muscles, and central nervous system) work together to deliver oxygen to the bloodstream and remove excess carbon dioxide from the body.

Upper airways

The upper airways include the nasopharynx (nose), oropharynx (mouth), laryngopharynx, and larynx. These structures warm, filter, and humidify inhaled air.

Lower airways

The lower airways begin with the trachea, or windpipe, which extends from the cricoid cartilage to the carina. The trachea then divides into the right and left mainstem bronchi, which continue to divide all the way down to the alveoli, the gas-exchange units of the lungs.

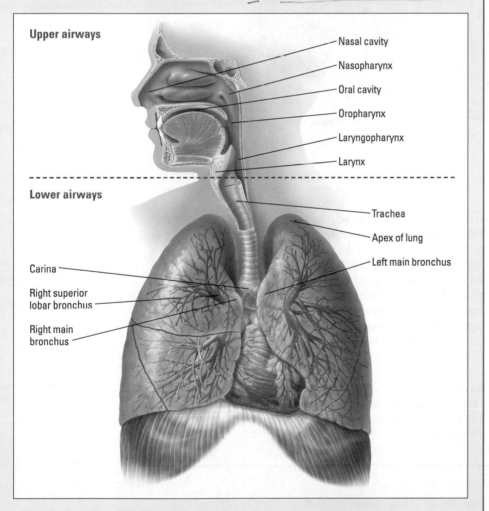

Upper airways

- Nasal cavity
- Nasopharynx
- Oral cavity
- Oropharynx
- Laryngopharynx
- Larynx

Lower airways

- Trachea
- Apex of lung
- Left main bronchus

Carina

Right superior lobar bronchus

Right main bronchus

A close look at a pulmonary airway

As illustrated below, each lobule or airway contains bronchioles and alveoli.

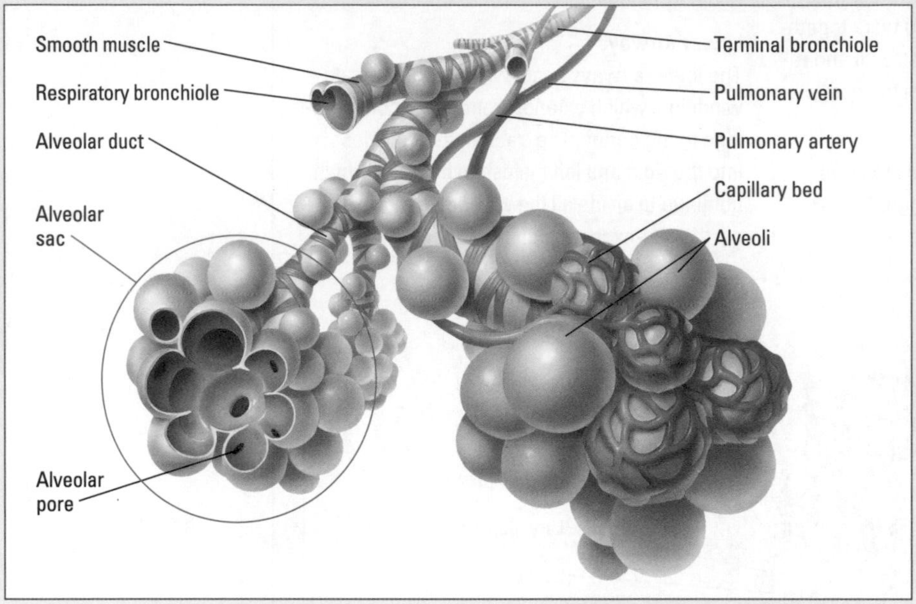

Smooth muscle

Respiratory bronchiole

Alveolar duct

Alveolar sac

Alveolar pore

Terminal bronchiole

Pulmonary vein

Pulmonary artery

Capillary bed

Alveoli

The mucociliary system produces mucus, which traps foreign particles. Foreign matter is then swept to the upper airway for expectoration. A breakdown in the epithelium of the lungs or the mucociliary system can cause the defense mechanisms to malfunction. This allows atmospheric pollutants and irritants to enter and cause inflammation to occur in the lungs.

Secretory immunity protects the lungs by releasing an antibody in the respiratory mucosal secretions that initiates an immune response against antigens contacting the mucosa.

Blocked again!

Like the upper airway, the lower airway can become partially or totally blocked as a result of inflammation, tumors, foreign bodies, bronchospasm, or trauma. This can lead to respiratory distress and failure.

Lungs

The lungs are air-filled, spongelike organs. They're divided into lobes (three lobes on the right, two lobes on the left). Lobes are further divided into lobules and segments.

Plunging into the lungs

The lungs contain about 300 million pulmonary alveoli, which are grapelike clusters of air-filled sacs at the ends of the respiratory passages. Here, gas exchange takes place by diffusion (the passage of gas molecules through respiratory membranes).

In diffusion, O_2 is passed to the blood for circulation through the body. At the same time, CO_2—a cellular waste product that's gathered by the blood as it circulates—is collected from the blood for disposal out of the body through the lungs.

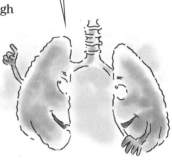

What's my secret? Millions of pulmonary alveoli that perform gas exchange.

All about alveoli

Alveoli consist of type I and type II epithelial cells:

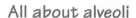 Type I cells form the alveolar walls, through which gas exchange occurs.

Type II cells produce surfactant, a lipid-type substance that coats the alveoli. During inspiration, the alveolar surfactant allows the alveoli to expand uniformly. During expiration, the surfactant prevents alveolar collapse.

Trading places: O_2 and CO_2

How much O_2 and CO_2 trade places in the alveoli? That depends largely on the amount of air in the alveoli (ventilation) and the amount of blood in the pulmonary capillaries (perfusion). The ratio of ventilation to perfusion is called the $\dot{V}/\dot{Q}$ ratio. The $\dot{V}/\dot{Q}$ ratio expresses the effectiveness of gas exchange.

For effective gas exchange, ventilation and perfusion must match as closely as possible. In normal lung function, the alveoli receive air at a rate of about 4 L/minute while the capillaries supply blood to the alveoli at a rate of about 5 L/minute, creating a $\dot{V}/\dot{Q}$ ratio of 4:5 or 0.8. (See *Understanding ventilation and perfusion*, page 72.)

Let's see...the $\dot{V}/\dot{Q}$ ratio is the ratio of ventilation to perfusion. It expresses the effectiveness of gas exchange.

Mismatch mayhem

A $\dot{V}/\dot{Q}$ mismatch, resulting from ventilation-perfusion dysfunction or altered lung mechanics, accounts for most of the impaired gas exchange in respiratory disorders. Ineffective gas exchange between the alveoli and the pulmonary capillaries can affect all body systems by altering the amount of O_2 delivered to living cells.

Ineffective gas exchange from an abnormality causes three outcomes:

shunting (reduced ventilation to a lung unit)

dead-space ventilation (reduced perfusion to a lung unit)

silent unit (combination of the above).

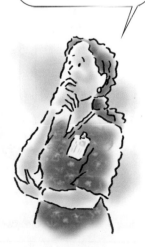

Now I get it!

Understanding ventilation and perfusion

Effective gas exchange depends on the relationship between ventilation and perfusion or the $\dot{V}/\dot{Q}$ ratio. The diagrams below show what happens when the $\dot{V}/\dot{Q}$ ratio is normal and abnormal.

Normal ventilation and perfusion

When ventilation and perfusion are matched, unoxygenated blood from the venous system returns to the right side of the heart through the pulmonary artery to the lungs, carrying carbon dioxide (CO_2). The arteries branch into the alveolar capillaries. Gas exchange takes place in the alveolar capillaries.

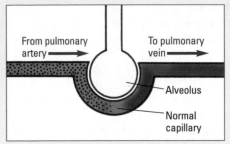

Inadequate perfusion (dead-space ventilation)

When the $\dot{V}/\dot{Q}$ ratio is high, as shown here, ventilation is normal, but alveolar perfusion is reduced or absent. Note the narrowed capillary, indicating poor perfusion. This commonly results from a perfusion defect, such as pulmonary embolism or a disorder that decreases cardiac output.

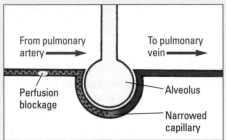

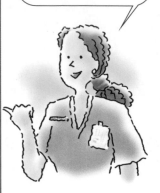

A high $\dot{V}/\dot{Q}$ ratio results from reduced or absent alveolar perfusion.

Inadequate ventilation (shunt)

When the $\dot{V}/\dot{Q}$ ratio is low, pulmonary circulation is adequate but not enough oxygen (O_2) is available to the alveoli for normal diffusion. A portion of the blood flowing through the pulmonary vessels doesn't become oxygenated.

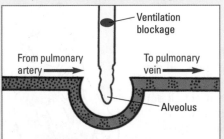

Inadequate ventilation and perfusion (silent unit)

The silent unit indicates an absence of ventilation and perfusion to the lung area. The silent unit may help compensate for a $\dot{V}/\dot{Q}$ imbalance by delivering blood flow to better-ventilated lung areas.

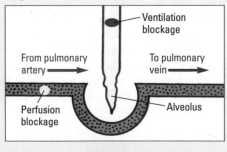

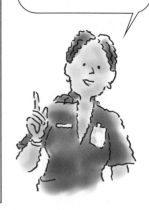

A silent unit can stem from several causes, including pulmonary embolism and chronic alveolar collapse.

Key Blood with CO_2 Blood with O_2 Blood with CO_2 and O_2

Don't shunt me out

Shunting causes the movement of unoxygenated blood from the right side of the heart to the left side of the heart. A shunt may occur from a physical defect that allows unoxygenated blood to bypass fully functioning alveoli. It may also result when airway obstruction prevents O_2 from reaching an adequately perfused area of the lung.

Respiratory disorders are commonly classified as shunt-producing if the $\dot{V}/\dot{Q}$ ratio falls below 0.8 and dead space–producing if the $\dot{V}/\dot{Q}$ ratio exceeds 0.8.

Dead calm

Dead-space ventilation occurs when alveoli don't have adequate blood supply for gas exchange to occur. This occurs with pulmonary emboli, pulmonary infarction, and cardiogenic shock.

The science of silence

A silent unit occurs when little or no ventilation and perfusion are present, such as in cases of pneumothorax and acute respiratory distress syndrome (ARDS).

Breathing mechanics

The amount of air that reaches the lungs carrying O_2 and then departs carrying CO_2 depends on three factors:

☞ lung volume and capacity

☞ compliance (the lungs' ability to expand)

☞ resistance to airflow. – opposition

Air apparent

Lung volume and capacity is the amount of air that's moved in and out of the lungs. Such conditions as polio and tuberculosis create lung changes that reduce the lungs' capacity for air.

No room for expansion

Changes in compliance can occur in either the lung or the chest wall. Destruction of the lung's elastic fibers, which occurs in ARDS, decreases lung compliance. The lungs become stiff, making breathing difficult. The alveolocapillary membrane may also be affected, causing hypoxia. Chest-wall compliance is affected by thoracic deformity, muscle spasm, and abdominal distention.

La pièce de résistance

Resistance refers to opposition to airflow. Changes in resistance may occur in the lung tissue, chest wall, or airways. Airway resistance accounts for about 80% of all respiratory system resistance. It's increased in such obstructive diseases as asthma, chronic bronchitis, and emphysema.

With increased resistance, a person has to work harder to breathe, especially during expiration, to compensate for narrowed airways and diminished gas exchange.

> The central nervous system's respiratory center is located in the lateral medulla oblongata of the brain stem.

Neurochemical control

The respiratory center of the central nervous system (CNS) is located in the lateral medulla oblongata of the brain stem. Impulses travel down the phrenic nerves to the diaphragm and then down the intercostal nerves to the intercostal muscles between the ribs. There, they change the rate and depth of respiration.

Getting to know your neurons

The respiratory center consists of different groups of neurons:
• The dorsal respiratory group of neurons determines the autonomic rhythm of respiration.
• The ventral respiratory group of neurons is inactive during normal respiration but becomes active when increased ventilatory effort is needed. It contains both inspiratory and expiratory neurons.
• The pneumotaxic center and apneustic center don't generate a rhythm but modulate an established rhythm. The pneumotaxic center affects the inspiratory effort by limiting the volume of air inspired. The apneustic center prevents excessive inflation of the lungs.

Factors of influence

Chemoreceptors respond to the hydrogen ion concentration (pH) of arterial blood, the partial pressure of arterial carbon dioxide ($Paco_2$), and the partial pressure of arterial oxygen (Pao_2). Central chemoreceptors respond indirectly to arterial blood by sensing changes in the pH of cerebrospinal fluid (CSF).

amt. of O_2 dissolved in the plasma

$Paco_2$ also helps regulate ventilation (by impacting the pH of CSF). If $Paco_2$ is high, the respiratory rate increases. If $Paco_2$ is low, the respiratory rate decreases.

On the peripheral

The respiratory center also receives information from peripheral chemoreceptors in the carotid and aortic bodies (small neurovascular structures in the carotid arteries and on either side of the aorta). These chemoreceptors respond to decreased Pao_2 and decreased pH. Either change results in increased respiratory drive within minutes.

Respiratory disorders

The respiratory disorders discussed in this section include:
- ARDS
- acute respiratory failure (ARF)
- asbestosis
- asthma
- chronic bronchitis
- cor pulmonale
- emphysema
- pneumonia
- pneumothorax
- pulmonary edema
- pulmonary embolism
- severe acute respiratory syndrome (SARS)
- tuberculosis.

Acute respiratory distress syndrome

ARDS is a form of pulmonary edema that can quickly lead to ARF. Also known as *shock, stiff, white, wet,* or *Da Nang lung,* ARDS may follow a direct or indirect lung injury. It's difficult to diagnose and can prove fatal within 48 hours of onset if not promptly diagnosed and treated. Mortality associated with ARDS remains at 50% to 70%.

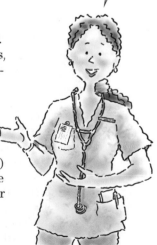

Shock, sepsis, and trauma are the most common causes of ARDS.

How it happens

Shock, sepsis, and trauma are the most common causes of ARDS. Trauma-related factors, such as fat emboli, pulmonary contusions, and multiple transfusions, may increase the likelihood that microemboli will develop.

Other causes of ARDS include:
- anaphylaxis
- aspiration of gastric contents
- diffuse pneumonia, especially viral pneumonia
- drug overdose (for example, heroin, aspirin, and ethchlorvynol)
- idiosyncratic drug reaction to ampicillin or hydrochlorothiazide
- inhalation of noxious gases (such as nitrous oxide, ammonia, or chlorine)
- near-drowning
- oxygen toxicity
- coronary artery bypass grafting
- hemodialysis
- leukemia

- acute miliary tuberculosis
- pancreatitis
- thrombotic thrombocytopenic purpura (embolism and thrombosis of the small blood vessels of the brain)
- uremia
- venous air embolism.

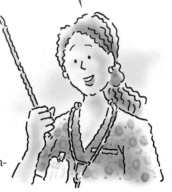

In ARDS, fluid builds up in the lungs, causing them to stiffen.

An account of fluid accumulation

In ARDS, fluid accumulates in the lungs' interstitium, alveolar spaces, and small airways, causing the lungs to stiffen. This impairs ventilation and reduces oxygenation of pulmonary capillary blood. (See *Alveolar changes in ARDS.*)

What to look for

ARDS initially produces rapid, shallow breathing and dyspnea within hours to days of the initial injury. As ARDS progresses, look for the following signs and symptoms:
- Hypoxemia develops, causing an increased drive for ventilation. Because of the effort required to expand the stiff lungs, intercostal and suprasternal retractions result.
- Fluid accumulation produces crackles and rhonchi. Worsening hypoxemia causes restlessness, apprehension, mental sluggishness, motor dysfunction, and tachycardia.
- Severe ARDS causes overwhelming hypoxemia. If uncorrected, this results in hypotension, decreased urine output, and respiratory and metabolic acidosis. Eventually, ventricular fibrillation or standstill may occur. (See *Treating ARDS*, page 78.)

What tests tell you

Arterial blood gas (ABG) analysis with the patient breathing room air initially shows a reduced PaO_2 (less than 60 mm Hg) and a decreased $PaCO_2$ (less than 35 mm Hg). Hypoxemia despite increased supplemental oxygen indicates the presence of an ARDS characteristic shunt. The resulting blood pH usually reflects respiratory alkalosis.

As ARDS worsens, ABG values show:
- respiratory acidosis—increasing $PaCO_2$ (more than 45 mm Hg)
- metabolic acidosis—decreasing bicarbonate (HCO_3^-) levels (less than 22 mEq/L)
- declining PaO_2 despite oxygen therapy
- declining oxygen saturation (SaO_2).

Other diagnostic tests include the following:
- Pulmonary artery catheterization identifies the cause of edema by measuring pulmonary artery wedge pressure (PAWP) (12 mm Hg or less in ARDS). Pulmonary artery mixed venous blood shows hypoxia.

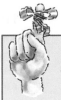

Memory jogger

To remember the progression of **ARDS**, use this mnemonic.

Assault to the pulmonary system

Respiratory distress

Decreased lung compliance

Severe respiratory failure

Now I get it!

Alveolar changes in ARDS

The alveoli undergo major changes in each phase of ARDS.

Phase 1
In *phase 1,* injury reduces normal blood flow to the lungs. Platelets aggregate and release histamine (H), serotonin (S), and bradykinin (B).

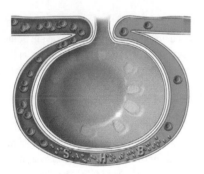

Phase 2
In *phase 2,* those substances—especially histamine—inflame and damage the alveolocapillary membrane, increasing capillary permeability. Fluids then shift into the interstitial space.

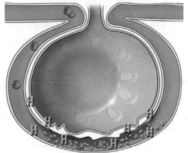

Phase 3
In *phase 3,* as capillary permeability increases, proteins and fluids leak out, increasing interstitial osmotic pressure and causing pulmonary edema.

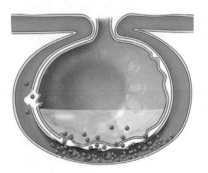

Phase 4
In *phase 4,* decreased blood flow and fluids in the alveoli damage surfactant and impair the cell's ability to produce more. As a result, alveoli collapse, impeding gas exchange and decreasing lung compliance.

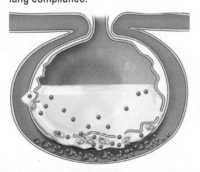

Phase 5
In *phase 5,* sufficient oxygen can't cross the alveolocapillary membrane, but carbon dioxide (CO_2) can and is lost with every exhalation. Oxygen (O_2) and CO_2 levels decrease in the blood.

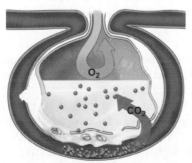

Phase 6
In *phase 6,* pulmonary edema worsens, inflammation leads to fibrosis, and gas exchange is further impeded.

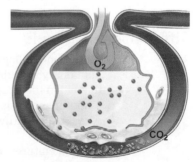

Battling illness

Treating ARDS

Therapy focuses on correcting the cause of acute respiratory distress syndrome (ARDS) and preventing progression of hypoxemia and respiratory acidosis. Supportive care consists of administering continuous positive airway pressure. However, this therapy alone seldom fulfills the patient's ventilatory requirements, so several other treatments are used.

Ventilation

The primary treatment for ARDS is intubation and mechanical ventilation to increase lung volume, open airways, and improve oxygenation. Positive end-expiratory pressure is also added to increase lung volume and open alveoli.

Maximizing mechanical ventilation

Two other techniques can maximize the benefits and minimize the risks of mechanical ventilation:

• Pressure-controlled inverse ratio ventilation reverses the conventional inspiration to expiration ratio and minimizes the risk of barotrauma. The mechanical breaths are pressure-limited.

• Permissive hypercapnia limits peak inspiratory pressure. Although carbon dioxide (CO_2) removal is compromised, no treatment is given for subsequent changes in blood hydrogen and oxygen (O_2) concentration.

Drugs

During mechanical ventilation, sedatives (such as propofol or midazolam), opioids, or neuromuscular blocking agents such as vecuronium may be ordered. These drugs minimize restlessness, O_2 consumption, and CO_2 production and facilitate ventilation.

When ARDS results from fat emboli or a chemical injury, a short course of high-dose corticosteroids may be given. Sodium bicarbonate may reverse severe metabolic acidosis, and fluids and vasopressors help maintain blood pressure. Nonviral infections require treatment with antimicrobial drugs.

Additional support

Supportive measures include diuretic therapy, correction of electrolyte and acid-base imbalances, prone positioning, and fluid restriction (even small increases in capillary pressures from I.V. fluids can greatly increase interstitial and alveolar edema).

• Serial chest X-rays in early stages show bilateral infiltrates. In later stages, they show lung fields with a ground-glass appearance and, with irreversible hypoxemia, "whiteouts" of both lung fields.
• Pulse oximetry shows decreasing SaO_2.

Differential diagnosis

A differential diagnosis rules out cardiogenic pulmonary edema, pulmonary vasculitis, and diffuse pulmonary hemorrhage. Tests that aid in the diagnosis include:

• sputum analysis, including Gram stain and culture and sensitivity tests, to identify organisms and help determine the disease process
• blood cultures to identify infectious organisms
• toxicology tests to screen for drug ingestion
• serum amylase tests to rule out pancreatitis.

Acute respiratory failure

When the lungs can't adequately maintain oxygenation or eliminate CO_2, ARF results, which can lead to tissue hypoxia. There are approximately 150,000 cases of ARF annually in the United States. Mortality ranges from 50% to 70%.

> When I can't adequately maintain oxygenation or eliminate carbon dioxide, ARF results.

How it happens

In patients with essentially normal lung tissue, ARF usually means a $Paco_2$ above 50 mm Hg and a Pao_2 below 50 mm Hg.

COPD has different values

These limits, however, don't apply to patients with chronic obstructive pulmonary disease (COPD), who usually have a consistently high $Paco_2$. In patients with COPD, only acute deterioration in ABG values with corresponding clinical deterioration, indicates ARF.

Conditions that can lead to ARF include:
- COPD
- bronchitis
- pneumonia
- bronchospasm
- ventilatory failure
- pneumothorax
- atelectasis
- cor pulmonale
- pulmonary edema
- pulmonary emboli
- CNS disease
- CNS depression—head trauma or use of sedatives, opioids, tranquilizers, or O_2.

If it isn't hypoventilation...

ARF results from impaired gas exchange. Conditions associated with alveolar hypoventilation (deficient movement of air into and out of the alveoli), $\dot{V}/\dot{Q}$ (ventilation-perfusion) mismatch, and intrapulmonary (right-to-left) shunting can cause ARF if left untreated. Decreased Sao_2 may result from alveolar hypoventilation, in which chronic airway obstruction reduces alveolar minute ventilation (the volume of air inhaled and exhaled in 60 seconds). Pao_2 levels fall and $Paco_2$ levels rise, resulting in hypoxemia.

Hypoventilation can result from a decrease in the respiratory rate or duration or inspiratory signal from the respiratory center, such as with CNS conditions, trauma, or CNS-depressant drugs. The most common cause of alveolar hypoventilation is airway obstruction, commonly seen with COPD (emphysema or bronchitis).

...then it's hypoxemia

Hypoxemia—$\dot{V}/\dot{Q}$ imbalance—most commonly occurs when such conditions as pulmonary embolism or ARDS interrupts normal gas exchange in a specific lung region. Too little ventilation with normal blood flow or too little blood flow with normal ventilation may cause the imbalance, resulting in decreased PaO_2 levels and, thus, hypoxemia.

The hypoxemia and hypercapnia characteristic of ARF stimulate strong compensatory responses by all body systems, including the respiratory system, cardiovascular system, and CNS. In response to hypoxemia, for example, the sympathetic nervous system triggers vasoconstriction and increases peripheral resistance and heart rate. Untreated $\dot{V}/\dot{Q}$ imbalances can lead to right-to-left shunting in which blood passes from the heart's right side to its left without being oxygenated.

Tissue hypoxemia also occurs in ARF, resulting in anaerobic metabolism and lactic acidosis. Respiratory acidosis is due to hypercapnia. Heart rate increases, stroke volume increases, and heart failure may occur. Cyanosis occurs because of increased amounts of unoxygenated blood. Hypoxia of the kidneys results in the release of erythropoietin from renal cells, which in turn causes the bone marrow to increase red blood cell (RBC) production—an attempt by the body to increase the blood's O_2-carrying capacity.

The body responds to hypercapnia with cerebral depression, hypotension, circulatory failure, and increased heart rate and cardiac output. Hypoxemia, hypercapnia, or both cause the brain's respiratory control center first to increase respiratory depth (tidal volume) and then to increase the respiratory rate. As ARF worsens, retractions may also occur.

What to look for

Specific symptoms vary with the underlying cause of ARF, and the following body systems may be affected:
• Respiratory system—Rate may be increased, decreased, or normal depending on the cause; respirations may be shallow or deep or alternate between the two. The patient may experience air hunger. Cyanosis may occur depending on hemoglobin level and arterial oxygenation. Auscultation of the chest may reveal crackles, rhonchi, wheezing, or diminished breath sounds.
• CNS—The patient may demonstrate restlessness, confusion, loss of concentration, irri-

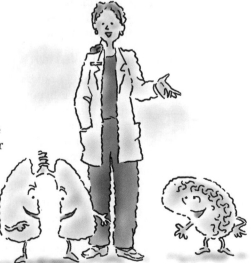

ARF affects the respiratory and central nervous systems as well as the cardiovascular system.

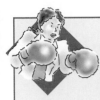

Battling illness

Treating ARF

Therapy for acute respiratory failure (ARF) focuses on correcting hypoxemia and preventing respiratory acidosis.

Oxygenation

These measures can be used to improve oxygenation in patients with ARF:
• deep breathing with pursed lips, if the patient isn't intubated and mechanically ventilated, to help keep airway patent
• incentive spirometry to increase lung volume
• oxygen therapy to promote oxygenation and raise partial pressure of arterial oxygen
• mechanical ventilation with an endotracheal or tracheostomy tube, if needed, to provide adequate oxygenation and reverse acidosis
• high-frequency ventilation, if the patient doesn't respond to treatment, to force the airways open, promoting oxygenation and preventing alveoli collapse.

Drugs

These drugs may be used in the treatment of ARF:
• antibiotics to treat infection
• bronchodilators to maintain airway patency
• corticosteroids to decrease inflammation
• positive inotropic agents to increase cardiac output
• vasopressors to maintain blood pressure
• diuretics to reduce edema and fluid overload
• opioids such as morphine to reduce respiratory rate and promote comfort by relieving anxiety
• anxiolytics such as lorazepam to reduce anxiety
• sedatives, such as propofol, if the patient requires mechanical ventilation and is having difficulty tolerating it
• fluid restriction to reduce volume and cardiac workload (for patients with ARF who have cor pulmonale).

---

tability, tremulousness, diminished tendon reflexes, papilledema, and coma.
• Cardiovascular system—Tachycardia, increased cardiac output, and mildly elevated blood pressure occur early in response to low PaO_2. With myocardial hypoxia, arrhythmias may develop. Pulmonary hypertension may cause increased pressure on the right side of the heart, distended neck veins, enlarged liver, and peripheral edema. (See *Treating ARF*.)

What tests tell you

These tests help identify ARF:
• ABG analysis shows deteriorating values and a pH below 7.35. Patients with COPD may have a lower than normal pH compared with previous levels.
• Chest X-rays identify pulmonary diseases or conditions, such as emphysema, atelectasis, lesions, pneumothorax, infiltrates, and effusions.
• Electrocardiography (ECG) can demonstrate ventricular arrhythmias (indicating myocardial hypoxia) or right ventricular hypertrophy (indicating cor pulmonale).
• Pulse oximetry reveals decreasing SaO_2.

• White blood cell (WBC) count detects the underlying infection.
• Abnormally low hemoglobin level and hematocrit signal blood loss, which indicates decreased O_2-carrying capacity.
• Pulmonary artery catheterization helps to distinguish pulmonary and cardiovascular causes of ARF and monitors hemodynamic pressures.

Asbestosis

Asbestosis is characterized by diffuse interstitial pulmonary fibrosis. Prolonged exposure to airborne asbestos particles causes pleural plaques and tumors of the pleura and peritoneum. Asbestosis may develop 15 to 20 years after the period of regular exposure to asbestos has ended. (See *A close look at asbestosis.*)

A carcinogenic coworker

Asbestos is a potent cocarcinogen, increasing a cigarette smoker's risk for lung cancer. An asbestos worker who smokes is 90 times more likely to develop lung cancer than a smoker who has never worked with asbestos.

How it happens

Asbestosis is caused by prolonged inhalation of asbestos fibers. People at high risk include workers in the mining, milling, construction, fireproofing, and textile industries. Asbestos is also used in paints, plastics, and brake and clutch linings.

Family members of asbestos workers may develop asbestosis from exposure to stray fibers shaken off the workers' clothing. The general public may be exposed to fibrous asbestos dust in deteriorating buildings or in waste piles from asbestos plants.

> Asbestosis occurs when lung spaces become filled with asbestos fibers.

The best info on asbestosis

Here's what happens in asbestosis:
• Inhaled asbestos fibers travel down the airway and penetrate respiratory bronchioles and alveolar walls.
• Fibers become encased in a brown, iron-rich, proteinlike sheath in sputum or lung tissue.
• Interstitial fibrosis may develop in lower lung zones, affecting lung parenchyma and the pleurae.

A close look at asbestosis

After years of exposure to asbestos, healthy lung tissue progresses from simple asbestosis to massive pulmonary fibrosis, as shown below.

Simple asbestosis

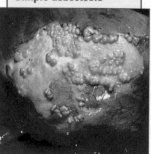

Progressive massive pulmonary fibrosis

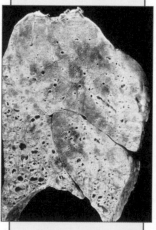

• Raised hyaline plaques may form in the parietal pleura, the diaphragm, and the pleura adjacent to the pericardium.

What to look for

Signs and symptoms of asbestosis include:
• dyspnea on exertion
• dyspnea at rest with extensive fibrosis
• severe, nonproductive cough in nonsmokers
• productive cough in smokers
• finger clubbing
• chest pain (typically pleuritic)
• recurrent respiratory tract infections
• pleural friction rub and crackles on auscultation
• decreased lung inflation
• recurrent pleural effusions
• decreased forced expiratory volume and vital capacity.

  Asbestosis may progress to pulmonary fibrosis with respiratory failure and cardiovascular complications, including pulmonary hypertension and cor pulmonale. (See *Treating asbestosis*.)

What tests tell you

These tests are used to diagnose asbestosis:
• Chest X-rays may show fine, irregular, linear, diffuse infiltrates. With extensive fibrosis, the lungs have a honeycomb or ground-glass appearance. Other findings include pleural thickening and calcification, bilateral obliteration of costophrenic angles and, in later disease stages, an enlarged heart with a classic "shaggy" border.
• Pulmonary function tests may identify decreased vital capacity, forced vital capacity (FVC), and total lung capacity; decreased or normal forced expiratory volume in 1 second (FEV_1); a normal ratio of FEV_1 to FVC; and reduced diffusing capacity for carbon monoxide when fibrosis destroys alveolar walls and thickens the alveolocapillary membrane.
• ABG analysis may reveal decreased Pao_2 and $Paco_2$ from hyperventilation.

The moral of the story: Inhaled asbestos fibers are bad news. Avoid them at all costs or wear an appropriate protective mask!

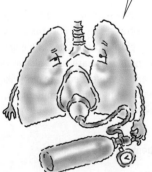

Asthma

Asthma is a chronic reactive airway disorder that can present as an acute attack. It causes episodic airway obstruction resulting from bronchospasms, increased mucus secretion, and mucosal edema.

For the long haul

Asthma is one type of COPD, a long-term pulmonary disease characterized by airflow resistance. Chronic bronchitis and emphysema (discussed on pages 88 and 94) are other types of COPD. (See *Understanding COPD.*)

It usually strikes early

Cases of asthma continue to rise. It currently affects an estimated 17 million Americans; children account for 4.8 million asthma sufferers in the United States. Twice as many boys than girls are affected.

It's a family affair

About one-third of patients develop asthma between ages 10 and 30. In this group, incidence is the same in both sexes. About one-third of all patients share the disease with at least one immediate family member.

How it happens

In asthma, bronchial linings overreact to various triggers, causing episodic smooth-muscle spasms that severely constrict the airways. Mucosal edema and thickened secretions further block the airways. (See *Understanding asthma.*)

Understanding COPD

Chronic obstructive pulmonary disease (COPD) refers to long-term pulmonary disorders characterized by air flow resistance. Such disorders include asthma, chronic bronchitis, and emphysema. Chronic bronchitis and emphysema are more closely related in cause, pathogenesis, and treatment and are more likely to occur together. Asthma is more acute and intermittent than chronic bronchitis or emphysema.

Predisposing factors

Factors that predispose a patient to COPD include:
• smoking
• recurrent or chronic respiratory infections
• allergies
• hereditary factors such as an inherited deficiency in alpha$_1$-protease inhibitor (an inhibitor to the enzyme protease).

Smoking ranks first

Smoking is the most important predisposing factor of COPD. It impairs ciliary action and macrophage function, causing inflammation in the airway, increased mucus production, alveolar destruction, and peribronchiolar fibrosis.

Now I get it!

Understanding asthma

During an asthma attack, muscles surrounding the bronchial tubes tighten (bronchospasm), narrowing the air passage and interrupting the normal flow of air into and out of the lungs. Airflow is further interrupted by an increase in mucus secretion, forming mucus plugs, and the swelling of the bronchial tubes.

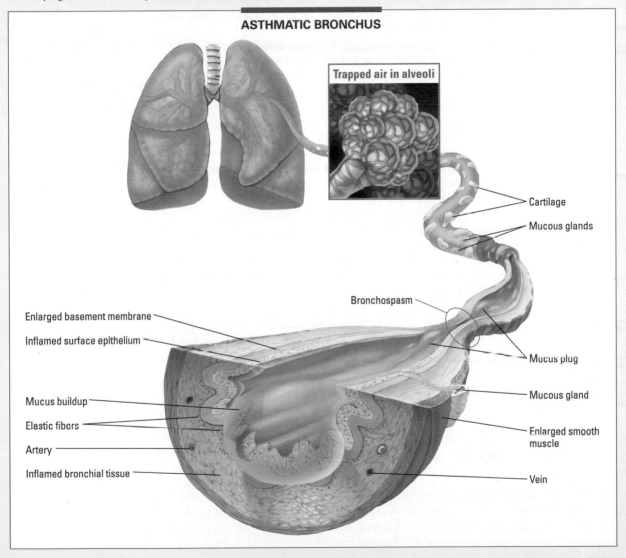

ASTHMATIC BRONCHUS

Trapped air in alveoli

Cartilage

Mucous glands

Bronchospasm

Enlarged basement membrane

Inflamed surface epithelium

Mucus plug

Mucous gland

Mucus buildup

Elastic fibers

Artery

Enlarged smooth muscle

Inflamed bronchial tissue

Vein

What causes the overreaction can be attributed to:

 genetics

 environment.

It's all in the genes

Genetically induced asthma is a sensitivity to specific external allergens, which include pollen, animal dander, house dust or mold, kapok or feather pillows, food additives containing sulfites, cockroach allergen (major allergen for inner-city children), and any other sensitizing substance.

Genetically induced asthma begins in childhood and is commonly accompanied by other hereditary allergies, such as eczema and allergic rhinitis.

Environmentally speaking

Environmentally induced asthma is a reaction to internal, nonallergenic factors. Most episodes occur after a severe respiratory tract infection, especially in adults. Other predisposing conditions include irritants, emotional stress, fatigue, endocrine changes, temperature and humidity variations, and exposure to noxious fumes, such as nitrogen dioxide, which is produced by tobacco smoking among family members and inadequately vented stoves and heating appliances.

Many asthmatics, especially children, have both genetically induced and environmentally induced asthma. (See *Asthma: A complex disease*.)

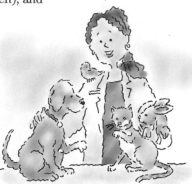

Genetically induced asthma is caused by sensitivity to specific external allergens.

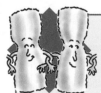

The genetic link

Asthma: A complex disease

More than one gene
Asthma is known as a complex inheritable disease. That means there are several genes that make a person susceptible to the disease, including genes on chromosomes 5, 6, 11, 12, and 14.

Chromosome 5
The role of these genes in the development of asthma isn't clear, but one of the most promising sites of study is chromosome 5. Even though researchers haven't specifically identified a gene from this site, they do know that the area is rich in genes coding for molecules that play a key role in the inflammatory response seen in asthma. Scientists continue to search for specific asthma genes.

What to look for

Signs and symptoms vary depending on the severity of a patient's asthma.

From mild...

Patients with mild asthma have adequate air exchange and are asymptomatic between attacks. *Mild asthma* is classified as either mild intermittent asthma or mild persistent asthma. With *mild intermittent asthma*, the patient experiences symptoms of cough, wheezing, chest tightness, or difficulty breathing less than twice per week. Flare-ups are brief but may vary in intensity. Nighttime symptoms occur less than twice per month.

In *mild persistent asthma*, symptoms of cough, wheezing, chest tightness, or difficulty breathing occur three to six times per week. Flare-ups may affect the patient's activity level. Nighttime symptoms occur three or four times per month.

...to not so bad...

Patients with *moderate persistent asthma* have normal or below-normal air exchange as well as signs and symptoms that include cough, wheezing, chest tightness, or difficulty breathing daily. Flare-ups may affect the patient's level of activity. Nighttime symptoms occur five or more times per month.

...to worse

Patients with *severe persistent asthma* have below-normal air exchange and experience continual symptoms of cough, wheezing, chest tightness, and difficulty breathing. Their activity level is greatly affected. Nighttime symptoms occur frequently.

Patients with any type of asthma may develop status asthmaticus, a severe acute attack that doesn't respond to conventional treatment. The patient will have signs and symptoms that include:
• marked respiratory distress
• marked wheezing or absent breath sounds
• pulsus paradoxus greater than 10 mm Hg
• chest wall contractions. (See *Treating asthma*, page 88.)

What tests tell you

These tests are used to diagnose asthma:
• Pulmonary function tests reveal signs of obstructive airway disease, low-normal or decreased vital capacity, and increased total lung and residual capacities. Pulmonary function may be normal between attacks. Pao_2 and $Paco_2$ are usually decreased, except in severe asthma, when $Paco_2$ may be normal or increased, indicating severe bronchial obstruction.
• Serum immunoglobulin (Ig) E levels may increase from an allergic reaction.

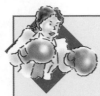

Battling illness

Treating asthma

The best treatment for asthma is prevention by identifying and avoiding precipitating factors, such as environmental allergens or irritants. Usually, such stimuli can't be removed entirely, so desensitization to specific antigens may be helpful, especially in children. Other common treatments are medication and oxygen (O_2).

Medication
These types of drugs are usually given:

Long-acting bronchodilators (salmeterol and formoterol) decrease bronchoconstriction, reduce bronchial airway edema, and increase pulmonary ventilation.

Corticosteroids (hydrocortisone and methylprednisolone) have the same effects as bronchodilators as well as anti-inflammatory and immunosuppressive effects. Inhaled corticosteroids are used in long-term control of asthma.

Leukotriene modifiers (montelukast, zafirlukast, and zileuton) are effective in reducing mucus formation and airway constriction.

Mast cell stabilizers (cromolyn and nedocromil), when given prophylactically, block the acute obstructive effects of antigen exposure.

Immunomodulators (omalizumab) change how the immune system reacts to asthma triggers and are used in long-term asthma control.

Oxygen
Low-flow humidified O_2 may be needed to treat dyspnea, cyanosis, and hypoxemia. The amount delivered is designed to maintain a partial pressure of arterial oxygen between 65 and 85 mm Hg, as determined by arterial blood gas studies. Mechanical ventilation is necessary if the patient doesn't respond to initial ventilatory support and drugs or develops respiratory failure.

• Complete blood count (CBC) with differential reveals increased eosinophil count.
• Chest X-rays can diagnose or monitor asthma's progress and may show hyperinflation with areas of atelectasis.
• ABG analysis detects hypoxemia and guides treatment.
• Skin testing may identify specific allergens. Test results are read in 1 to 2 days to detect an early reaction and again after 4 to 5 days to reveal a late reaction.
• Bronchial challenge testing evaluates the clinical significance of allergens identified by skin testing.
• Pulse oximetry may show a reduced SaO_2 level.

Chronic bronchitis

Chronic bronchitis, a form of COPD, is inflammation of the bronchi caused by irritants or infection.

In chronic bronchitis, hypersecretion of mucus and chronic productive cough last for 3 months of the year and occur for at least 2 consecutive years. The distinguishing characteristic of bronchitis is obstruction of airflow caused by mucus.

How it happens

Chronic bronchitis occurs when irritants are inhaled for a prolonged period. The result is resistance in the small airways and severe $\dot{V}/\dot{Q}$ imbalance that decreases arterial oxygenation.

Patients have a diminished respiratory drive, so they usually hypoventilate. Chronic hypoxia causes the kidneys to produce erythropoietin. This stimulates excessive RBC production, leading to polycythemia. Hemoglobin levels are high, but the amount of reduced hemoglobin that comes in contact with O_2 is low; therefore, cyanosis is evident. (See *Mucus buildup in chronic bronchitis.*)

Now I get it!

Mucus buildup in chronic bronchitis

In chronic bronchitis, excessive mucus production obstructs the small airways.

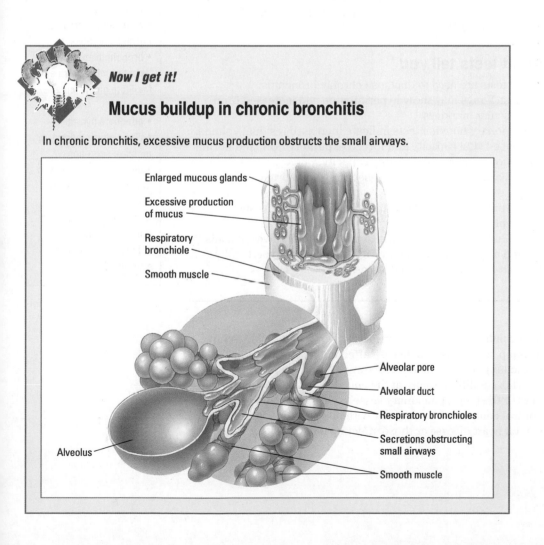

What to look for

Signs and symptoms of advanced chronic bronchitis include:
- productive cough
- dyspnea
- cyanosis
- use of accessory muscles for breathing
- pulmonary hypertension.

The pressure is on

As pulmonary hypertension continues, right ventricular end-diastolic pressure increases. This leads to cor pulmonale (right ventricular hypertrophy with right-sided heart failure). Heart failure results in increased venous pressure, liver engorgement, epigastric distress, S_3 gallop, and dependent edema. (See *Treating chronic bronchitis*.)

What tests tell you

These tests are used to diagnose chronic bronchitis:
- Chest X-rays may show hyperinflation and increased bronchovascular markings.
- Pulmonary function tests indicate increased residual volume, decreased vital capacity and forced expiratory flow, and normal static compliance and diffusing capacity.
- ABG analysis displays decreased Pao_2 and normal or increased $Paco_2$.
- Sputum culture may reveal many microorganisms and neutrophils.
- ECG may show atrial arrhythmias; peaked P waves in leads II, III, and aV_F; and, occasionally, right ventricular hypertrophy.
- Pulse oximetry shows a decreased Sao_2 level.

Battling illness

Treating chronic bronchitis

The most effective treatment for chronic bronchitis is to avoid air pollutants and, if the patient is a smoker, to stop smoking. Other treatments include:
- antibiotics to treat recurring infections
- bronchodilators to relieve bronchospasm and facilitate mucus clearance
- adequate hydration
- chest physiotherapy to mobilize secretions
- nebulizer treatments to loosen and mobilize secretions
- corticosteroids to combat inflammation
- diuretics for edema
- oxygen for hypoxia.

Cor pulmonale

In cor pulmonale, hypertrophy and dilation of the right ventricle develop secondary to a disease affecting the structure or function of the lungs or associated structures.

This condition occurs at the end stage of various chronic disorders of the lungs, pulmonary vessels, chest wall, and respiratory control center. It doesn't occur with disorders stemming from congenital heart disease or those affecting the left side of the heart.

The core facts about cor pulmonale

Cor pulmonale causes about 25% of all types of heart failure. About 85% of patients with cor pulmonale also have COPD, and about 25% of patients with bronchial COPD eventually develop cor pulmonale. It's most common in smokers and in middle-age and elderly men; however, incidence in women is rising.

> Cor pulmonale causes about 25% of all types of heart failure.

How it happens

Cor pulmonale may result from:
• disorders that affect the pulmonary parenchyma
• pulmonary diseases that affect the airways such as COPD
• vascular diseases, such as vasculitis, pulmonary emboli, or external vascular obstruction resulting from a tumor or aneurysm
• chest wall abnormalities, including such thoracic deformities as kyphoscoliosis and pectus excavatum (funnel chest)
• neuromuscular disorders, such as muscular dystrophy and poliomyelitis
• external factors, such as obesity or living at a high altitude.

With a heavy heart (it's working harder)

In cor pulmonale, pulmonary hypertension increases the heart's workload. To compensate, the right ventricle hypertrophies to force blood through the lungs. As long as the heart can compensate for the increased pulmonary vascular resistance, signs and symptoms reflect only the underlying disorder.

What to look for

In early stages of cor pulmonale, patients are most likely to report:
• chronic productive cough
• exertional dyspnea
• wheezing respirations
• fatigue and weakness.
    As the compensatory mechanism begins to fail, larger amounts of blood remain in the right ventricle at the end of diastole, causing ventricular dilation. As cor pulmonale progresses, these additional symptoms occur:
• dyspnea at rest
• tachypnea
• orthopnea
• dependent edema
• distended neck veins
• hepatomegaly (enlarged, tender liver)

- hepatojugular reflux (jugular vein distention induced by pressing over the liver)
- right upper quadrant discomfort
- tachycardia
- decreased cardiac output
- weight gain.

Chest examination reveals characteristics of the underlying lung disease.

Getting complicated

In response to hypoxia, the bone marrow produces more RBCs, causing polycythemia. The blood's viscosity increases, which further aggravates pulmonary hypertension. This increases the right ventricle's workload, causing right-sided heart failure.

Eventually, cor pulmonale may lead to biventricular failure, edema, ascites, and pleural effusions. Polycythemia increases the risk of thromboembolism. (See *Understanding cor pulmonale*.)

Because cor pulmonale occurs late in the course of COPD and other irreversible diseases, prognosis is poor. (See *Treating cor pulmonale*, page 94.)

What tests tell you

These tests are used to diagnose cor pulmonale:
- Pulmonary artery catheterization shows increased right ventricular and pulmonary artery pressures, resulting from increased pulmonary vascular resistance. Both right ventricular systolic and pulmonary artery systolic pressures are greater than 30 mm Hg, and pulmonary artery diastolic pressure is greater than 15 mm Hg.
- Echocardiography or angiography demonstrates right ventricular enlargement.
- Chest X-rays reveal large central pulmonary arteries and right ventricular enlargement.
- ABG analysis detects decreased PaO_2 (usually less than 70 mm Hg and never more than 90 mm Hg).
- Pulse oximetry shows a reduced SaO_2 level.
- ECG discloses arrhythmias, such as premature atrial and ventricular contractions and atrial fibrillation during severe hypoxia. It may also show right bundle-branch block, right axis deviation, prominent P waves, and an inverted T wave in right precordial leads.
- Pulmonary function tests reflect underlying pulmonary disease.
- Magnetic resonance imaging (MRI) measures right ventricular mass, wall thickness, and ejection fraction.
- Cardiac catheterization measures pulmonary vascular pressures.
- Hematocrit is typically over 50%.

Now I get it!

Understanding cor pulmonale

Three types of disorders are responsible for cor pulmonale:

restrictive pulmonary disorders, such as fibrosis or obesity

obstructive pulmonary disorders such as chronic obstructive pulmonary disease

primary vascular disorders such as recurrent pulmonary emboli.

These disorders share a common pathway to the formation of cor pulmonale. Hypoxic constriction of pulmonary blood vessels and obstruction of pulmonary blood flow lead to increased pulmonary resistance, which progresses to cor pulmonale.

```
                    Pulmonary disorder

    Anatomic alterations in the pulmonary blood vessels and
              functional alterations in the lungs

            Increased pulmonary vascular resistance

                  Pulmonary hypertension

                Right ventricular hypertrophy

                     Cor pulmonale

                Right-sided heart failure
```

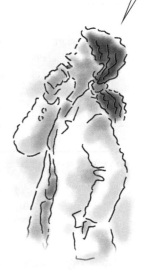

Three different types of disorders may cause cor pulmonale, but all share a common pathway.

• Serum hepatic enzyme levels show an elevated level of aspartate aminotransferase with hepatic congestion and decreased liver function.
• Serum bilirubin levels may be elevated if liver dysfunction and hepatomegaly are present.

Battling illness

Treating cor pulmonale

Therapy for the patient with cor pulmonale has three aims:

 reducing hypoxemia and pulmonary vasoconstriction

increasing exercise tolerance

correcting the underlying condition when possible.

Bed rest, drug therapy, and more
Treatment includes:
• bed rest
• antibiotics for an underlying respiratory tract infection
• oral calcium channel blockers, such as nifedipine, nicardipine, amlodipine, and diltiazem for vasodilation
• potent pulmonary artery vasodilator, such as diazoxide, nitroprusside, or hydralazine, to treat primary pulmonary hypertension

• I.V. prostacyclin therapy to dilate blood vessels and reduce clotting by stopping platelet aggregation
• endolithin receptor antagonists such as bosentan to reduce vasoconstriction
• continuous administration of low concentrations of oxygen to decrease polycythemia and tachypnea
• mechanical ventilation in acute disease
• low-sodium diet with restricted fluid
• phlebotomy to decrease red blood cell mass and anticoagulation with small doses of heparin to decrease the risk of thromboembolism.

What lies underneath
Treatment may vary, depending on the underlying cause. For example, the patient may need a tracheotomy if he has an upper airway obstruction. He may require corticosteroids if he has vasculitis or an autoimmune disorder.

Emphysema

A form of COPD, emphysema is the abnormal, permanent enlargement of the acini accompanied by destruction of the alveolar walls. Obstruction results from tissue changes, rather than mucus production, which is the case in asthma and chronic bronchitis.

Losing elasticity

The distinguishing characteristic of emphysema is airflow limitation caused by lack of elastic recoil in the lungs.

How it happens

Emphysema may be caused by a deficiency of $alpha_1$-protease inhibitor or by cigarette smoking.

In emphysema, recurrent inflammation is associated with the release of proteolytic enzymes (enzymes that promote splitting of proteins by hydrolysis of peptide bonds)

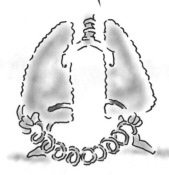

Now that I have emphysema, I seem to lack the spring in my step!

Now I get it!

Air trapping in emphysema

After alveolar walls are damaged or destroyed, they can't support and keep the airways open. The alveolar walls then lose their capability of elastic recoil. Collapse then occurs on expiration, as shown here.

Normal expiration
Note normal recoil and the open bronchiole.

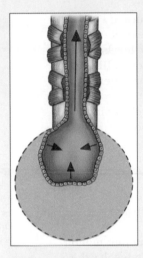

Impaired expiration
Note decreased elastic recoil and a narrowed bronchiole.

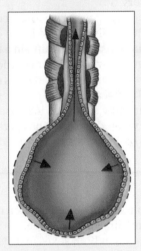

from lung cells. This causes irreversible enlargement of the air spaces distal to the terminal bronchioles. Enlargement of air spaces destroys the alveolar walls, which results in a breakdown of elasticity and loss of fibrous and muscle tissues, making the lungs less compliant. (See *Air trapping in emphysema.*)

What to look for

Signs and symptoms of emphysema include:
- dyspnea on exertion (initial symptom)
- barrel-shaped chest from lung overdistention
- prolonged expiration because accessory muscles are used for inspiration and abdominal muscles are used to force air out of the lungs
- decreased breath sounds.

Hidden by hyperventilation?

Because minimal V̇/Q̇ imbalance occurs, hyperventilation keeps blood gases within a normal range until late in the disease. (See *Treating emphysema.*)

Battling illness

Treating emphysema

Patients with emphysema need counseling on avoiding smoking and air pollution. Additional treatment includes:
- bronchodilators, such as beta-adrenergic blockers, albuterol, and ipratropium to reverse bronchospasm and promote mucociliary clearance
- mucolytics to thin secretions and aid mucus expectoration
- antibiotics to treat respiratory tract infections
- immunizations to prevent influenza and pneumococcal pneumonia
- adequate hydration
- chest physiotherapy to mobilize secretions
- oxygen therapy at low concentrations to increase patient's partial pressure of arterial oxygen to 55 to 65 mm Hg
- lung volume reduction surgery to allow more functional lung tissue to expand and the diaphragm to return to its normally elevated position
- corticosteroids to reduce inflammation.

What tests tell you

The following tests are used to diagnose emphysema:
- Chest X-rays in advanced disease may show a flattened diaphragm, reduced vascular markings at the lung periphery, over-aeration of the lungs, a vertical heart, enlarged anteroposterior chest diameter, and large retrosternal air space.
- Pulmonary function tests indicate increased residual volume and total lung capacity, reduced diffusing capacity, and increased inspiratory flow.
- ABG analysis usually shows reduced PaO_2 and normal $PaCO_2$ until late in the disease. Late in the disease, $PaCO_2$ is elevated. As the body compensates to maintain a normal pH, HCO_3^- levels rise.
- ECG may reveal tall, symmetrical P waves in leads II, III, and aV_F; vertical QRS axis; and signs of right ventricular hypertrophy late in the disease.
- CBC usually shows an increased hemoglobin level late in the disease when the patient has persistent severe hypoxia.
- Pulse oximetry may show a reduced SaO_2 level.

Pneumonia

Pneumonia is an acute infection of the lung parenchyma that commonly impairs gas exchange.

It occurs in both sexes and at all ages. More than four million cases of pneumonia occur annually in the United States. It's the leading cause of death from infectious disease.

The prognosis is good for patients with normal lungs and adequate immune systems. However, bacterial pneumonia is the leading cause of death in debilitated patients.

How it happens

Pneumonia is classified three ways:

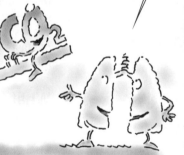

Origin—Pneumonia may be viral, bacterial, fungal, or protozoal in origin.

Location—Bronchopneumonia involves distal airways and alveoli; lobar pneumonia involves part of a lobe or an entire lobe.

Type—Primary pneumonia results from inhalation or aspiration of a pathogen, such as bacteria or a virus, and includes pneumococcal and viral pneumonia; secondary pneumonia may follow lung damage from a noxious chemical or other insult or may result from hematogenous spread of bacteria; aspiration pneumonia results from inhalation of foreign matter, such as vomitus or food particles, into the bronchi.

Colonial expansion

In general, the lower respiratory tract can be exposed to pathogens by inhalation, aspiration, vascular dissemination, or direct contact with contaminated equipment such as suction catheters. After pathogens get inside, they begin to colonize and infection develops.

Stasis report

In bacterial pneumonia, which can occur in any part of the lungs, an infection initially triggers alveolar inflammation and edema. This produces an area of low ventilation with normal perfusion. Capillaries become engorged with blood, causing stasis. As the alveolocapillary membrane breaks down, alveoli fill with blood and exudate, resulting in atelectasis (lung collapse).

In severe bacterial infections, the lungs look heavy and liver-like—reminiscent of ARDS.

Virus attack!

In viral pneumonia, the virus first attacks bronchiolar epithelial cells. This causes interstitial inflammation and desquamation. The virus also invades bronchial mucous glands and goblet cells. It then spreads to the alveoli, which fill with blood and fluid. In advanced infection, a hyaline membrane may form. Like bacterial infections, viral pneumonia clinically resembles ARDS. (See *Looking at lobar pneumonia and bronchopneumonia*, page 98.)

Subtracting surfactant

In aspiration pneumonia, inhalation of gastric juices or hydrocarbons triggers inflammatory changes and also inactivates surfactant over a large area. Decreased surfactant leads to alveolar collapse. Acidic gastric juices may damage the airways and alveoli. Particles containing aspirated gastric juices may obstruct the airways and reduce airflow, leading to secondary bacterial pneumonia.

Risky business

Certain predisposing factors increase the risk of pneumonia. For bacterial and viral pneumonia, these include:
- chronic illness and debilitation
- cancer (particularly lung cancer)
- abdominal and thoracic surgery
- atelectasis
- colds or other viral respiratory infections

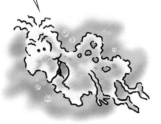

I can sneak into the lower respiratory tract through inhalation, aspiration, or vascular dissemination or through contaminated equipment.

Looking at lobar pneumonia and bronchopneumonia

Pneumonia can involve the distal airways, alveoli, part of a lobe, or an entire lobe.

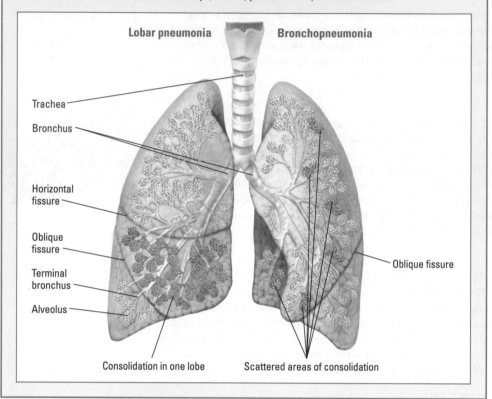

Lobar pneumonia — Bronchopneumonia

Trachea

Bronchus

Horizontal fissure

Oblique fissure

Terminal bronchus

Alveolus

Oblique fissure

Consolidation in one lobe

Scattered areas of consolidation

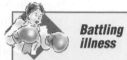

Battling illness

Treating pneumonia

The patient with pneumonia needs antimicrobial therapy based on the causative agent. Reevaluation should be done early in treatment.

Supportive measures include:
• humidified oxygen therapy for hypoxia
• bronchodilator therapy
• antitussives
• mechanical ventilation for respiratory failure
• positive end-expiratory pressure ventilation to maintain adequate oxygenation for patients with severe pneumonia on mechanical ventilation
• high-calorie diet and adequate fluid intake
• bed rest
• analgesic to relieve pleuritic chest pain.

• chronic respiratory disease, such as COPD, bronchiectasis, or cystic fibrosis
• influenza
• smoking
• malnutrition
• alcoholism
• sickle cell disease
• tracheostomy
• exposure to noxious gases
• aspiration
• immunosuppressive therapy
• premature birth.

Aspiration pneumonia is more likely to occur in elderly or debilitated patients, those receiving nasogastric tube feedings, and those with an impaired gag reflex, poor oral hygiene, or a decreased level of consciousness. (See *Treating pneumonia*.)

What to look for

The clinical manifestations of different types of pneumonia vary.
(See *Distinguishing among types of pneumonia.*)

Distinguishing among types of pneumonia

The characteristics and prognosis of the different types of pneumonia vary.

Type	Characteristics	Type	Characteristics
Viral		**Viral** *(continued)*	
Influenza	• Prognosis poor even with treatment • 50% mortality from cardiopulmonary collapse • Cough (initially nonproductive; later, purulent sputum), marked cyanosis, dyspnea, high fever, chills, substernal pain and discomfort, moist crackles, frontal headache, myalgia	Chickenpox (varicella pneumonia)	• Uncommon in children but present in 30% of adults with varicella • Characteristic rash, cough, dyspnea, cyanosis, tachypnea, pleuritic chest pain, and hemoptysis and rhonchi 1 to 6 days after onset of rash
Adenovirus	• Insidious onset • Generally affects young adults • Good prognosis; usually clears with no residual effects • Sore throat, fever, cough, chills, malaise, small amounts of mucoid sputum, retrosternal chest pain, anorexia, rhinitis, adenopathy, scattered crackles, and rhonchi	Cytomegalovirus	• Difficult to distinguish from other non-bacterial pneumonias • In adults with healthy lung tissue, resembles mononucleosis and is generally benign; in neonates, occurs as devastating multisystemic infection; in immuno-compromised hosts, varies from clinically inapparent to fatal infection • Fever, cough, shaking chills, dyspnea, cyanosis, weakness, and diffuse crackles
Respiratory syncytial virus	• Most prevalent in infants and children • Complete recovery in 1 to 3 weeks; may cause death in premature infants younger than age 6 months • Listlessness, irritability, tachypnea with retraction of intercostal muscles, slight sputum production, fever, severe malaise, possible cough or croup, and fine, moist crackles	**Bacterial**	
		Streptococcus	• Sudden onset of a single, shaking chill, and sustained temperature of 102° to 104° F (38.9° to 40° C); commonly preceded by upper respiratory tract infection
Measles (rubeola)	• Typically more severe in adults than in children • Fever, dyspnea, cough, small amounts of sputum, rash, cervical adenopathy, and profusely runny nose	*Klebsiella*	• More likely in patients with chronic alcoholism, pulmonary disease, and diabetes • Fever and recurrent chills; cough producing rusty, bloody, viscous sputum (currant jelly); cyanosis of lips and nail beds from hypoxemia; shallow, grunting respirations

(continued)

Distinguishing among types of pneumonia *(continued)*

Type	Characteristics
***Bacterial** (continued)*	
Staphylococcus	• Commonly occurs in patients with viral illness, such as influenza or measles, and in those with cystic fibrosis • Temperature of 102° to 104° F (38.9° to 40° C), recurrent shaking chills, bloody sputum, dyspnea, tachypnea, and hypoxemia

Type	Characteristics
Aspiration	
	• Results from vomiting and aspiration of gastric or oropharyngeal contents into trachea and lungs • Noncardiogenic pulmonary edema possible with damage to respiratory epithelium from contact with gastric acid • Subacute pneumonia possible with cavity formation • Lung abscess possible if foreign body present • Crackles, dyspnea, cyanosis, hypotension, and tachycardia

> The clinical manifestations of different types of pneumonia vary.

What tests tell you

These tests are used to diagnose pneumonia:
• Chest X-rays confirm the diagnosis by disclosing infiltrates.
• Sputum specimen, Gram stain, and culture and sensitivity tests help differentiate the type of infection and the drugs that are effective in treatment.
• WBC count indicates leukocytosis in bacterial pneumonia and a normal or low count in viral or mycoplasmal pneumonia.
• Blood cultures reflect bacteremia and are used to determine the causative organism.
• ABG levels vary, depending on the severity of pneumonia and the underlying lung state.
• Bronchoscopy or transtracheal aspiration allows the collection of material for culture.
• Pulse oximetry may show a reduced SaO_2 level.

Pneumothorax

Pneumothorax is an accumulation of air in the pleural cavity that leads to partial or complete lung collapse. When the amount of air between the visceral and parietal pleurae increases, increasing tension in the pleural cavity can cause the lung to progressively collapse. In some cases, venous return to the heart is impeded, causing a life-threatening condition called *tension pneumothorax*.

Spontaneous or traumatic?

Pneumothorax is classified as either traumatic or spontaneous. *Traumatic pneumothorax* may be further classified as *open* (sucking chest wound) or *closed* (blunt or penetrating trauma). Note that an open (penetrating) wound may cause closed pneumothorax if communication between the atmosphere and the pleural space seals itself off. *Spontaneous pneumothorax*, which is also considered closed, can be further classified as *primary* (idiopathic) or *secondary* (related to a specific disease).

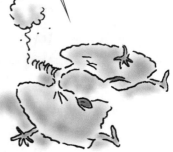

When air accumulates in my pleural cavity, I begin to collapse.

How it happens

The causes of pneumothorax vary according to classification.

Traumatic pneumothorax

A penetrating injury, such as a stab wound, a gunshot wound, or an impaled object, may cause traumatic open pneumothorax, traumatic closed pneumothorax, or hemothorax (accumulation of blood in the pleural cavity).

Blunt trauma from a car accident, a fall, or a crushing chest injury may also cause traumatic closed pneumothorax or hemothorax.

Traumatic pneumothorax may also result from:
• insertion of a central line
• thoracic surgery
• thoracentesis
• pleural or transbronchial biopsy
• tracheotomy.

Tension pneumothorax can develop from either spontaneous or traumatic pneumothorax. (See *Understanding tension pneumothorax*, page 102.)

A change in atmosphere

Open pneumothorax results when atmospheric air (positive pressure) flows directly into the pleural cavity (negative pressure). As the air pressure in the pleural cavity becomes positive, the lung collapses on the affected side. Lung collapse leads to decreased total lung capacity. The patient then develops $\dot{V}/\dot{Q}$ imbalance leading to hypoxia.

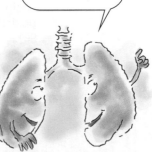

Pneumothorax for us can be an open or shut case.

A leak within the lung

Closed pneumothorax occurs when air enters the pleural space from within the lung. This causes increased pleural pressure and prevents lung expansion during inspiration. It may be called *traumatic pneumothorax* when blunt chest trauma causes lung tissue to rupture, resulting in air leakage.

Now I get it!

Understanding tension pneumothorax

In tension pneumothorax, air accumulates intrapleurally and can't escape. Intrapleural pressure rises, collapsing the ipsilateral lung.

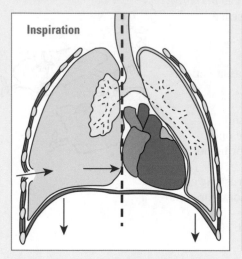

Inspiration

On inspiration, the mediastinum shifts toward the unaffected lung, impairing ventilation.

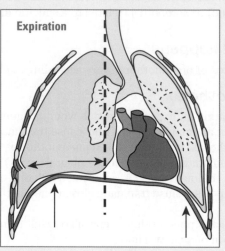

Expiration

On expiration, the mediastinal shift distorts the vena cava and reduces venous return.

Rupture!

Spontaneous pneumothorax is a type of closed pneumothorax. It's more common in men and in older patients with chronic pulmonary disease. However, it also occurs in healthy young adults. The usual cause is rupture of a subpleural bleb (a small cystic space) at the surface of the lung. This causes air leakage into the pleural spaces; then the lung collapses, causing decreased total lung capacity, vital capacity, and lung compliance—leading, in turn, to hypoxia. The total amount of lung collapse can range from 5% to 95%.

What to look for

Although the causes of traumatic and spontaneous pneumothorax vary greatly, the effects are similar. The cardinal signs and symptoms of pneumothorax include:
• sudden, sharp, pleuritic pain exacerbated by chest movement, breathing, and coughing

- asymmetric chest wall movement
- shortness of breath
- cyanosis
- hyperresonance or tympany heard with percussion
- respiratory distress.
      The signs and symptoms of open pneumothorax also include:
- absent breath sounds on the affected side
- chest rigidity on the affected side
- tachycardia
- subcutaneous emphysema (air in the tissues) causing crackling beneath the skin upon palpation.
      Tension pneumothorax produces the most severe respiratory symptoms, including:
- decreased cardiac output
- hypotension
- compensatory tachycardia
- tachypnea
- lung collapse due to air or blood in the intrapleural space
- mediastinal shift and tracheal deviation to the opposite side
- cardiac arrest. (See *Treating pneumothorax*.)

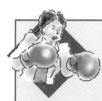

Battling illness

Treating pneumothorax

Treatment of pneumothorax depends on its type.

Spontaneous

Treatment is usually conservative for spontaneous pneumothorax when there's:

- no sign of increased pleural pressure
- lung collapse less than 30%
- no dyspnea or indication of physiologic compromise.

      Such treatment consists of bed rest; careful monitoring of blood pressure, pulse, and respiratory rate; pulse oximetry; oxygen administration; and, possibly, aspiration of air with a large-bore needle attached to a syringe.

      If more than 30% of the lung collapses, a thoracostomy tube is typically placed in the second intercostal space in the mid-clavicular line to try to reexpand the lung. The tube then connects to an underwater seal or to low-pressure suction. If blood is present in the pleural space, a second thoracostomy tube is placed in the fourth, fifth, or sixth intercostal space to drain the blood. Treatment for recurring spontaneous pneumothorax is thoracotomy and pleurectomy, which causes the lung to adhere to the parietal pleura.

Traumatic

Traumatic pneumothorax requires thoracostomy tube insertion and chest drainage and may also require surgical repair.

Tension

Tension pneumothorax is a medical emergency. If the tension in the pleural space isn't relieved, the patient will die from inadequate cardiac output or hypoxemia. A large-bore needle is inserted into the pleural space through the second intercostal space. If large amounts of air escape through the needle after insertion, the needle is left in place until a thoracostomy tube can be inserted.

What tests tell you

These tests are used to diagnose pneumothorax:
• Chest X-rays confirm the diagnosis by revealing air in the pleural space and, possibly, a mediastinal shift. Sequential chest X-rays show whether thoracostomy was effective in resolving pneumothorax.
• ABG studies may show hypoxemia, possibly with respiratory acidosis and hypercapnia. SaO_2 levels may decrease at first but typically return to normal within 24 hours.
• Pulse oximetry reveals hypoxemia.

Pulmonary edema

Pulmonary edema is a common complication of cardiac disorders. It's marked by accumulated fluid in the extravascular spaces of the lung. It may occur as a chronic condition or develop quickly and rapidly become fatal.

How it happens

Pulmonary edema may result from left-sided heart failure caused by arteriosclerotic, cardiomyopathic, hypertensive, or valvular heart disease.

Off balance

Normally, pulmonary capillary hydrostatic pressure, capillary oncotic pressure, capillary permeability, and lymphatic drainage are in balance. This prevents fluid infiltration to the lungs. When this balance changes, or the lymphatic drainage system is obstructed, pulmonary edema results.

If colloid osmotic pressure decreases, the hydrostatic force that regulates intravascular fluids is lost because nothing opposes it. Fluid flows freely into the interstitium and alveoli, impairing gas exchange and leading to pulmonary edema. (See *How pulmonary edema develops.*)

What to look for

Signs and symptoms vary with the stage of pulmonary edema. In the early stages, look for:
• dyspnea on exertion
• paroxysmal nocturnal dyspnea
• orthopnea
• cough
• mild tachypnea
• increased blood pressure
• dependent crackles

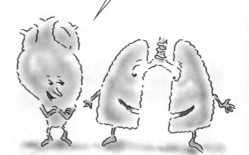

Let's face it. We have to depend on each other.

Now I get it!

How pulmonary edema develops

In pulmonary edema, diminished function of the left ventricle causes blood to pool there and in the left atrium. Eventually, blood backs up into the pulmonary veins and capillaries.

Increasing capillary hydrostatic pressure pushes fluid into the interstitial spaces and alveoli. The illustrations below show a normal alveolus and the effects of pulmonary edema.

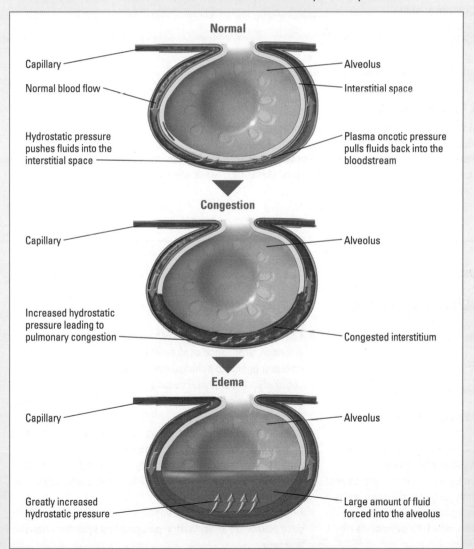

Normal

Capillary

Normal blood flow

Hydrostatic pressure pushes fluids into the interstitial space

Alveolus

Interstitial space

Plasma oncotic pressure pulls fluids back into the bloodstream

Congestion

Capillary

Increased hydrostatic pressure leading to pulmonary congestion

Alveolus

Congested interstitium

Edema

Capillary

Greatly increased hydrostatic pressure

Alveolus

Large amount of fluid forced into the alveolus

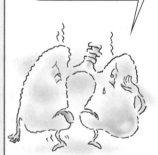

Note that when gas exchange is impaired, oxygen can't get to tissues.

- jugular vein distention
- diastolic S_3 gallop
- tachycardia.

    As tissue hypoxia and decreased cardiac output occur, you'll see:
- labored, rapid respiration
- more diffuse crackles
- cough producing frothy, bloody sputum
- increased tachycardia
- arrhythmias
- cold, clammy skin
- diaphoresis
- cyanosis
- falling blood pressure
- thready pulse. (See *Treating pulmonary edema.*)

What tests tell you

Clinical features of pulmonary edema permit a working diagnosis. These diagnostic tests are used to confirm the disease:
- ABG analysis usually shows hypoxia with variable $Paco_2$, depending on the patient's degree of fatigue. Metabolic acidosis may be revealed.

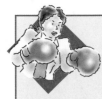

Battling illness

Treating pulmonary edema

Treatment for pulmonary edema has three aims:

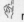 reducing extravascular fluid

  improving gas exchange and myocardial function

  correcting the underlying disease, if possible.

    Treatments include:
- high concentrations of oxygen (O_2) administered by nasal cannula (the patient usually can't tolerate a mask)
- assisted ventilation to improve O_2 delivery to the tissues and acid-base balance for persistently low arterial oxygen levels
- diuretics, such as furosemide, ethacrynic acid, and bumetanide, to increase urination, which helps mobilize extravascular fluid

- positive inotropic agents, such as digoxin, milrinone, and inamrinone, to enhance contractility in myocardial dysfunction
- pressor agents to enhance contractility and promote vasoconstriction in peripheral vessels
- antiarrhythmics for arrhythmias related to decreased cardiac output
- arterial vasodilators, such as nitroprusside, to decrease peripheral vascular resistance, preload, and afterload
- morphine to reduce anxiety and dyspnea and dilate the systemic venous bed, promoting blood flow from pulmonary circulation to the periphery
- human B-type natriuretic peptide, such as nesiritide, to reduce pulmonary artery wedge pressure and systemic arterial pressure.

• Chest X-rays show diffuse haziness of the lung fields and, usually, cardiomegaly and pleural effusion.
• Pulse oximetry may reveal decreasing SaO_2 levels.
• Pulmonary artery catheterization identifies left-sided heart failure and helps rule out ARDS.
• ECG may show previous or current myocardial infarction (MI).

Pulmonary embolism

Pulmonary embolism is an obstruction of the pulmonary arterial bed by a dislodged thrombus, heart valve growths, or a foreign substance. It strikes an estimated 6 million adults each year in the United States, resulting in 100,000 deaths.

May not produce symptoms, or may be fatal

Although pulmonary infarction that results from embolism may be so mild as to produce no symptoms, massive embolism (more than a 50% obstruction of pulmonary arterial circulation) and the accompanying infarction can be rapidly fatal.

How it happens

Pulmonary embolism generally results from dislodged thrombi originating in the leg veins or pelvis. More than one-half of such thrombi arise in the deep veins of the legs.
    Predisposing factors include:
• long-term immobility
• chronic pulmonary disease
• heart failure
• atrial fibrillation
• thrombophlebitis
• polycythemia vera
• thrombocytosis
• autoimmune hemolytic anemia
• sickle cell disease
• varicose veins
• recent surgery
• advanced age
• pregnancy
• lower-extremity fractures or surgery
• burns
• obesity
• vascular injury
• cancer
• I.V. drug abuse
• hormonal contraceptives.

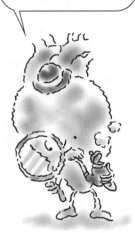

I do believe that pulmonary embolism generally results from dislodged thrombi originating in the leg veins or pelvis.

Floating fragments

Thrombus formation results directly from vascular wall damage, venostasis, or hypercoagulability of the blood. Trauma, clot dissolution, sudden muscle spasm, intravascular pressure changes, or a change in peripheral blood flow can cause the thrombus to loosen or fragment. Then the thrombus—now called an *embolus*—floats to the heart's right side and enters the lung through the pulmonary artery. There, the embolus may dissolve, continue to fragment, or grow.

A growing problem

By occluding the pulmonary artery, the embolus prevents alveoli from producing enough surfactant to maintain alveolar integrity. As a result, alveoli collapse and atelectasis develops. If the embolus enlarges, it may clog most or all of the pulmonary vessels and cause death. (See *Looking at pulmonary emboli.*)

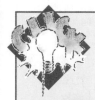

Now I get it!

Looking at pulmonary emboli

This illustration shows multiple emboli in pulmonary artery branches and a larger embolus that has resulted in an infarcted area in the lung.

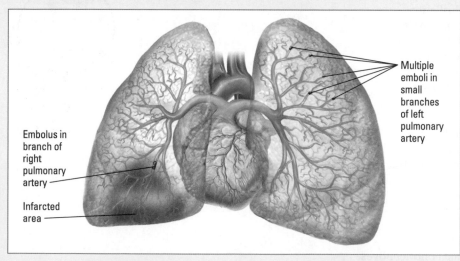

Multiple emboli in small branches of left pulmonary artery

Embolus in branch of right pulmonary artery

Infarcted area

What to look for

Total occlusion of the main pulmonary artery is rapidly fatal; smaller or fragmented emboli produce symptoms that vary with the size, number, and location of the emboli. Usually, the first symptom of pulmonary embolism is dyspnea, which may be accompanied by anginal or pleuritic chest pain.

Other clinical features include:
- tachycardia
- "air hunger"
- feeling of impending doom
- productive cough (sputum may be blood-tinged)
- low-grade fever
- pleural effusion.

Less common signs include:
- massive hemoptysis
- splinting of the chest
- leg edema
- cyanosis, syncope, and distended neck veins (with a large embolus).

In addition, pulmonary embolism may cause pleural friction rub, signs of circulatory collapse (weak, rapid pulse and hypotension), and hypoxia (restlessness and anxiety). (See *Treating pulmonary embolism.*)

Battling illness

Treating pulmonary embolism

Treatment of pulmonary embolism is designed to:
- maintain adequate cardiovascular and pulmonary function during resolution of the obstruction
- prevent embolus recurrence.

Heparin and nonpharmacologic therapies

Because most emboli resolve within 10 to 14 days, treatment consists of oxygen therapy, as needed, and anticoagulation with heparin to inhibit new thrombus formation. Heparin therapy is monitored with daily coagulation studies (partial thromboplastin time). Nonpharmacologic therapies include pneumatic compression devices.

Fibrinolytic therapy

Patients with massive pulmonary embolism and shock may need fibrinolytic therapy with streptokinase or alteplase to enhance fibrinolysis of the pulmonary emboli and remaining thrombi. Emboli that cause hypotension may require the use of vasopressors.

Surgery

Surgery is performed on patients who can't take anticoagulants (because of recent surgery or blood dyscrasias), or who have recurrent emboli during anticoagulant therapy. Surgery consists of vena caval ligation or insertion of a device (umbrella filter) to filter blood returning to the heart and lungs.

What tests tell you

The patient history should reveal predisposing conditions for pulmonary embolism as well as risk factors, including long car or plane trips, cancer, pregnancy, hypercoagulability, and previous deep vein thromboses or pulmonary emboli.

These tests support the diagnosis of pulmonary embolism:
• Chest X-rays help to rule out other pulmonary diseases.
• Lung scan shows perfusion defects in areas beyond occluded vessels; however, it doesn't rule out microemboli.
• Pulmonary angiography is the most definitive test, but it poses some risk to the patient. Its use depends on the uncertainty of the diagnosis and the need to avoid unnecessary anticoagulant therapy in a high-risk patient.
• ECG is inconclusive, but helps distinguish pulmonary embolism from MI.
• Auscultation occasionally reveals a right ventricular S_3 gallop and increased intensity of a pulmonic component of S_2. Also, crackles and a pleural rub may be heard at the embolism site.
• ABG measurements showing decreased PaO_2 and $PaCO_2$ are characteristic, but don't always occur.
• If pleural effusion is present, thoracentesis may rule out empyema, which indicates pneumonia.

Severe acute respiratory syndrome

SARS, a viral respiratory illness caused by a coronavirus, was first reported in Asia in February 2003. According to the World Health Organization (WHO), a total of 8,422 people worldwide became sick with SARS during the 2003 outbreak. Of these, 916 died. In the United States, 192 cases were reported; all of these patients recovered.

How it happens

The SARS virus incubates for 2 to 10 days. It seems to spread by close person-to-person contact. The coronavirus that causes SARS is thought to be transmitted by respiratory droplets produced when an infected person coughs or sneezes. Droplet spread occurs when droplets from the cough or sneeze of an infected person are propelled a short distance (typically up to 3 feet) through the air and deposited on the mucous membranes of the mouth, nose, or eyes of a person who is nearby. The virus can also spread when a person touches a surface or object contaminated with infectious droplets and then touches his mouth, nose, or eyes. (See *Looking at a SARS virion.*)

> The SARS virus incubates for 2 to 10 days. It seems to spread by close person-to-person contact.

Looking at a SARS virion

The SARS virion (A) attaches to receptors on the host cell membrane and releases enzymes (called *absorption*) (B) that weaken the membrane and enable the SARS virion to penetrate the cell. The SARS virion removes the protein coating that protects its genetic material (C), replicates (D), and matures, and then escapes from the cell by budding from the plasma membrane (E). The infection then can spread to other host cells.

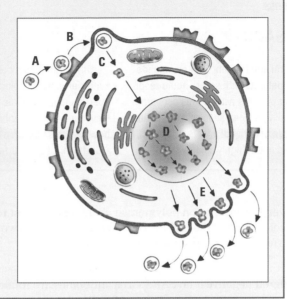

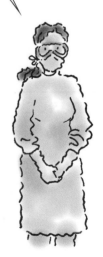

Droplet spread is probably SARS' mode of transmission.

What to look for

SARS mimics many other respiratory diseases. It begins with a high fever (usually a temperature greater than 100.4° F [38° C]), chills, and achiness. Patients develop respiratory symptoms 4 to 7 days after the onset of fever. Respiratory symptoms can be mild to severe and include dry cough, shortness of breath, hypoxemia, and pneumonia. Up to 20% of patients develop diarrhea. (See *Treating SARS*, page 112.)

What tests tell you

The following information can be used to diagnosis SARS:
• Patient history is one of the most valuable sources of information when diagnosing suspected SARS. The diagnosis is fairly certain if the patient traveled to an area with documented SARS cases or has had close contact within the past 10 days with a person suspected of having SARS.
• Chest X-ray reveals hazy opacities and ground-glass appearance that progresses to bilateral consolidation within 24 to 48 hours.
• Suspect SARS in patients with severe atypical pneumonia.
• The SARS virus may be detected in nasopharyngeal or oropharyngeal secretions, blood, or stool.
   The WHO developed three types of diagnostic tests for SARS, including:

Battling illness

Treating SARS

The Centers for Disease Control and Prevention recommends using the same treatment for patients with severe acute respiratory syndrome (SARS) as for patients with serious community-acquired pneumonia, including oxygen support, as needed. Some experts advocate the use of antiviral agents, such as oseltamivir or ribavirin. Steroid use is highly controversial.

Other treatments being studied include:
• interferon beta to block the virus from entering the cell; however, stopping the virus may require 10 times the normal dose
• cysteine protease inhibitors to inhibit SARS virus replication; however, this has been effective in only 30% of cases
• Surfaxin, a liquid surfactant.

 reverse transcription polymerase chain reaction test to detect ribonucleic acid of the SARS virus. To confirm SARS, two tests on two different specimens must be positive.

serum tests to detect antibodies IgM and IgG. The test result is considered negative if no SARS virus antibodies are found in serum obtained more than 28 days after the onset of symptoms.

cell culture test.

A positive result for any of these tests confirms the diagnosis of SARS, but negative results don't necessarily rule out the diagnosis.

Tuberculosis

Tuberculosis is an infectious disease that primarily affects the lungs but can invade other body systems as well. In tuberculosis, pulmonary infiltrates accumulate, cavities develop, and masses of granulated tissue form within the lungs. Tuberculosis may occur as an acute or a chronic infection.

The American Lung Association estimates that active tuberculosis afflicts 5.2 of every 100,000 people in the United States, which is a 43.5% decrease over the past 10 years. Tuberculosis is 63% more common in men and four times as common in non-whites.

Too many people, not enough air

Incidence is highest in people who live in crowded, poorly ventilated, unsanitary conditions, such as prisons, tenement houses, and homeless shelters. Others at high risk for tuberculosis include alcoholics, I.V. drug abusers, elderly people, and those who are immunocompromised.

How it happens

Tuberculosis results from exposure to *Mycobacterium tuberculosis* and, sometimes, other strains of mycobacteria. Here's what happens:

• *Transmission*—An infected person coughs or sneezes, spreading infected droplets. When someone without immunity inhales these droplets, the bacilli are deposited in the lungs.

• *Immune response*—The immune system responds by sending leukocytes, and inflammation results. After a few days, leukocytes are replaced by macrophages. Bacilli are then ingested by the macrophages and carried off by the lymphatics to the lymph nodes.

• *Tubercle formation*—Macrophages that ingest the bacilli fuse to form epithelioid cell tubercles, tiny nodules surrounded by lymphocytes. Within the lesion, caseous necrosis develops and scar tissue encapsulates the tubercle. The organism may be killed in the process.

• *Dissemination*—If the tubercles and inflamed nodes rupture, the infection contaminates the surrounding tissue and may spread through the blood and lymphatic circulation to distant sites. This process is called *hematogenous dissemination*. (See *Understanding tuberculosis invasion*, page 114.)

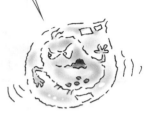

I'm flying in a droplet, looking for someone to land on.

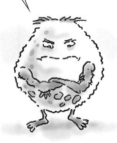

No doubt, the immune system will try to wipe me out.

What to look for

After exposure to *M. tuberculosis*, roughly 5% of infected people develop active tuberculosis within 1 year. They may complain of a low-grade fever at night, a productive cough that lasts longer than 3 weeks, and symptoms of airway obstruction from lymph node involvement.

In other infected people, microorganisms cause a latent infection. The host's immunologic defense system may destroy the bacillus. Alternatively, the encapsulated bacilli may live within the tubercle. It may lie dormant for years, reactivating later to cause active infection.

Adding insult to injury

Tuberculosis can cause massive pulmonary tissue damage, with inflammation and tissue necrosis eventually leading to respiratory failure. Bronchopleural fistulas can develop from lung tissue damage, resulting in pneumothorax. The disease can also lead to hemorrhage, pleural effusion, and pneumonia. Small mycobacterial foci can infect other body organs, including the kidneys, skeleton, and CNS.

With proper treatment, the prognosis for a patient with tuberculosis is usually excellent. (See *Treating tuberculosis*, page 114.)

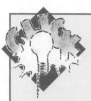

Now I get it!

Understanding tuberculosis invasion

After infected droplets are inhaled, they enter the lungs and are deposited either in the lower part of the upper lobe or in the upper part of the lower lobe. Leukocytes surround the droplets, which leads to inflammation. As part of the inflammatory response, some mycobacteria are carried off in the lymphatic circulation by the lymph nodes.

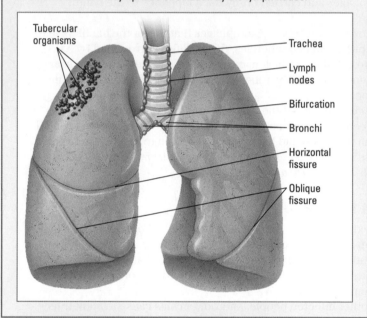

Tubercular organisms

Trachea

Lymph nodes

Bifurcation

Bronchi

Horizontal fissure

Oblique fissure

What tests tell you

These tests are used to diagnose tuberculosis:
• Chest X-rays show nodular lesions, patchy infiltrates (mainly in upper lobes), cavity formation, scar tissue, and calcium deposits.
• A tuberculin skin test reveals infection at some point but doesn't indicate active disease.
• Stains and cultures of sputum, CSF, urine, drainage from abscesses, or pleural fluid show heat-sensitive, nonmotile, aerobic, acid-fast bacilli.
• Computed tomography or MRI scans allow the evaluation of lung damage and may confirm a difficult diagnosis.

Battling illness

Treating tuberculosis

The usual treatment is daily oral doses of isoniazid or rifampin, with ethambutol added in some cases, for at least 9 months. After 2 to 4 weeks, the disease is no longer infectious, and the patient can resume normal activities while continuing to take medication.

The patient with atypical mycobacterial disease or drug-resistant tuberculosis may require second-line drugs, such as capreomycin, streptomycin, para-aminosalicylic acid, pyrazinamide, and cycloserine.

The rise of resistant strains
Many patients find it difficult to follow this lengthy treatment regimen. Therefore, the incidence of noncompliance is high. This has led to the development of resistant strains of tuberculosis in recent years.

• Bronchoscopy shows inflammation and altered lung tissue. It may also be performed to obtain sputum if the patient can't produce an adequate sputum specimen.

Ruling out the copycats

Several of these tests may be needed to distinguish tuberculosis from other diseases that mimic it, such as lung cancer, lung abscess, pneumoconiosis, and bronchiectasis.

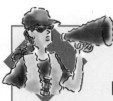

That's a wrap!

Respiratory system review

Understanding the respiratory system
Major function of the respiratory system is gas exchange.

Components consist of two lungs, conducting airways, and associated blood vessels.

During ventilation:
• air is taken into the body by inhalation (inspiration) and travels through respiratory passages to the lungs.

During perfusion:
• O_2 in the lungs replaces CO_2 in the blood
• CO_2 is expelled from the body on exhalation (expiration).

Conducting airways
Conduction airways allow air into and out of structures within the lung that perform gas exchange and consist of the:
• nose
• mouth
• pharynx
• larynx.

Conduction airways in the lower airway consist of:
• trachea
• right and left mainstem bronchi
• five secondary bronchi
• bronchioles.

Breathing mechanisms
Three factors regulate the amount of air that reaches the lungs carrying O_2 and departs with CO_2:
• lung volume and capacity
• compliance (the lungs' ability to expand)
• resistance to airflow.

Neurochemical control
The respiratory center, located in the lateral medulla oblongata of the brain stem, consists of three different groups of neurons:
• dorsal respiratory neurons
• ventral respiratory neurons
• pneumotaxic center and apneustic center.

Chemoreceptors
Factors that influence respiration are called *chemoreceptors* that respond to the:
• hydrogen ion concentration (pH) of arterial blood
• $Paco_2$
• Pao_2.

Functions of pH, $Paco_2$, and Pao_2:
• $Paco_2$ regulates ventilation by impacting the pH of cerebrospinal fluid.
• If $Paco_2$ is high and Pao_2 and pH are low, respiratory rate increases.

(continued)

Respiratory system review (continued)

Respiratory disorders

• *ARDS*—form of pulmonary edema that can quickly lead to acute respiratory failure
• *ARF*—condition in which the lungs can't adequately maintain oxygenation to eliminate CO_2, which can lead to tissue hypoxia
• *Asbestosis*—condition characterized by diffuse interstitial pulmonary fibrosis
• *Asthma*—form of COPD that's a chronic reactive airway disorder that can present as an acute attack
• *Chronic bronchitis*—form of COPD that's an inflammation of the bronchi caused by resistance in small airways from prolonged irritant inhalation
• *Cor pulmonale*—condition that develops secondary to a disease that affects the structure or function of the lungs or associated structures

• *Emphysema*—form of COPD that's the abnormal, permanent enlargement of the acini accompanied by destruction of the alveolar walls
• *Pneumonia*—acute infection of the lung parenchyma that impairs gas exchange
• *Pneumothorax*—accumulation of air in the pleural cavity that leads to partial or complete lung collapse
• *Pulmonary edema*—common complication of cardiac disorders that's marked by accumulated fluid in the extravascular spaces of the lung
• *Pulmonary embolism*—obstruction of the pulmonary arterial bed caused by a dislodged thrombus, heart valve growths, or a foreign substance
• *SARS*—viral respiratory illness caused by a coronavirus
• *Tuberculosis*—infectious disease that primarily affects the lungs but can invade other body systems

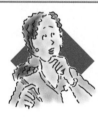

Quick quiz

1.   Which PAWP is one of the hallmark signs of ARDS?
        A.   12 mm Hg
        B.   16 mm Hg
        C.   18 mm Hg
        D.   20 mm Hg

Answer: A. Patients with ARDS have a PAWP of 12 mm Hg or less because their pulmonary edema isn't cardiac in nature. An elevated pressure indicates pulmonary edema related to heart failure.

2. Asthma is caused by:
   A. sensitivity to specific allergens.
   B. severe respiratory tract infection.
   C. emotional stress.
   D. fatigue.

Answer: A. Asthma may result from sensitivity to specific external allergens, including pollen, animal dander, house dust, cockroach allergens, and mold. Although a severe respiratory tract infection may precede an attack and emotional stress and fatigue may aggravate asthma, these factors don't cause the disease.

3. Tuberculosis is transmitted through:
   A. the fecal-oral route.
   B. contact with blood.
   C. contact with urine.
   D. inhalation of infected droplets.

Answer: D. Transmission occurs when an infected person coughs or sneezes, spreading infected droplets.

4. Patients with cor pulmonale usually also have which other respiratory disorder?
   A. Tuberculosis
   B. Emphysema
   C. COPD
   D. SARS

Answer: C. About 85% of patients with cor pulmonale also have COPD; about 25% of patients with bronchial COPD eventually develop cor pulmonale.

5. Tuberculosis of the kidneys is spread by which method?
   A. Homogenous dissemination
   B. Hematogenous dissemination
   C. Exogenous dissemination
   D. Endogenous dissemination

Answer: B. Hematogenous dissemination; it's the process by which the tubercles and inflamed nodes rupture and spread through the blood and lymphatic circulation to distant sites.

6. What's one of the first symptoms of SARS?
   A. Dry cough
   B. Shortness of breath
   C. Hypoxemia
   D. High fever

Answer: D. SARS typically begins with a high fever, chills, and achiness. Respiratory symptoms develop 4 to 7 days later; they can be mild to severe and include dry cough, shortness of breath, hypoxemia, and pneumonia.

7. Which type of pneumonia is most prevalent in infants and children?

  A. Cytomegalovirus
  B. Varicella
  C. Respiratory syncytial virus (RSV)
  D. Influenza

Answer: C. Pneumonia caused by RSV is most prevalent in infants and children.

Scoring

☆☆☆   If you answered all seven items correctly, excellent! When it comes to understanding the respiratory system, no one can accuse you of being full of hot air.

☆☆   If you answered five or six items correctly, swell up with pride! You inhaled the chapter and exhaled right answers.

☆   If you answered fewer than five items correctly, that's life. Take a deep breath and get ready for chapter 4 on the neurologic system.

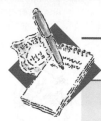

4

Neurologic system

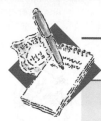

Just the facts

In this chapter, you'll learn:

♦ the structures of the neurologic system

♦ how the neurologic system works

♦ causes, pathophysiology, diagnostic tests, and treatments for several common neurologic disorders.

Understanding the neurologic system

The neurologic, or nervous, system is the body's communication network. It coordinates and organizes the functions of all other body systems. This intricate network has two main divisions:
• The central nervous system (CNS), made up of the brain and spinal cord, is the body's control center.
• The peripheral nervous system (PNS), containing cranial and spinal nerves, provides communication between the CNS and remote body parts.

The fundamental unit

The neuron, or nerve cell, is the nervous system's fundamental unit. This highly specialized conductor cell receives and transmits electrochemical nerve impulses. Delicate, threadlike nerve fibers called *axons* and *dendrites* extend from the central cell body and transmit signals. Axons carry impulses away from the cell body; dendrites carry impulses to the cell body. Most neurons have multiple dendrites but only one axon. Neuroglial cells, which outnumber neurons, provide support, nourishment, and protection for neurons.

The body's information superhighway

This intricate network of interlocking receptors and transmitters, along with the brain and spinal cord, forms a living computer that

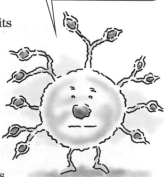

Glad to meet you. I'm a neuron, the basic unit of the nervous system.

controls and regulates every mental and physical function. From birth to death, the nervous system efficiently organizes the body's affairs, controlling the smallest actions, thoughts, and feelings.

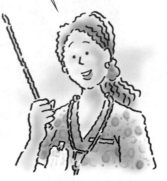

The nervous system is a wonderful thing. Its many parts are well coordinated and interact constantly.

Central nervous system

The CNS consists of the brain and the spinal cord. The fragile brain and spinal cord are protected by the bony skull and vertebrae, cerebrospinal fluid (CSF), and three membranes—the dura mater, the arachnoid mater, and the pia mater.

They all "mater"

The *dura mater*, which forms the outermost protective layer, is a tough, fibrous, leatherlike tissue composed of two layers, the endosteal dura and the meningeal dura. The endosteal dura forms the periosteum of the skull and is continuous with the lining of the vertebral canal, whereas the meningeal dura, a thick membrane, covers the brain, dipping between the brain tissue and providing support and protection.

The *arachnoid mater*, which forms the middle protective layer, is a thin, delicate, fibrous membrane that loosely hugs the brain and spinal cord. The arachnoid mater is avascular.

The *pia mater* is the innermost protective layer of connective tissue that covers and contours the spinal tissue and brain. The pia mater is vascular.

Space exploration

The epidural space lies between the skull and the dura mater. Between the dura mater and the arachnoid mater is the subdural space. Between the arachnoid mater and the pia mater is the subarachnoid space. Within the subarachnoid space and the brain's four ventricles is CSF, a liquid composed of water and traces of organic materials (especially protein), glucose, and minerals. This fluid protects the brain and spinal tissue from jolts and blows.

Cerebrum

The cerebrum, the largest part of the brain, houses the nerve center that controls sensory and motor activities and intelligence. The outer layer, the cerebral cortex, consists of neuron cell bodies (gray matter). The inner layer consists of axons (white matter) plus basal ganglia, which control motor coordination and steadiness.

The right controls the left; the left controls the right

The cerebrum is divided into the right and left hemispheres. Because motor impulses descending from the brain cross in the medulla, the right hemisphere controls the left side of the body and the left hemisphere controls the right side of the body. Several fissures divide the cerebrum into lobes. Each lobe has a specific function. (See *A close look at lobes and fissures*.)

A call to order

The thalamus, a relay center in the cerebrum, further organizes cerebral function by transmitting impulses to and from appropri-

---

A close look at lobes and fissures

Several fissures divide the cerebrum into hemispheres and lobes:
• The fissure of Sylvius, or the lateral sulcus, separates the temporal lobe from the frontal and parietal lobes.
• The fissure of Rolando, or the central sulcus, separates the frontal lobes from the parietal lobe.
• The parieto-occipital fissure separates the occipital lobe from the two parietal lobes.

To each lobe, a function
Each lobe has a specific function:
• The frontal lobe controls voluntary muscle movements and contains motor areas such as

the one for speech (Broca's motor speech area). It's the center for personality, behavioral functions, intellectual functions (such as judgment, memory, and problem solving), autonomic functions, and emotional responses.
• The temporal lobe is the center for taste, hearing, smell, and interpretation of spoken language.
• The parietal lobe coordinates and interprets sensory information from the opposite side of the body.
• The occipital lobe interprets visual stimuli.

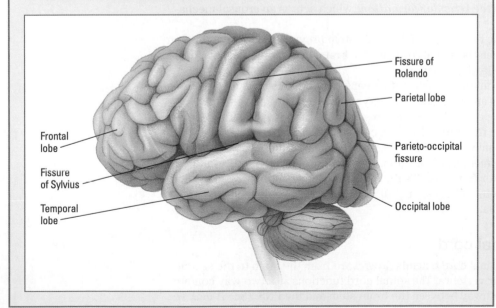

Fissure of Rolando

Parietal lobe

Parieto-occipital fissure

Occipital lobe

Frontal lobe

Fissure of Sylvius

Temporal lobe

I'm rather proud of my cerebrum and its two cerebral hemispheres. It controls sensory and motor activities as well as intelligence.

ate areas of the cerebrum. The thalamus is also responsible for primitive emotional responses such as fear and for distinguishing pleasant stimuli from unpleasant ones.

The multi-tasker

The hypothalamus, located beneath the thalamus, is an autonomic center with connections to the brain, spinal cord, autonomic nervous system, and pituitary gland. It regulates temperature control, appetite, blood pressure, breathing, sleep patterns, and peripheral nerve discharges that occur with behavioral and emotional expression. It also partially controls pituitary gland secretion and stress reaction.

Cerebellum and brain stem

Other main parts of the brain are the cerebellum and the brain stem.

Tell 'em about the cerebellum

The cerebellum lies beneath the cerebrum, at the base of the brain. It coordinates muscle movements, controls posture, and maintains equilibrium.

A gem of a stem

The brain stem includes the midbrain, pons, and medulla oblongata. It houses cell bodies for most of the cranial nerves. Along with the thalamus and hypothalamus, it makes up a nerve network called the *reticular formation*, which acts as an arousal mechanism.

The three parts of the brain stem provide two-way conduction between the spinal cord and the brain. In addition, they perform the following functions:
• The midbrain is the reflex center for the third and fourth cranial nerves and mediates pupillary reflexes and eye movements.
• The pons helps regulate respirations. It's also the reflex center for the fifth through eighth cranial nerves and mediates chewing, taste, saliva secretion, hearing, and equilibrium.
• The medulla oblongata influences cardiac, respiratory, and vasomotor functions. It's the center for the vomiting, coughing, and hiccuping reflexes. Cranial nerves IX, X, and XII emerge from the medulla.

Spinal cord

The spinal cord extends downward from the brain to the second lumbar vertebra. The spinal cord functions as a two-way conductor pathway between the brain stem and the PNS. (See *A look inside the spinal cord.*)

A look inside the spinal cord

This cross section of the spinal cord shows an H-shaped mass of gray matter divided into horns, which consist primarily of neuron cell bodies.

Cell bodies in the posterior or dorsal horn primarily relay information. Cell bodies in the anterior or ventral horn are needed for voluntary or reflex motor activity.

The illustration below shows the major components of the spinal cord.

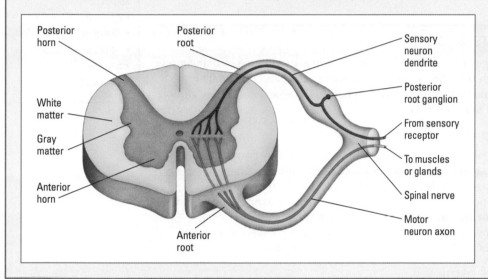

A gray area

The spinal cord contains a mass of gray matter divided into horns, which consist mostly of neuron cell bodies. The horns of the spinal cord relay sensations and are needed for voluntary or reflex motor activity.

The outside of the horns is surrounded by white matter consisting of myelinated nerve fibers grouped in vertical columns called *tracts*.

Tract record

The sensory, or ascending, tracts carry sensory impulses up the spinal cord to the brain, whereas motor, or descending, tracts carry motor impulses down the spinal cord.

The brain's motor impulses reach a descending tract and continue to the PNS via upper motor neurons (also called *cranial motor neurons*).

Upper motor neurons in the brain conduct impulses from the brain to the spinal cord. Upper motor neurons form two major systems:
• The pyramidal system, or corticospinal tract, is responsible for fine, skilled movements of skeletal muscle.
• The extrapyramidal system, or extracorticospinal tract, is responsible for the control of gross motor movements.

Lower motor neurons or spinal motor neurons conduct impulses that originate in upper motor neurons to the muscles.

Peripheral nervous system

Messages transmitted through the spinal cord reach outlying areas through the PNS. The PNS originates in 31 pairs of spinal nerves arranged in segments and attached to the spinal cord. (See *How spinal nerves are numbered.*)

A route with two roots

Spinal nerves are attached to the spinal cord by two roots:
• The anterior, or ventral, root consists of motor fibers that relay impulses from the spinal cord to the glands and muscles.
• The posterior, or dorsal, root consists of sensory fibers that relay information from receptors to the spinal cord.

A swollen area of the posterior root, the posterior root ganglion, is made up of sensory neuron cell bodies.

Ramifications of rami

After leaving the vertebral column, each spinal nerve separates into branches called *rami*, which distribute peripherally with extensive overlapping. This overlapping reduces the chance of lost sensory or motor function from interruption of a single spinal nerve.

Who's in control here?

The PNS can be divided into the somatic nervous system and the autonomic nervous system. The somatic nervous system regulates voluntary motor control. The autonomic nervous system helps regulate the body's internal environment through involuntary control of organ systems.

Balancing act

The autonomic nervous system controls involuntary body functions, such as digestion, respirations, and cardiovascular function. It's usually divided into two antagonistic systems that balance each other to support homeostasis:

How spinal nerves are numbered

Spinal nerves are numbered according to their point of origin in the spinal cord:
• 8 cervical: C1 to C8
• 12 thoracic: T1 to T12
• 5 lumbar: L1 to L5
• 5 sacral: S1 to S5
• 1 coccygeal.

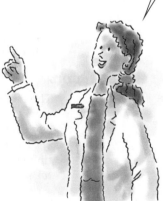

The autonomic nervous system operates without conscious control as the caretaker of the body.

- The sympathetic nervous system controls energy expenditure, especially in stressful situations, by releasing the adrenergic catecholamine norepinephrine.
- The parasympathetic nervous system helps conserve energy by releasing the cholinergic neurohormone acetylcholine.

So much to know about the somatic system

The somatic nervous system, composed of somatic nerve fibers, conducts impulses from the CNS to skeletal muscles. It's typically referred to as the voluntary nervous system because it allows the individual to consciously control skeletal muscles.

Neurologic disorders

In this section, you'll find information on some common neurologic disorders:
- Alzheimer's disease
- amyotrophic lateral sclerosis (ALS)
- epilepsy
- Guillain-Barré syndrome
- meningitis
- multiple sclerosis (MS)
- myasthenia gravis
- Parkinson's disease
- stroke.

Alzheimer's disease

Alzheimer's disease is a progressive degenerative disorder of the cerebral cortex. It accounts for more than one-half of all cases of dementia. Cortical degeneration is most marked in the frontal lobes, but atrophy occurs in all areas of the cortex.

A growing problem

An estimated 4.5 million Americans have Alzheimer's disease. This number has more than doubled since 1980. One in 10 individuals older than age 65 and nearly one-half of those older than age 85 are affected.

Because this is a primary progressive dementia, the prognosis is poor. Most patients die 2 to 20 years after the onset of symptoms. The average duration of the illness before death is 8 years.

Sometimes it's all in the family

Researchers recognize two forms of Alzheimer's disease: familial and sporadic. In familial Alzheimer's, genes directly cause the disease. These cases are very rare and have been identified in a relatively small number of families, with many people in multiple generations affected. (See *Genes and Alzheimer's disease.*)

Sometimes it's sporadic

In sporadic Alzheimer's, the most common form of the disease, genes don't cause the disease, but may influence the risk of developing the disease. The incidence of sporadic Alzheimer's disease is less predictable than the familial type and occurs in fewer family members. (See *Tissue changes in Alzheimer's disease.*)

How it happens

The cause of Alzheimer's disease is unknown, but four factors are thought to contribute:
• neurochemical factors, such as deficiencies in the neurotransmitters acetylcholine, somatostatin, substance P, and norepinephrine

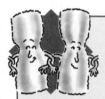

The genetic link

Genes and Alzheimer's disease

Familial Alzheimer's disease

According to the Alzheimer's Association, in this form of Alzheimer's disease, the affected person has inherited an abnormal mutation in one of three genes—PS1, PS2, or APP. An individual who carries one of the mutated genes has a 50% chance of passing the gene onto his children. Those who inherit the mutated gene will most likely develop Alzheimer's disease.

Although it isn't fully understood how these mutations cause the disease, they all influence beta-amyloid production.

Sporadic Alzheimer's disease

Sporadic Alzheimer's disease doesn't develop with a mutation in one particular gene. Instead, slight variations in genes may influence whether someone is more or less susceptible to the disease.

APOE

The most researched gene in sporadic Alzheimer's disease is APOE, which is responsible for the production of a protein that transports cholesterol and other fats throughout the body. The protein may also be involved in the structure and function of the outer wall of a brain cell.

APOE has three common forms—APOE–epsilon 2, APOE–epsilon 3, and APOE–epsilon 4. A person inherits one form of the gene from each parent. The form associated with sporadic Alzheimer's disease is APOE–epsilon 4. People who carry at least one of this type of gene are at a higher risk for developing Alzheimer's disease. Studies have shown that 35% to 50% of people with Alzheimer's disease have at least one copy of this form of the gene. People who have two copies of the gene are at even higher risk and, when they develop the disease, typically show symptoms at a younger age.

Now I get it!

Tissue changes in Alzheimer's disease

The illustrations below show the progressive tissue changes that occur in Alzheimer's disease.

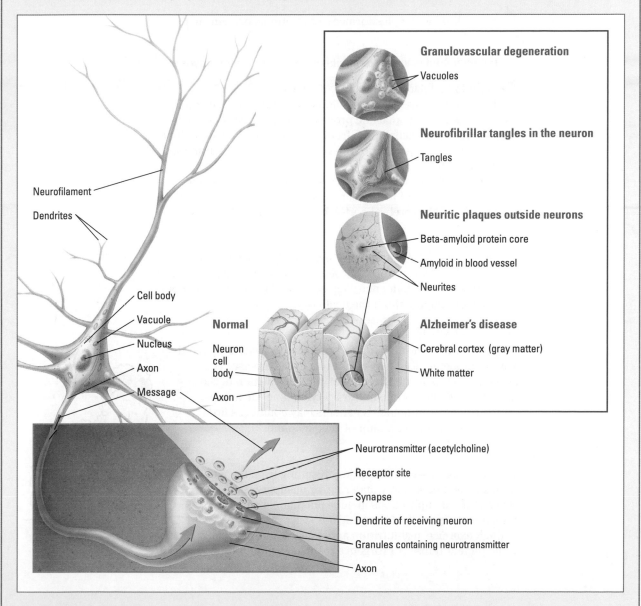

Neurofilament

Dendrites

Cell body

Vacuole

Nucleus

Axon

Message

Normal

Neuron cell body

Axon

Granulovascular degeneration

Vacuoles

Neurofibrillar tangles in the neuron

Tangles

Neuritic plaques outside neurons

Beta-amyloid protein core

Amyloid in blood vessel

Neurites

Alzheimer's disease

Cerebral cortex (gray matter)

White matter

Neurotransmitter (acetylcholine)

Receptor site

Synapse

Dendrite of receiving neuron

Granules containing neurotransmitter

Axon

- viral factors such as slow-growing CNS viruses
- trauma
- genetic factors.

An issue of brain tissue

The brain tissue of Alzheimer's patients has three distinguishing features:

neurofibrillary tangles formed out of fibrous proteins in the neurons

beta-amyloid plaques (deposits of protein-like substances)

granulovascular degeneration of neurons.

The disease causes degeneration of neuropils (dense complexes of interwoven cytoplasmic processes of nerve cells and neuroglial cells), especially in the frontal, parietal, and occipital lobes. It also causes enlargement of the ventricles (cavities within the brain filled with CSF).

Early cerebral changes include formation of microscopic plaques, consisting of a core surrounded by fibrous tissue. Later on, atrophy of the cerebral cortex becomes strikingly evident.

The part plaques play

If a patient has a large number of beta-amyloid plaques, his dementia will be more severe. The amyloid in the plaques may exert neurotoxic effects. Evidence suggests that plaques play an important part in bringing about the death of neurons.

Absence of acetylcholine

Problems with neurotransmitters and the enzymes associated with their metabolism may play a role in the disease. The severity of dementia is directly related to reduction of the amount of the neurotransmitter acetylcholine. On autopsy, the brains of Alzheimer's patients may contain as little as 10% of the normal amount of acetylcholine.

Getting complicated

Complications may include injury resulting from the patient's violent behavior, wandering, or unsupervised activity. Other complications include pneumonia and other infections, especially if the patient doesn't receive enough exercise; malnutrition and dehydration, especially if the patient refuses or forgets to eat; and aspiration.

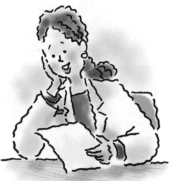

Defining characteristics of Alzheimer's are noted on autopsy.

What to look for

Alzheimer's disease has an insidious onset. At first, changes are barely perceptible, but they gradually lead to serious problems. Patient history is almost always obtained from a family member or caregiver.

Early changes may include forgetfulness, subtle memory loss without loss of social skills or behavior patterns, difficulty learning and retaining new information, inability to concentrate, and deterioration in personal hygiene and appearance. As the disease progresses, signs and symptoms indicate a degenerative disorder of the frontal lobe. They may include:

• difficulty with abstract thinking and activities that require judgment
• progressive difficulty in communicating
• severe deterioration of memory, language, and motor function progressing to coordination loss and an inability to speak or write
• repetitive actions
• restlessness, wandering
• irritability, depression, mood swings, paranoia, hostility, and combativeness
• nocturnal awakenings
• disorientation. (See *Treating Alzheimer's disease.*)

Battling illness

Treating Alzheimer's disease

No cure for Alzheimer's disease exists. Although current drugs can't alter the progressive loss of brain cells, the drugs listed below may help minimize or stabilize symptoms.

Drug therapy
• Cholinesterase inhibitors, such as donepezil, rivastigmine, and galantamine, prevent the breakdown of acetylcholine, a chemical messenger in the brain that's important for memory and other thinking skills. The drugs work to keep levels of acetylcholine high, even while the cells that produce it continue to become damaged or die.
• Memantine, an uncompetitive low-to-moderate affinity N-methyl-D-aspartate receptor antagonist, is sometimes pre-

scribed. It appears to work by regulating the activity of glutamate, one of the brain's chemicals that's involved in information processing, storing, and retrieval.
• Vitamin E supplements are commonly prescribed because they may help defend the brain against damage.

Possible vaccine
Many clinical trials are currently under way for the treatment of Alzheimer's disease, including a vaccine that would stimulate the immune system to recognize and attack the beta-amyloid plaques that occur with the disease.

The proof is in the...

Neurologic examination confirms many of the problems revealed during the history. In addition, it commonly reveals an impaired sense of smell (usually an early symptom), an inability to recognize and understand the form and nature of objects by touching them, gait disorders, and tremors. The patient will also have a positive snout reflex; in response to a tap or stroke of the lips or the area just under the nose, the patient grimaces or puckers his lips.

In the final stages, urinary or fecal incontinence, twitching, and seizures commonly occur.

What tests tell you

Alzheimer's disease can't be confirmed until death, when an autopsy reveals pathologic findings.

These tests help rule out other disorders:
• Positron emission tomography (PET) scan measures the metabolic activity of the cerebral cortex and may help confirm early diagnosis.
• Computed tomography (CT) scan may show more brain atrophy than occurs in normal aging.
• Magnetic resonance imaging (MRI) evaluates the condition of the brain and rules out intracranial lesions as the source of dementia.
• EEG evaluates the brain's electrical activity and may show brain wave slowing late in the disease. It also helps to differentiate tumors, abscesses, and other intracranial lesions that might cause symptoms.
• CSF analysis helps determine whether signs and symptoms stem from a chronic neurologic infection.
• Cerebral blood flow studies may detect abnormalities in blood flow to the brain.

Amyotrophic lateral sclerosis

Commonly called *Lou Gehrig's disease,* after the New York Yankee first baseman who died of the disorder, ALS is the most common of the motor neuron diseases causing muscular atrophy. Other motor neuron diseases include progressive muscular atrophy and progressive bulbar palsy. Onset occurs between ages 40 and 70. A chronic, progressively debilitating disease, ALS is rapidly fatal.

All about ALS

More than 30,000 Americans have ALS; about 5,000 new cases are diagnosed each year, with men affected three times more com-

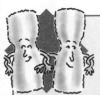

The genetic link

ALS breakthrough

The good news

The first and most important breakthrough so far in amyotrophic lateral sclerosis (ALS) genetic research was the discovery of mutations in the SOD1 gene. This mutation is seen in about 20% of patients with familial ALS.

...and the not so good news

Initially, researchers were very excited about this discovery; however, they soon learned that the mutation was quite complex. Researchers understand how the gene functions, but the mutation is an acquisition of a toxic property. That means that the gene gains a function, rather than losing its normal function. Researchers are perplexed about what that gain of function is. Therefore, genetic studies continue.

monly than women. The exact cause of ALS is unknown, but 5% to 10% of ALS cases have a genetic component. In genetic cases, ALS is an autosomal dominant trait and affects men and women equally. (See *ALS breakthrough.*)

ALS and other motor neuron diseases may result from:
• a slow-acting virus
• nutritional deficiency related to a disturbance in enzyme metabolism
• metabolic interference in nucleic acid production by the nerve fibers
• autoimmune disorders that affect immune complexes in the renal glomerulus and basement membrane.

Precipitating factors for acute deterioration include trauma, viral infection, and physical exhaustion.

How it happens

In ALS, the nerve cells that control the muscles, known as *motor neurons*, are destroyed. These motor neurons, which are located in the anterior gray horns of the spinal column and the motor nuclei of the lower brain stem, die. As the cells die, the muscle fibers that they supply atrophy. The loss of motor neurons may occur in both the upper and the lower motor neuron systems. The patient's signs and symptoms develop according to the affected motor neurons because specific neurons activate specific muscle fibers.

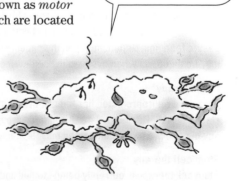

I apologize for lying down on the job, but this ALS hurts us motor neurons!

What to look for

Muscle weakness, the primary or hallmark sign of ALS, is seen in 60% of those patients affected. Patients with ALS develop fasciculations (involuntary twitching or contraction of muscles), accompanied by atrophy and weakness, especially in the muscles of the forearms and hands. Other signs and symptoms include:

- impaired speech
- difficulty chewing and swallowing
- difficulty breathing
- choking
- excessive drooling
- depression
- inappropriate laughing
- crying spells. (See *Treating ALS*.)

What tests tell you

These tests help confirm the diagnosis:
- Electromyography helps show nerve damage instead of muscle damage.
- Muscle biopsy helps rule out muscle disease.
- CSF analysis reveals increased protein content in one-third of patients.
- A thorough neurologic examination is needed to rule out other diseases of the neuromuscular system.

Battling illness

Treating ALS

Treatment of amyotrophic lateral sclerosis (ALS) aims to control symptoms and provide emotional, psychological, and physical support. Patients who experience difficulty swallowing may require gastric feedings. Depending upon the patient's wishes, tracheotomy and mechanical ventilation may be an option when hypoventilation develops.

Drug therapy
Riluzole, a neuroprotector, has been shown to slow the deterioration of motor neurons in the early stages of ALS. Baclofen, dantrolene, or diazepam may be given to control spasticity. Quinine therapy may be prescribed for painful muscle cramps.

Stem cell therapy
Stem cell therapy is currently being studied and shows great promise in the treatment of ALS.

Epilepsy

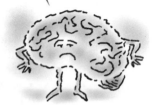

I've got those abnormal electrical discharge blues.

Also known as *seizure disorder*, epilepsy is a brain condition characterized by recurrent seizures. Seizures are paroxysmal events associated with abnormal electrical discharges of neurons in the brain. The discharge may trigger a convulsive movement, an interruption of sensation, an alteration in level of consciousness (LOC), or a combination of these symptoms. In most patients, epilepsy doesn't affect intelligence.

From young to old

This condition affects people of all ages, races, and ethnic backgrounds. More than 2.5 million Americans are living with epilepsy. Every year, 181,000 Americans develop seizures for the first time. The condition appears most commonly in early childhood and advanced age. About 80% of patients have good seizure control with strict adherence to prescribed treatment.

How it happens

A group of neurons may lose afferent stimulation (ability to transmit impulses from the periphery toward the CNS) and function as an epileptogenic focus. These neurons are hypersensitive and easily activated. In response to changes in the cellular environment, the neurons become hyperactive and fire abnormally.

Don't know why

About one-half of epilepsy cases are idiopathic. No specific cause can be found, and the patient has no other neurologic abnormality. In other cases, however, possible causes of epilepsy include:
• genetic abnormalities, such as tuberous sclerosis (tumors and sclerotic patches in the brain) and phenylketonuria (inability to convert phenylalanine into tyrosine)
• perinatal injuries
• metabolic abnormalities, such as hyponatremia, hypocalcemia, hypoglycemia, and pyridoxine deficiency
• brain tumors or other space-occupying lesions of the cortex
• infections, such as meningitis, encephalitis, or brain abscess
• traumatic injury, especially if the dura mater has been penetrated
• ingestion of toxins, such as mercury, lead, or carbon monoxide
• stroke
• hereditary abnormalities (some seizure disorders appear to run in families)
• fever.

All fired up

This is what happens during a seizure:
- The electronic balance at the neuronal level is altered, causing the neuronal membrane to become susceptible to activation.
- Increased permeability of the cytoplasmic membranes helps hypersensitive neurons fire abnormally. Abnormal firing may be activated by hyperthermia, hypoglycemia, hyponatremia, hypoxia, or repeated sensory stimulation.
- When the intensity of a seizure discharge has progressed sufficiently, it spreads to adjacent brain areas. The midbrain, thalamus, and cerebral cortex are most likely to become epileptogenic.
- Excitement feeds back from the primary focus and to other parts of the brain.
- The discharges become less frequent until they stop.

I'm hypersensitive by nature—and a change in my environment can really make me hyperactive.

Getting complicated

Depending on the type of seizure, injury may result from a fall at the onset of a seizure or afterward, when the patient is confused. Injury may also result from the rapid, jerking movements that occur during or after a seizure. Anoxia can occur due to airway occlusion by the tongue, aspiration of vomit, or traumatic injury. A continuous seizure state known as *status epilepticus* can cause respiratory distress and even death. (See *Understanding status epilepticus* and *Electrical impulses in seizures*.)

What to look for

Signs and symptoms of epilepsy vary depending on the type and cause of the seizure. (See *Understanding types of seizures*, page 136.)

Understanding status epilepticus

Status epilepticus is a continuous seizure state that must be interrupted by emergency measures. It can occur during all types of seizures. For example, generalized tonic-clonic status epilepticus is a continuous generalized tonic-clonic seizure without an intervening return of consciousness.

Always an emergency
Status epilepticus is accompanied by respiratory distress. It can result from withdrawal of antiepileptic medications, hypoxic or metabolic encephalopathy, acute head trauma, or septicemia secondary to encephalitis or meningitis.

Acting fast
Emergency treatment usually consists of lorazepam, phenytoin, or phenobarbital; I.V. dextrose 50% when seizures are secondary to hypoglycemia; and I.V. thiamine in patients with chronic alcoholism or who are undergoing withdrawal.

Electrical impulses in seizures

The spread of electrical impulses is different in each type of seizure.

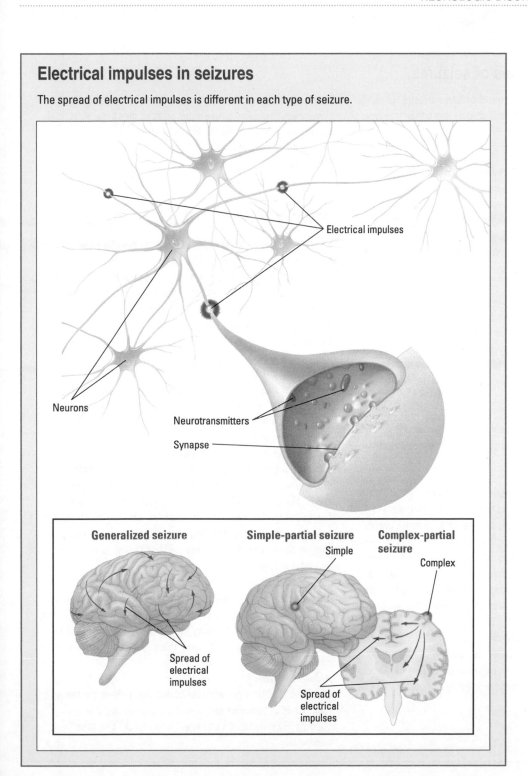

Understanding types of seizures

Use these guidelines to understand different seizure types. Remember that patients may be affected by more than one type of seizure.

Partial seizures

Arising from a localized area in the brain, partial seizure activity may spread to the entire brain, causing a generalized seizure. Several types and subtypes of partial seizures exist:
- simple partial, which includes jacksonian and sensory
- complex partial
- secondarily generalized partial seizure (partial onset leading to generalized tonic-clonic seizure).

Jacksonian seizure

A jacksonian seizure begins as a localized motor seizure, characterized by a spread of abnormal activity to adjacent areas of the brain. The patient experiences a stiffening or jerking in one extremity, accompanied by a tingling sensation in the same area. Although the patient in a jacksonian seizure seldom loses consciousness, the seizure may progress to a generalized tonic-clonic seizure.

Sensory seizure

Symptoms of a sensory seizure include hallucinations, flashing lights, tingling sensations, vertigo, déjà vu, and smelling a foul odor.

Complex partial seizure

Signs and symptoms of a complex partial seizure are variable but usually include purposeless behavior, including a glassy stare, picking at clothes, aimless wandering, lip-smacking or chewing motions, and unintelligible speech. An aura may occur first, and seizures may last from a few seconds to 20 minutes. Afterward, mental confusion may last for several minutes, and an observer may mistakenly suspect alcohol or drug intoxication or psychosis. The patient has no memory of his actions during the seizure.

Secondarily generalized seizure

A secondarily generalized seizure can be simple or complex and can progress to a generalized seizure. An aura may occur first, with loss of consciousness occurring immediately or 1 to 2 minutes later.

Generalized seizures

Generalized seizures cause a generalized electrical abnormality within the brain. Types include:
- absence or petit mal
- myoclonic
- generalized tonic-clonic
- akinetic.

Absence seizure

Absence seizure occurs most commonly in children. It usually begins with a brief change in the level of consciousness, signaled by blinking or rolling of the eyes, a blank stare, and slight mouth movements. The patient retains his posture and continues preseizure activity without difficulty. Seizures last from 1 to 10 seconds, and impairment is so brief that the patient may be unaware of it. However, if not properly treated, these seizures can recur up to 100 times per day and progress to a generalized tonic-clonic seizure.

Myoclonic seizure

Also called *bilateral massive epileptic myoclonus,* myoclonic seizure is marked by brief, involuntary muscular jerks of the body or extremities, which may occur in a rhythmic manner, and a brief loss of consciousness.

Generalized tonic-clonic seizure

Typically, a generalized tonic-clonic seizure begins with a loud cry, caused by air rushing from the lungs through the vocal cords. The patient falls to the ground, losing consciousness. The body stiffens (tonic phase) and then alternates between episodes of muscle spasm and relaxation (clonic phase). Tongue biting, incontinence, labored breathing, apnea, and cyanosis may also occur.

The seizure stops in 2 to 5 minutes, when abnormal electrical conduction of the neurons is completed. Afterward, the patient regains consciousness but is somewhat confused. He may have difficulty talking and may have drowsiness, fatigue, headache, muscle soreness, and arm or leg weakness. He may fall into a deep sleep afterward.

Akinetic seizure

Characterized by a general loss of postural tone and a temporary loss of consciousness, akinetic seizure occurs in young children. Sometimes it's called a "drop attack" because the child falls.

It isn't always clear

Physical findings may be normal if the patient doesn't have a seizure during assessment and the cause is idiopathic. If the seizure is caused by an underlying problem, the patient's history and physical examination should uncover related signs and symptoms.

In many cases, the patient's history shows that seizures are unpredictable and unrelated to activities. Occasionally, a patient may report precipitating factors. For example, the seizures may always take place at a certain time, such as during sleep, or after a particular circumstance, such as lack of sleep or emotional stress. He may also report nonspecific symptoms, such as headache, mood changes, lethargy, and myoclonic jerking up to several hours before a seizure. (See *Treating epilepsy*.)

Aura report

Some patients report an aura a few seconds or minutes before a generalized seizure. An aura signals the beginning of abnormal electrical discharges within a focal area of the brain. Typical auras include:

- a pungent smell
- nausea or indigestion
- a rising or sinking feeling in the stomach
- a dreamy feeling
- an unusual taste
- a visual disturbance such as a flashing light.

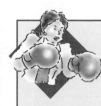

Battling illness

Treating epilepsy

Treatment for epilepsy seeks to reduce the frequency of seizures or prevent their occurrence.

Drug therapy
Drug therapy is specific to the type of seizure. The most commonly prescribed drugs for generalized tonic-clonic and complex partial seizures are phenytoin, carbamazepine, phenobarbital, and primidone, administered individually. Valproic acid, clonazepam, and ethosuximide are commonly prescribed for absence seizures. Lamotrigine is also given as adjunct therapy for partial seizures.

Surgery
If drug therapy fails, treatment may include surgical removal of a demonstrated focal lesion to try to stop seizures. Surgery is also performed when epilepsy results from an underlying problem, such as an intracranial tumor, a brain abscess or cyst, or vascular abnormalities.

What tests tell you

These tests are used to diagnose epilepsy:
• EEG showing paroxysmal abnormalities may confirm the diagnosis by providing evidence of continuing seizure tendency. A negative EEG doesn't rule out epilepsy because paroxysmal abnormalities occur intermittently. EEG also helps determine the prognosis and can help classify the disorder.
• CT scan and MRI provide density readings of the brain and may indicate abnormalities in internal structures.

Other tests include serum glucose and calcium studies, skull X-rays, lumbar puncture, brain scan, and cerebral angiography.

Guillain-Barré syndrome

Guillain-Barré syndrome is an acute, autoimmune, rapidly progressive, potentially fatal syndrome. It's associated with segmented demyelination of peripheral nerves. It may also be called *acute demyelinating polyneuropathy*.

This syndrome occurs equally in both sexes, usually occurring between ages 30 and 50. It affects about 1 out of every 100,000 people. As a result of better symptom management, 80% to 90% of patients recover with few or no residual symptoms.

Going through the phases

The clinical course of Guillain-Barré syndrome has three phases:

The acute phase begins when the first definitive symptom develops and ends 1 to 3 weeks later, when no further deterioration is noted.

The plateau phase lasts for several days to 2 weeks.

The recovery phase, believed to coincide with remyelination and axonal process regrowth, can last from 4 months to 3 years.

How it happens

The precise cause of Guillain-Barré syndrome is unknown, but it's thought to be a cell-mediated, immunologic attack on peripheral nerves in response to a virus. Risk factors include surgery, rabies or swine influenza vaccination, viral illness, Hodgkin's disease or another malignant disease, and lupus erythematosus.

We're under attack! Inflammation and degenerative changes in both our sensory and motor nerve roots cause sensory and motor impairment simultaneously!

Danger! Demyelination!

An immunologic reaction causes segmental demyelination of the peripheral nerves, which prevents normal transmission of electrical impulses along the sensorimotor nerve roots.

The myelin sheath, which covers the nerve axons and conducts electrical impulses along the nerve pathways, degenerates for unknown reasons. With degeneration comes inflammation, swelling, and patchy demyelination. (See *Peripheral nerve demyelination in Guillain-Barré syndrome.*)

As myelin is destroyed, the nodes of Ranvier, located at the junctures of the myelin sheaths, widen. This delays and impairs impulse transmission along the dorsal and ventral nerve roots.

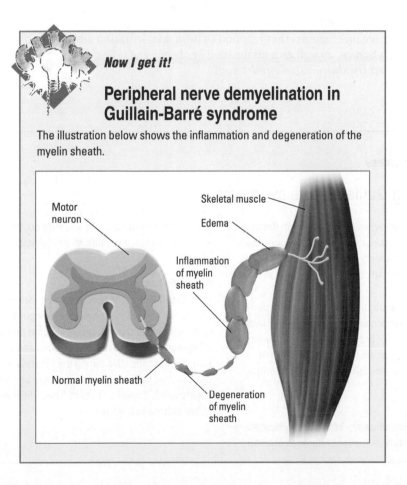

Now I get it!

Peripheral nerve demyelination in Guillain-Barré syndrome

The illustration below shows the inflammation and degeneration of the myelin sheath.

Motor neuron

Skeletal muscle

Edema

Inflammation of myelin sheath

Normal myelin sheath

Degeneration of myelin sheath

What to look for

Impairment of dorsal nerve roots affects sensory function, so the patient may experience tingling and numbness. Impairment of ventral nerve roots affects motor function, so the patient may experience muscle weakness, immobility, and paralysis.

Other signs and symptoms include muscle stiffness and pain, sensory loss, loss of position sense, and diminished or absent deep tendon reflexes.

Symptoms usually follow an ascending pattern, beginning in the legs and progressing to the arms, trunk, and face. In mild forms, only cranial nerves may be affected. In some patients, muscle weakness may be absent.

Respiratory risk

The disorder commonly affects respiratory muscles. If the patient dies, it's usually from respiratory complications. Paralysis of the internal and external intercostal muscles leads to a reduction in functional breathing. Vagus nerve paralysis causes a loss of the protective mechanisms that respond to bronchial irritation and foreign bodies, as well as a diminished or absent gag reflex. (See *Treating Guillain-Barré syndrome.*)

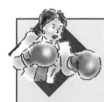

Battling illness

Treating Guillain-Barré syndrome

Most patients seek treatment when the disease is in the acute stage. Treatment is primarily supportive and may require endotracheal intubation or tracheotomy if the patient has difficulty clearing secretions and mechanical ventilation if he has respiratory problems.

Continuous electrocardiographic monitoring is necessary to identify the autonomic symptoms such as cardiac arrhythmias. Atropine may be used for bradycardia. Marked hypotension may require volume replacement and administration of vasopressors, such as dopamine, phenylephrine, or norepinephrine.

A spontaneous recovery

Most patients recover spontaneously. Intensive physical therapy starts as soon as voluntary movement returns to skeletal muscles, to prevent muscle and joint contractures. However, a small percentage of patients are left with some residual disability.

Alternative approaches

High-dose I.V. immune globulin and plasmapheresis may shorten recovery time. Plasmapheresis temporarily reduces circulating antibodies through removal of the patient's blood, centrifugation of blood to remove plasma, and subsequent reinfusion. It's most effective during the first few weeks of the disease, and patients need less ventilatory support if treatment begins within 2 weeks of onset. The patient may receive three to five plasma exchanges.

What tests tell you

These tests are used to diagnose Guillain-Barré syndrome:
• CSF analysis may show a normal white blood cell (WBC) count, an elevated protein count and, in severe disease, increased CSF pressure. The CSF protein level begins to rise several days after the onset of signs and symptoms, peaking in 4 to 6 weeks, probably because of widespread inflammatory disease of the nerve roots.
• Electromyography may demonstrate repeated firing of the same motor unit instead of widespread sectional stimulation.
• Electrophysiologic testing may reveal marked slowing of nerve conduction velocities.

Meningitis

In meningitis, the brain and spinal cord meninges become inflamed. Inflammation may involve all three meningeal membranes: the dura mater, the arachnoid mater, and the pia mater and the underlying cortex. Blood flow to the brain is reduced. Tissues swell, causing increased intracranial pressure (ICP).

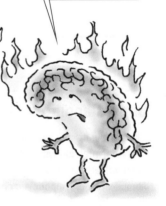

Oh no! In meningitis, my meninges become inflamed.

Knowledge is power

The prognosis for patients with meningitis is good and complications are rare, especially if the disease is recognized early and the infecting organism responds to antibiotics. However, mortality in untreated meningitis is 70% to 100%. The prognosis is poorer for infants and elderly people.

How it happens

The origin of meningeal inflammation may be:
• bacterial
• viral
• protozoal
• fungal.
    The most common causes of meningitis are bacterial and viral. Bacterial infection may be due to *Neisseria meningitidis*, *Haemophilus influenzae*, *Streptococcus pneumoniae*, or *Escherichia coli*. Sometimes, no causative organism can be found.

Blame it on bacteria

Bacterial meningitis is one of the most serious infections that may affect infants and children. In most patients, the infection that causes meningitis is secondary to another bacterial infection, such as bacteremia (especially from pneumonia, empyema, osteomyelitis, and endocarditis), sinusitis, otitis media, encephalitis, myelitis, or brain abscess. Respiratory infections increase the risk of bacterial meningitis. Meningitis may also follow a skull fracture, a penetrating head wound, lumbar puncture, ventricular shunting, or other neurosurgical procedures.

Sabotage in the subarachnoid space

Bacterial meningitis occurs when bacteria enter the subarachnoid space and cause an inflammatory response. Usually, organisms enter the nervous system after invading and infecting another region of the body. The organisms gain access to the subarachnoid space and the CSF, where they cause irritation of the tissues bathed by the fluid.

The viral version

Meningitis caused by a virus is called *aseptic viral meningitis*. Aseptic viral meningitis may result from a direct infection or secondary to disease, such as mumps, herpes, measles, or leukemia. Usually, symptoms are mild and the disease is self-limiting. (See *Understanding aseptic viral meningitis*.)

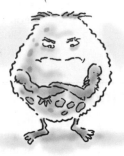

Bacterial meningitis begins when I enter the subarachnoid space.

Understanding aseptic viral meningitis

A benign syndrome, aseptic viral meningitis results from infection with enteroviruses (most common), arboviruses, herpes simplex virus, mumps virus, or lymphocytic choriomeningitis virus.

First, a fever

Signs and symptoms of viral meningitis usually begin suddenly with a temperature up to 104° F (40° C), drowsiness, confusion, stupor, and slight neck or spine stiffness when the patient bends forward. The patient history may reveal a recent illness.

Other signs and symptoms include headache, nausea, vomiting, abdominal pain, poorly defined chest pain, and sore throat.

What virus is this anyway?

A complete patient history and knowledge of seasonal epidemics are key to differentiating among the many forms of aseptic viral meningitis. Negative bacteriologic cultures and cerebrospinal fluid (CSF) analysis showing pleocytosis (a greater than normal number of cells in the CSF) and increased protein suggest the diagnosis. Isolation of the virus from CSF confirms it.

Begin with bed rest

Treatment for aseptic viral meningitis includes bed rest, maintenance of fluid and electrolyte balance, analgesics for pain, and exercises to combat residual weakness. Careful handling of excretions and good hand-washing technique prevent the spread of the disease, although isolation isn't necessary.

Risky business

Infants, children, and elderly people have the highest risk of developing meningitis. Other risk factors include malnourishment, immunosuppression (for example, from radiation therapy), and CNS trauma. (See *Meningeal inflammation in meningitis.*)

Getting complicated

Potential complications of meningitis include:
- vision impairment
- optic neuritis
- cranial nerve palsies
- deafness
- personality changes
- headache
- paresis or paralysis
- endocarditis
- coma
- vasculitis
- cerebral infarction.

Now I get it!

Meningeal inflammation in meningitis

The illustration below shows normal meninges and how the meninges become inflamed in meningitis.

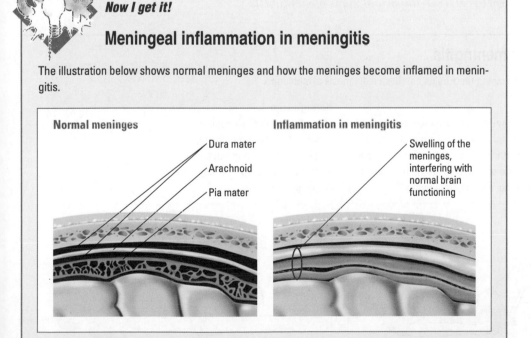

Normal meninges
- Dura mater
- Arachnoid
- Pia mater

Inflammation in meningitis
- Swelling of the meninges, interfering with normal brain functioning

Complications in infants and children may also include:

- sensory hearing loss
- epilepsy
- mental retardation
- hydrocephalus
- subdural effusions.

What to look for

The cardinal signs and symptoms of meningitis are those of infection and increased ICP:

- headache
- stiff neck and back
- malaise
- photophobia
- chills
- fever
- vomiting
- twitching
- seizures
- altered LOC, such as confusion or delirium.
    Signs and symptoms in infants and children may also include:
- fretfulness
- bulging of the fontanels (infants)
- refusal to eat. (See *Important signs of meningitis*.)

Important signs of meningitis

A positive response to the following tests helps establish a diagnosis of meningitis.

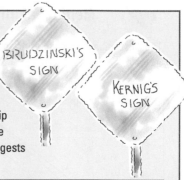

Brudzinski's sign
Place the patient in a dorsal recumbent position; then put your hands behind his neck and bend it forward. Pain and resistance may indicate neck injury or arthritis. But if the patient also involuntarily flexes the hips and knees, chances are he has meningeal irritation and inflammation, a sign of meningitis.

Kernig's sign
Place the patient in a supine position. Flex his leg at the hip and knee; then straighten the knee. Pain or resistance suggests meningitis.

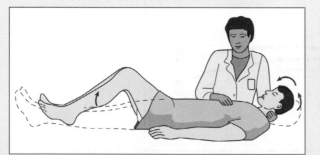

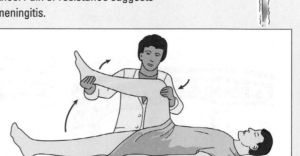

Patient history is key

Findings vary depending on the type and severity of meningitis. In pneumococcal meningitis, the patient history may uncover a recent lung, ear, or sinus infection or endocarditis. It may also reveal alcoholism, sickle cell disease, basal skull fracture, recent splenectomy, or organ transplant. In meningitis caused by *H. influenzae*, the patient history may reveal a recent respiratory tract or ear infection. In meningococcal meningitis, you may see a petechial, purpuric, or ecchymotic rash on the patient's lower body.

It's so irritating

Signs of meningeal irritation are nuchal rigidity, exaggerated and symmetrical deep tendon reflexes, opisthotonos (a spasm in which the back and extremities arch backward so that the body rests on the head and heels), and positive Brudzinski's and Kernig's signs. (See *Treating meningitis.*)

What tests tell you

These tests are used to diagnose meningitis:
• Lumbar puncture shows elevated CSF pressure, cloudy or milky CSF, a high protein level, positive Gram stain and culture that usually identifies the infecting organism (unless it's a virus), and depressed CSF glucose concentration. The Xpert EV test isolates

---

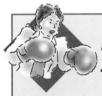

Battling illness

Treating meningitis

Treatment for meningitis includes medications, vigorous supportive care, and treatment of coexisting conditions, such as pneumonia and endocarditis.

Antibiotics and more antibiotics
Usually, I.V. antibiotics are given for at least 2 weeks, followed by oral antibiotics. The most common antibiotics are penicillin G, ampicillin, or nafcillin. If the patient is allergic to penicillin, tetracycline, chloramphenicol, or kanamycin are used.

Prophylactic antibiotics may also be used after ventricular shunting procedures, skull fractures, or penetrating head wounds, but this use is controversial.

Other drugs used in treatment include mannitol to decrease cerebral edema, an I.V. anticonvulsant to prevent seizures, a sedative to reduce restlessness, and aspirin or acetaminophen to relieve headache and fever. Note: aspirin should not be used in children under the age of 12 due to an increased incidence of Reye's syndrome and aspirin use.

Supportive measures
Supportive measures include bed rest, hypothermia, and fluid therapy to prevent dehydration. Isolation is necessary if nasal cultures are positive.

and amplifies viral genetic material in a patient's CSF and identifies infection resulting from the enterovirus responsible for approximately 90% of all viral meningitis cases.
- Chest X-rays are important because they may reveal pneumonitis or lung abscess, tubercular lesions, or granulomas secondary to fungal infection.
- Sinus and skull X-rays may help identify the presence of cranial osteomyelitis, paranasal sinusitis, or skull fracture.
- WBC count usually indicates leukocytosis and abnormal serum electrolyte levels.
- CT scan rules out cerebral hematoma, hemorrhage, or tumor.
- Blood cultures identify the causative agent in bacteremia.

Multiple sclerosis

MS results from progressive demyelination of the white matter of the brain and spinal cord, leading to widespread neurologic dysfunction. The structures usually involved are the optic and oculomotor nerves and the spinal nerve tracts. The disorder doesn't affect the PNS.

Demyelination is the loss of myelin sheath material essential in nerve impulse transmission.

The ups and downs of MS

Characterized by exacerbations and remissions, MS is a major cause of chronic disability in people between ages 18 and 40. The incidence is highest in women, in northern urban areas, in higher socioeconomic groups, and in people with a family history of the disease.

The prognosis varies. The disease may progress rapidly, causing death in a few months or disability by early adulthood. However, about 70% of patients lead active, productive lives with prolonged remissions.

How it happens

The exact cause of MS is unknown. It may be caused by a slow-acting viral infection, an autoimmune response of the nervous system, or an allergic response. Other possible causes include trauma, anoxia, toxins, nutritional deficiencies, vascular lesions, and anorexia nervosa, all of which may help destroy axons and the myelin sheath.

In addition, emotional stress, overwork, fatigue, pregnancy, or an acute respiratory tract infection may precede the onset of this illness. Genetic factors may also play a part.

Dots of demyelination

MS affects the white matter of the brain and spinal cord by causing scattered demyelinated lesions that prevent normal neurologic conduction. After the myelin is destroyed, neuroglial tissue in the white matter of the CNS proliferates, forming hard yellow plaques of scar tissue. Proliferation of neuroglial tissue is called *gliosis*. (See *Understanding myelin breakdown*.)

Now I get it!

Understanding myelin breakdown

Myelin plays a key role in speeding electrical impulses to the brain for interpretation. The myelin sheath is a lipoprotein complex formed of glial cells. It protects the neuron's long nerve fiber (axon) much like the insulation on an electrical wire. Because of its high electrical resistance and weak ability to store an electrical charge, the myelin sheath permits conduction of nerve impulses from one node of Ranvier to the next.

Effects of injury

Myelin can be injured by hypoxemia, toxic chemicals, vascular insufficiency, or autoimmune responses. When this occurs, the myelin sheath becomes inflamed and the membrane layers break down into smaller components. These components become well-circumscribed plaques filled with microglial elements, macroglia, and lymphocytes. This process is called *demyelination*.

The damaged myelin sheath impairs normal conduction, causing partial loss or dispersion of the action potential and consequent neurologic dysfunction.

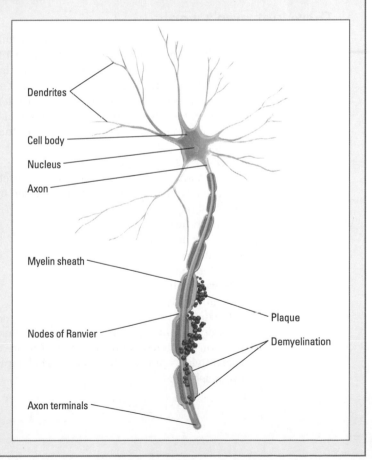

Dendrites

Cell body

Nucleus

Axon

Myelin sheath

Plaque

Nodes of Ranvier

Demyelination

Axon terminals

Interrupting an impulse

Scar tissue damages the underlying axon fiber so that nerve conduction is disrupted. The symptoms of MS caused by demyelination become irreversible as the disease progresses. However, remission may result from healing of demyelinated areas by sclerotic tissue.

What to look for

Signs and symptoms of MS depend on these four factors:

 the extent of myelin destruction

 the site of myelin destruction

the extent of remyelination

the adequacy of subsequent restored synaptic transmission.

There just aren't words

Symptoms may be unpredictable and difficult for the patient to describe. They may be transient or may last for hours or weeks. Usually, the patient history reveals two initial symptoms: vision problems (caused by an optic neuritis) and sensory impairment such as paresthesia. After the initial episode, findings may vary. They may include blurred vision or diplopia, emotional lability (from involvement of the white matter of the frontal lobes), and dysphagia.

Other signs and symptoms include:
• poorly articulated speech (caused by cerebellar involvement)
• muscle weakness and spasticity (caused by lesions in the corticospinal tracts)
• hyperreflexia
• urinary problems
• intention tremor
• gait ataxia
• bowel problems
• cognitive dysfunction
• fatigue
• paralysis, ranging from monoplegia to quadriplegia
• vision problems, such as scotoma (an area of lost vision in the visual field), optic neuritis, and ophthalmoplegia (paralysis of the eye muscles).

Getting complicated

Complications include injuries from falls, urinary tract infections, constipation, joint contractures, pressure ulcers, rectal distention, and pneumonia. (See *Treating MS.*)

What tests tell you

Diagnosing MS may take years because of remissions. These tests help diagnose the disease:
• MRI is the most sensitive method of detecting lesions and is also used to evaluate disease progression. More than 90% of patients show lesions when this test is performed.
• CSF analysis reveals elevated immunoglobulin G levels but normal total protein levels. This elevation is significant only when serum gamma globulin levels are normal, and it reflects hyperactivity of the immune system due to chronic demyelination. The WBC count may be slightly increased.
• Evoked potential studies demonstrate slowed conduction of nerve impulses in 80% of patients.
• CT scan may disclose lesions within the brain's white matter.
• Neuropsychological tests may help rule out other disorders.
• EEG shows abnormalities in one-third of patients.

Battling illness

Treating MS

Treatment for multiple sclerosis (MS) aims to shorten exacerbations and, if possible, relieve neurologic deficits so the patient can resume a near-normal lifestyle.

Drug options
Because MS may have allergic and inflammatory causes, corticotropin, prednisone, or dexamethasone is used to reduce edema of the myelin sheath during exacerbations, relieving symptoms and hastening remissions. However, these drugs don't prevent future exacerbations.

Currently, the preferred treatment during an acute attack is a short course of methylprednisolone, with or without a short prednisone taper. Interferon beta-1a or interferon beta-1b may also be given to decrease the frequency of relapses. How these drugs achieve their effect isn't clearly understood.

Interferon beta-1b, a naturally occurring antiviral and immunoregulatory agent derived from human fibroblasts, is thought to attach to membrane receptors and cause cellular changes, including increased protein synthesis.

Other useful drugs include chlordiazepoxide to mitigate mood swings, baclofen or dantrolene to relieve spasticity, and bethanechol or oxybutynin to relieve urine retention and minimize urinary frequency and urgency.

Supportive measures
During acute exacerbations, supportive measures include bed rest, massage, prevention of fatigue and pressure ulcers, bowel and bladder training, treatment of bladder infections with antibiotics, physical therapy, and counseling.

Myasthenia gravis

Myasthenia gravis produces sporadic, progressive weakness and abnormal fatigue of voluntary skeletal muscles. These effects are exacerbated by exercise and repeated movement.

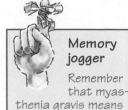

A menace to muscles

Myasthenia gravis usually affects muscles in the face, lips, tongue, neck, and throat, which are innervated by the cranial nerves—however, it can affect any muscle group. Eventually, muscle fibers may degenerate, and weakness (especially of the head, neck, trunk, and limb muscles) may become irreversible. When the disease involves the respiratory system, it may be life-threatening.

Myasthenia gravis affects 14 people per 100,000 and occurs at any age. The most common age of onset in women is from 20 to 30; for men, ages 70 to 80. Previously, the disease affected more women than men, but now, because of their increasing life span, males are affected more commonly than women.

The ups and downs

The disease follows an unpredictable course with periodic exacerbations and remissions. Spontaneous remissions occur in about 25% of patients. No cure exists but, thanks to drug therapy, patients may lead relatively normal lives except during exacerbations.

How it happens

The cause of myasthenia gravis is unknown. It commonly accompanies autoimmune disorders and disorders of the thymus. In fact, 15% of patients with myasthenia gravis have thymomas.

We interrupt this transmission...

For some reason, the patient's blood cells and thymus gland produce antibodies that block, destroy, or weaken the neuroreceptors that transmit nerve impulses, causing a failure in transmission of nerve impulses at the neuromuscular junction. (See *What happens in myasthenia gravis*.)

What to look for

Signs and symptoms of myasthenia gravis vary, depending on the muscles involved and the severity of the disease. However, in all cases, muscle weakness is progressive, and eventually some muscles may lose function entirely.

Now I get it!

What happens in myasthenia gravis

During normal neuromuscular transmission, a motor nerve impulse travels to a motor nerve terminal, stimulating the release of a chemical neurotransmitter called *acetylcholine.* When acetylcholine diffuses across the synapse, receptor sites in the motor end plate react and depolarize the muscle fiber. The depolarization spreads through the muscle fiber, causing muscle contraction.

Those darn antibodies

In myasthenia gravis, antibodies attach to the acetylcholine receptor sites. They block, destroy, and weaken these sites, leaving them insensitive to acetylcholine, thereby blocking neuromuscular transmission.

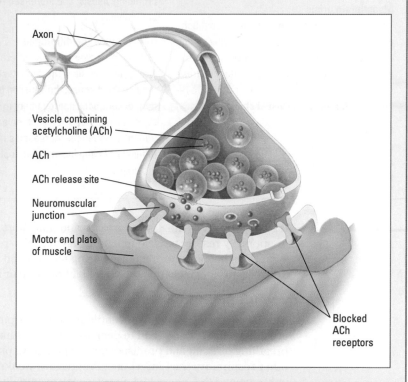

Axon

Vesicle containing acetylcholine (ACh)

ACh

ACh release site

Neuromuscular junction

Motor end plate of muscle

Blocked ACh receptors

Common signs and symptoms include:
- extreme muscle weakness
- fatigue
- ptosis
- diplopia
- difficulty chewing and swallowing
- sleepy, masklike expression
- drooping jaw
- bobbing head
- arm or hand muscle weakness.
    (See *Two types of crisis*, page 152.)

Listen to your patient

The patient may report that she must tilt her head back to see properly. She usually notes that symptoms are milder on awaken-

Two types of crisis

A patient with myasthenia gravis can undergo a crisis in one of two ways.

Myasthenia crisis

This type of crisis can be caused by too much anticholinesterase medication. In a myasthenia crisis, the patient has increased symptoms of myasthenia gravis such as respiratory distress, hypoxia, tachycardia, decreased protective reflexes (gag reflex), and visual changes.

Cholinergic crisis

A cholinergic crisis is caused by too much anticholinesterase medication. The patient in a cholinergic crisis will show side effects of the anticholinesterase medications such as hypotension, bradycardia, diarrhea, abdominal cramping, miosis, and increased respiratory secretions.

How to know the difference

The diagnostic test used to differentiate the two types of crisis is the same test used to diagnose the disease: the Tensilon test. If the patient experiences improvement in the symptoms, the diagnosis is myasthenia crisis. If the patient experiences increased salivation and difficulty swallowing, the diagnosis is cholinergic crisis.

---

ing and worsen as the day progresses and that short rest periods temporarily restore muscle function. She may also report that symptoms become more intense during menses and after emotional stress, prolonged exposure to sunlight or cold, or infections.

If respiratory muscles are involved

Auscultation may reveal hypoventilation if the respiratory muscles are involved. This may lead to decreased tidal volume, making breathing difficult and predisposing the patient to pneumonia and other respiratory tract infections. Progressive weakness of the diaphragm and the intercostal muscles may eventually lead to myasthenic crisis (an acute exacerbation that causes severe respiratory distress). (See *Treating myasthenia gravis*.)

What tests tell you

These tests are used to diagnose myasthenia gravis:
• Tensilon test confirms diagnosis by temporarily improving muscle function after an I.V. injection of edrophonium or, occasionally, neostigmine. However, long-standing ocular muscle dysfunction may not respond. This test also differentiates a myasthenic crisis from a cholinergic crisis.
• Electromyography measures the electrical potential of muscle cells and helps differentiate nerve disorders from muscle disorders. In myasthenia gravis, the amplitude of motor unit potential falls off with continued use. Muscle contractions decrease with each test, reflecting fatigue.

Battling illness

Treating myasthenia gravis

The main treatment for myasthenia gravis is anticholinesterase drugs, such as neostigmine and pyridostigmine. These drugs counteract fatigue and muscle weakness and restore about 80% of muscle function. However, they become less effective as the disease worsens. Corticosteroids may also help to relieve symptoms.

Options and alternatives

If medications aren't effective, some patients undergo plasmapheresis to remove acetylcholine-receptor antibodies and temporarily lessen the severity of symptoms. Patients with thymomas require thymectomy, which leads to remission in adult-onset disease in about 40% of patients if done within 2 years after diagnosis.

Yikes! It's an emergency!

Myasthenic crisis necessitates immediate hospitalization. Endotracheal intubation and mechanical ventilation, combined with vigorous suctioning to remove secretions, usually bring improvement in a few days. Because anticholinesterase drugs aren't effective in myasthenic crisis, they're discontinued until respiratory function improves.

- Nerve conduction studies measure the speed at which electrical impulses travel along a nerve and also help distinguish nerve disorders from muscle disorders.
- Chest X-ray or CT scan may identify a thymoma.

Parkinson's disease

Parkinson's disease produces progressive muscle rigidity, loss of muscle movement *(akinesia)*, and involuntary tremors. The patient's condition may deteriorate for more than 10 years. Eventually, aspiration pneumonia or some other infection causes death.

Parkinson's disease is one of the most common crippling diseases in the United States. It affects more men than women and usually occurs in middle age or later, striking 1 in every 100 people over age 60.

How it happens

In most cases, the cause of Parkinson's disease is unknown. However, some cases result from exposure to toxins, such as manganese dust and carbon monoxide, that destroy cells in the substantia nigra of the brain.

A defect in the dopamine pathway...

Parkinson's disease affects the extrapyramidal system, which influences the initiation, modulation, and completion of movement. The extrapyramidal system includes the corpus striatum, globus pallidus, and substantia nigra.

In Parkinson's disease, a dopamine deficiency occurs in the basal ganglia, the dopamine-releasing pathway that connects the substantia nigra to the corpus striatum.

...causes an imbalance of neurotransmitters

Reduction of dopamine in the corpus striatum upsets the normal balance between the inhibitory dopamine and excitatory acetylcholine neurotransmitters. This prevents affected brain cells from performing their normal inhibitory function within the CNS and causes most parkinsonian symptoms.

(See *Neurotransmitter action in Parkinson's disease.*)

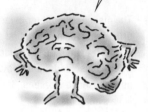

A deficiency of dopamine isn't good news...

Now I get it!

Neurotransmitter action in Parkinson's disease

Degeneration of the dopaminergic neurons and loss of available dopamine lead to rigidity, tremors, and bradykinesia.

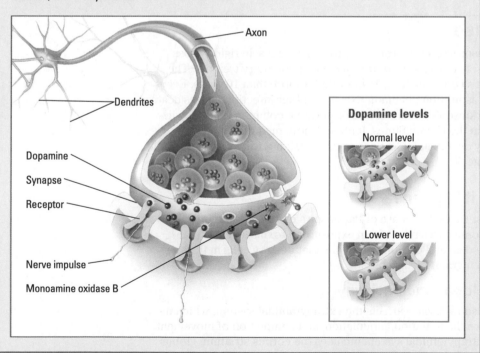

Axon

Dendrites

Dopamine

Synapse

Receptor

Nerve impulse

Monoamine oxidase B

Dopamine levels

Normal level

Lower level

What to look for

Important signs of Parkinson's disease include:

- muscle rigidity
- akinesia
- a unilateral "pill-roll" tremor.

Muscle rigidity results in resistance to passive muscle stretching, which may be uniform (lead-pipe rigidity) or jerky (cogwheel rigidity).

Akinesia causes gait and movement disturbances. The patient walks with his body bent forward, takes a long time initiating movement when performing a purposeful action, pivots with difficulty, and easily loses his balance.

Akinesia may also cause other signs that include:

- masklike facial expression
- blepharospasm, in which the eyelids stay closed.

"Pill-roll" tremor is insidious. It begins in the fingers, increases during stress or anxiety, and decreases with purposeful movement and sleep. (See *Treating Parkinson's disease*, page 156.)

And there's more

Other signs and symptoms of Parkinson's disease include:

- a high-pitched, monotone voice
- drooling
- dysarthria (impaired speech due to a disturbance in muscle control)
- dysphagia (difficulty swallowing)
- fatigue
- muscle cramps in the legs, neck, and trunk
- oily skin
- increased perspiration
- insomnia
- mood changes.

Getting complicated

Common complications of Parkinson's disease include injury from falls, food aspiration due to impaired swallowing, urinary tract infections, and skin breakdown due to increased immobility.

What tests tell you

Diagnosis of Parkinson's disease is based on the patient's age, history, and signs and symptoms, so laboratory tests are generally of little value. However, urinalysis may reveal decreased dopamine levels, and CT scan or MRI may rule out other disorders such as intracranial tumors.

Battling illness

Treating Parkinson's disease

Treatment for Parkinson's disease aims to relieve symptoms and keep the patient functional as long as possible. It consists of drugs, physical therapy, and stereotactic neurosurgery in extreme cases.

Looking to levodopa and other drugs

Drug therapy usually includes levodopa, a dopamine replacement that's most effective in the first few years after it's initiated. It's given in increasing doses until signs and symptoms are relieved or adverse reactions develop. Because adverse effects can be serious, levodopa is commonly given along with carbidopa to halt peripheral dopamine synthesis. Bromocriptine may be given as an additive to reduce the levodopa dose.

When levodopa is ineffective or too toxic, anticholinergics, such as trihexyphenidyl or benztropine, and antihistamines, such as diphenhydramine, are given. Anticholinergics may be used to control tremors and rigidity. They may also be used in combination with levodopa. Antihistamines may help decrease tremors because of their central anticholinergic and sedative effects.

Amantadine, an antiviral agent, is used early in treatment to reduce rigidity, tremors, and akinesia. Patients with mild disease are given deprenyl to slow the progression of the disease and ease symptoms. Tricyclic antidepressants may be given to decrease depression.

Stalevo, the new drug that combines carbidopa, levodopa, and entacapone, is used when carbidopa and levodopa are no longer effective throughout the dosing interval. The added component entacapone prolongs the time that levodopa is active in the brain.

Deep brain stimulation

In the past, pallidotomy and thalamotomy were the only available surgical options. However, deep brain stimulation is now the preferred surgical option. With deep brain stimulation, electrodes are implanted into the targeted brain area. These electrodes are connected to wires attached to an impulse generator that's implanted under the collarbone. The electrodes control symptoms on the opposite side of the body by sending electrical impulses to the brain.

Physical therapy

Physical therapy helps maintain the patient's normal muscle tone and function. It includes both active and passive range-of-motion exercises, routine daily activities, walking, and baths and massage to help relax muscles.

Stroke

Previously known as *cerebrovascular accident*, stroke is a sudden impairment of cerebral circulation in one or more of the blood vessels supplying the brain. It interrupts or diminishes oxygen supply, causing serious damage or necrosis in brain tissues.

The sooner, the better

The sooner circulation returns to normal after stroke, the better chances are for complete recovery. About one-half of those who survive remain permanently disabled and suffer another stroke within weeks, months, or years.

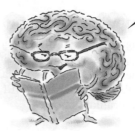

Oh, no! Says here that in stroke, circulation is impaired in the vessels that supply me with blood.

Statistically speaking

Stroke is the third most common cause of death in the United States and the most common cause of neurologic disability. It strikes about 700,000 people each year, and one-half of them die as a result. Although it mostly affects older adults, it can strike people of any age. Black men have a higher risk than other population groups.

Transient, progressive, or completed

Stroke is classified according to how it progresses:
• Transient ischemic attack (TIA), the least severe type, is caused by a temporary interruption of blood flow, usually in the carotid and vertebrobasilar arteries. (See *Understanding TIA*.)
• Progressive stroke, also called *stroke-in-evolution* or *thrombus-in-evolution*, begins with a slight neurologic deficit and worsens in a day or two.
• Completed stroke, the most severe type, causes maximum neurologic deficits at the onset.

Memory jogger

Here are some key points to remember about TIAs:

T: Temporary episode that clears within 12 to 24 hours.

I: It's usually considered a warning sign of Impending stroke.

A: Aspirin and Anticoagulant given during a TIA may minimize the risk of thrombosis.

Understanding TIA

A transient ischemic attack (TIA) is a recurrent episode of neurologic deficit, lasting from seconds to hours, that clears within 12 to 24 hours. It's usually considered a warning sign of an impending thrombotic stroke. In fact, TIAs have been reported in 50% to 80% of patients who've had a cerebral infarction from thrombosis. The age of onset varies, but incidence rises dramatically after age 50 and is highest among blacks and men.

Interrupting blood flow

In TIA, microemboli released from a thrombus may temporarily interrupt blood flow, especially in the small distal branches of the brain's arterial tree. Small spasms in those arterioles may precede TIA and also impair blood flow.

A transient experience

The most distinctive characteristics of TIAs are the transient duration of neurologic deficits and the complete return of normal function. The signs and symptoms of TIA correlate with the location of the affected artery. They include double vision, unilateral blindness, staggering or uncoordinated gait, unilateral weakness or numbness, falling because of weakness in the legs, dizziness, and speech deficits, such as slurring or thickness.

Preventing a complete stroke

During an active TIA, treatment aims to prevent a completed stroke and consists of aspirin (or other antiplatelet medications) or anticoagulants to minimize the risk of thrombosis. After or between attacks, preventive treatment includes carotid endarterectomy or cerebral microvascular bypass.

How it happens

Factors that increase the risk of stroke include:

- history of TIA
- atherosclerosis
- hypertension
- arrhythmias, especially atrial fibrillation
- electrocardiogram changes
- rheumatic heart disease
- diabetes mellitus
- gout
- orthostatic hypotension
- cardiac enlargement
- high serum triglyceride levels
- lack of exercise
- hormonal contraceptive use
- drug abuse
- smoking
- family history of cerebrovascular disease
- sickle cell disease.

Ranking stroke causes

Major causes of stroke include:

 thrombosis

 embolism

 hemorrhage.

First and foremost

Thrombosis is the most common cause of stroke in middle-aged and elderly people. It usually results from an obstruction in the extracerebral vessels, but sometimes it's intracerebral. The risk increases with obesity, smoking, hormonal contraceptive use, and surgery.

Second to none

The second most common cause of stroke, embolism is a blood vessel occlusion caused by a fragmented clot, a tumor, fat, bacteria, or air. It can occur at any age, especially in patients with a history of rheumatic heart disease, endocarditis, posttraumatic valvular disease, or atrial fibrillation or other cardiac arrhythmias. It also occurs after open-heart surgery. Embolism usually develops rapidly—in 10 to 20 seconds—and without warning. The left middle cerebral artery is usually the embolus site. (See *Ischemic stroke.*)

Now I get it!

Ischemic stroke

The illustrations below show common sites of cardiac thrombosis and the resulting sites of embolism and infarction.

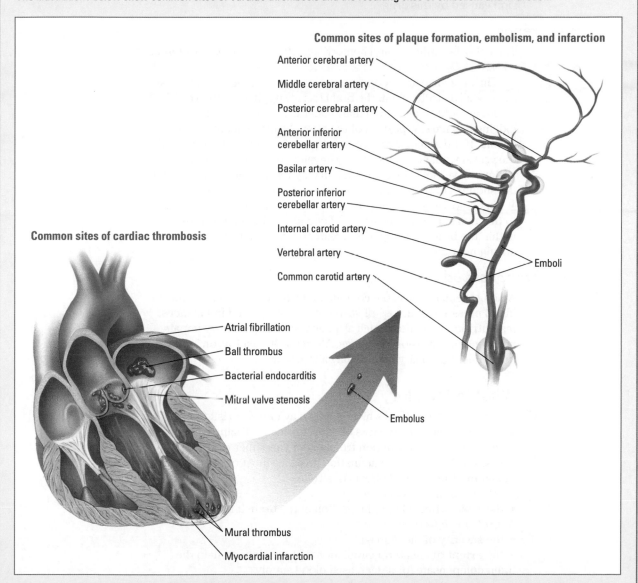

Common sites of plaque formation, embolism, and infarction

Anterior cerebral artery

Middle cerebral artery

Posterior cerebral artery

Anterior inferior cerebellar artery

Basilar artery

Posterior inferior cerebellar artery

Internal carotid artery

Vertebral artery

Common carotid artery

Emboli

Common sites of cardiac thrombosis

Atrial fibrillation

Ball thrombus

Bacterial endocarditis

Mitral valve stenosis

Embolus

Mural thrombus

Myocardial infarction

Last but not least

Hemorrhage, the third most common cause of stroke, may also occur suddenly at any age. It arises from chronic hypertension or aneurysms, which cause a sudden rupture of a cerebral artery. Increasing cocaine use by younger people has also increased the number of hemorrhagic strokes because of the severe hypertension caused by this drug.

Damage report

Thrombosis, embolus, and hemorrhage affect the body in different ways.

Thrombosis causes congestion and edema in the affected vessel as well as ischemia in the brain tissue supplied by the vessel.

An embolus cuts off circulation in the cerebral vasculature by lodging in a narrow portion of the artery, causing necrosis and edema. If the embolus is septic and the infection extends beyond the vessel wall, encephalitis may develop. If the infection stays within the vessel wall, an aneurysm may form, which could lead to the sudden rupture of an artery, or cerebral hemorrhage.

In hemorrhage, a brain artery bursts, diminishing blood supply to the area served by the artery. Blood also accumulates deep within the brain, causing even greater damage by further compromising neural tissue.

Getting complicated

Among the many possible complications of stroke are unstable blood pressure from loss of vasomotor control, fluid imbalances, malnutrition, infections such as pneumonia, and sensory impairment, including vision problems. Altered LOC, aspiration, contractures, and pulmonary emboli may also occur.

What to look for

When taking the patient's history, you may uncover risk factors for stroke. You may observe loss of consciousness, dizziness, or seizures. Obtain information from a family member or friend if necessary. Neurologic examination provides most of the information about the physical effects of stroke.

Physical findings depend on:
• the artery affected and the portion of the brain it supplies (see *Neurologic deficits in stroke*)
• the severity of the damage
• the extent of collateral circulation that develops to help the brain compensate for a decreased blood supply.

Neurologic deficits in stroke

In stroke, functional loss reflects damage to the brain area normally perfused by the occluded or ruptured artery. Whereas one patient may experience only mild hand weakness, another may develop unilateral paralysis. Hypoxia and ischemia may produce edema that affects distal parts of the brain, causing further neurologic deficits. The signs and symptoms that accompany stroke at different sites are described below.

Site	Signs and symptoms
Middle cerebral artery	• Aphasia • Dysphasia • Dyslexia (reading problems) • Dysgraphia (inability to write) • Visual field cuts • Hemiparesis on the affected side, which is more severe in the face and arm than in the leg
Internal carotid artery	• Headaches • Weakness • Paralysis • Numbness • Sensory changes • Monocular visual disturbance or loss • Altered level of consciousness • Bruits over the carotid artery • Aphasia • Dysphasia • Ptosis

Site	Signs and symptoms
Anterior cerebral artery	• Confusion • Weakness • Numbness on the affected side (especially in the arm) • Paralysis of the contralateral foot and leg with accompanying footdrop • Incontinence • Poor coordination • Impaired motor and sensory functions • Personality changes, such as flat affect and distractibility
Vertebral or basilar artery	• Mouth and lip numbness • Dizziness • Weakness on the affected side • Vision deficits, such as color blindness, lack of depth perception, and diplopia • Poor coordination • Dysphagia • Slurred speech • Amnesia • Ataxia
Posterior cerebral artery	• Visual field cuts • Sensory impairment • Dyslexia • Coma • Blindness from ischemia in the occipital area

Reflecting on reflexes

Assessment of motor function and muscle strength commonly shows a loss of voluntary muscle control and hemiparesis or hemiplegia on one side of the body. In the initial phase, flaccid paralysis with decreased deep tendon reflexes may occur. These reflexes return to normal after the initial phase, accompanied by an increase in muscle tone and, in some cases, muscle spasticity on the affected side.

Sensory impairment: Slight to severe

Vision testing usually reveals reduced vision or blindness on the affected side of the body and, in patients with left-sided hemiplegia, problems with visual-spatial relations. Sensory assessment may reveal sensory losses, ranging from slight impairment of touch to the inability to perceive the position and motion of body parts. The patient also may have difficulty interpreting visual, tactile, and auditory stimuli.

Whose side are you on, anyway?

If the stroke occurs in the brain's left hemisphere, it produces signs and symptoms on the right side of the body. If it occurs in the right hemisphere, signs and symptoms appear on the left side. However, a stroke that damages cranial nerves produces signs on the same side as the damage. (See *Treating stroke.*)

> Remember that my right hemisphere controls the left side of the body and my left hemisphere controls the right side of the body.

What tests tell you

These tests are used to diagnose stroke:
• Cerebral angiography details disruption or displacement of the cerebral circulation by occlusion or hemorrhage. It's the test of choice for examining the entire cerebral circulation.
• Digital subtraction angiography evaluates the patency of the cerebral vessels and identifies their position in the head and neck. It also detects and evaluates lesions and vascular abnormalities.
• CT scan detects structural abnormalities, edema, and lesions, such as nonhemorrhagic infarction and aneurysms. It differentiates stroke from other disorders, such as primary metastatic tumor and subdural, intracerebral, or epidural hematoma. Patients with TIA commonly have a normal CT scan.
• PET scan provides data on cerebral metabolism and cerebral blood flow changes, especially in ischemic stroke.
• Single-photon emission tomography identifies cerebral blood flow and helps diagnose cerebral infarction.
• MRI and magnetic resonance angiography evaluate the lesion's location and size. MRI doesn't distinguish hemorrhage, tumor, or infarction as well as a CT scan, but it provides superior images of the cerebellum and brain stem.
• Transcranial Doppler studies evaluate the velocity of blood flow through major intracranial vessels, which can indicate the vessels' diameter.

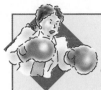

Battling illness

Treating stroke

Medical treatment for stroke commonly includes physical rehabilitation, dietary and drug regimens to help decrease risk factors, and measures to help the patient adapt to specific deficits, such as speech impairment and paralysis.

Drug therapy
Drugs commonly used for stroke therapy include:
• thrombolytic therapy such as recombinant tissue plasminogen activator given within the first 3 hours of an ischemic stroke to restore circulation to the affected brain tissue and limit the extent of brain injury
• anticonvulsants such as phenytoin to treat or prevent seizures
• stool softeners such as docusate to avoid straining, which increases intracranial pressure
• corticosteroids such as dexamethasone to minimize cerebral edema
• anticoagulants, such as heparin, warfarin, and ticlopidine, to reduce the risk of thrombotic stroke
• analgesics such as codeine to relieve headache that may follow hemorrhagic stroke.

Surgery
Depending on the stroke's cause and extent, the patient may also undergo surgery. A craniotomy may be done to remove a hematoma, an endarterectomy to remove atherosclerotic plaque from the inner arterial wall, or extracranial-intracranial bypass to circumvent an artery that's blocked by occlusion or stenosis. Ventricular shunts may be necessary to drain cerebrospinal fluid if hydrocephalus occurs.

• Cerebral blood flow studies measure blood flow to the brain and help detect abnormalities.
• Ophthalmoscopy may show signs of hypertension and atherosclerotic changes in the retinal arteries.
• EEG may detect reduced electrical activity in an area of cortical infarction and is especially useful when CT scan results are inconclusive. It can also differentiate seizure activity from stroke.
• Oculoplethysmography indirectly measures ophthalmic blood flow and carotid artery blood flow.

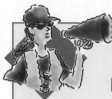

That's a wrap!

Neurologic system review

Understanding the neurologic system

The neurologic system is the body's communication network. It coordinates and organizes the functions of all other body systems. There are two divisions of this network:

• The CNS, made up of the brain and spinal cord, is the body's control center.

• The PNS, containing cranial and spinal nerves, provides communication between the CNS and remote body parts.

CNS

• Protects the brain and spinal cord by the skull and vertebrae, cerebrospinal fluid, and three membranes—the dura mater, the arachnoid mater, and the pia mater.

• Houses the nerve center, called the *cerebrum,* that controls sensory and motor activities and intelligence.

• Transmits impulses to and from the cerebrum by the thalamus and maintains connections to the brain, spinal cord, autonomic nervous system, and pituitary gland by the hypothalamus.

• Coordinates muscle movements, controls posture, and maintains equilibrium by the cerebellum and the brain stem.

• Relays sensations that are needed for voluntary or reflex motor activity through the spinal cord.

PNS

• Originates in 31 pairs of spinal nerves arranged in segments and attached to the spinal cord.

• Divided into the somatic nervous system, which regulates voluntary motor control, and the autonomic nervous system, which helps to regulate the body's internal environment through involuntary control of the organ systems.

Neurologic disorders

• *Alzheimer's disease*—progressive degenerative disorder of the cerebral cortex

• *Amyotrophic lateral sclerosis*—most common of the motor neuron diseases causing muscular atrophy

• *Epilepsy*—brain condition characterized by recurrent seizures

• *Guillain-Barré syndrome*—acute, rapidly progressive, potentially fatal syndrome that's associated with segmented demyelination of the peripheral nerves

• *Multiple sclerosis*—results from progressive demyelination of the white matter of the brain and spinal cord, leading to widespread neurologic dysfunction

• *Meningitis*—condition that causes inflammation of the brain and spinal cord meninges

• *Myasthenia gravis*—condition that produces sporadic, progressive weakness and abnormal fatigue of the voluntary skeletal muscles

• *Parkinson's disease*—produces progressive muscle rigidity, loss of muscle movement, and involuntary tremors

• *Stroke*—sudden impairment of cerebral circulation in one or more of the blood vessels supplying the brain

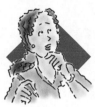

Quick quiz

1. Which type of epileptic seizure involves loss of consciousness, both tonic and clonic phases, tongue biting, and incontinence?

    A.   Simple partial seizure
    B.   Absence seizure
    C.   Generalized tonic-clonic seizure
    D.   Jacksonian seizure

Answer: C. A generalized tonic-clonic seizure stops in 2 to 5 minutes, when abnormal electrical conduction of the neurons is completed.

2. The major causes of stroke are:

    A.   smoking, drug abuse, and high cholesterol levels.
    B.   genetic and metabolic abnormalities.
    C.   brain and spinal cord tumors.
    D.   thrombosis, embolism, and hemorrhage.

Answer: D. Thrombosis is the most common cause of stroke; then embolism and hemorrhage, in that order.

3. Brudzinski's sign and Kernig's sign are two tests that help diagnose which neurologic disorder?

    A.   Stroke
    B.   Meningitis
    C.   Epilepsy
    D.   ALS

Answer: B. A positive response to one or both tests indicates meningeal irritation seen with meningitis.

4. Which neurologic disorder is characterized by progressive degeneration of the cerebral cortex?

    A.   Alzheimer's disease
    B.   Epilepsy
    C.   Guillain-Barré syndrome
    D.   Myasthenia gravis

Answer: A. Symptoms of Alzheimer's disease range from recent memory loss to debilitating dementia.

5. MS is characterized by:
    A. progressive demyelination of the white matter of the CNS.
    B. impairment of cerebral circulation.
    C. deficiency of the neurotransmitter dopamine.
    D. beta-amyloid plaques.

Answer: A. Patches of demyelination cause widespread neurologic dysfunction.

Scoring

☆☆☆   If you answered all five items correctly, unbelievable! Your dedication to dendrites and dopamine is downright unnerving.

☆☆   If you answered four items correctly, congratulations! We are honored to extend congratulations not only to you but to both lobes of your cerebrum.

☆   If you answered fewer than four items correctly, stay cool. We'll just chalk it up to one of those "lapses in the synapses."

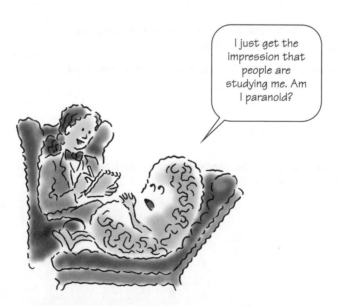

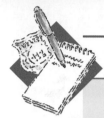

5

Gastrointestinal system

Just the facts

In this chapter, you'll learn:

♦ the structures of the gastrointestinal system and related organs

♦ how the gastrointestinal system functions

♦ pathophysiology, signs and symptoms, diagnostic tests, and treatments for common gastrointestinal disorders.

Understanding the gastrointestinal system

The gastrointestinal (GI) system is the body's food processing complex. It performs the critical task of supplying essential nutrients to fuel the other organs and body systems.

The GI system has two major components. They include:

☞ the GI tract, or alimentary canal

☞ the accessory glands and organs.

A GI-ant sphere of influence

A malfunction along the GI tract or in one of the accessory glands or organs can produce far-reaching metabolic effects, which may become life-threatening. (See *A close look at the GI system*, page 168.)

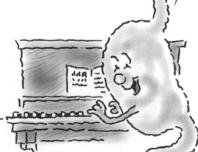

I'm a key player in the GI system where food is processed into fuel for other organs and body systems.

GI tract

The GI tract is basically a hollow, muscular tube that begins in the mouth and ends at the anus. It includes the:
• mouth
• esophagus
• stomach

A close look at the GI system

This illustration shows the organs of the GI tract and several accessory organs.
The GI tract also includes the mouth and epiglottis.

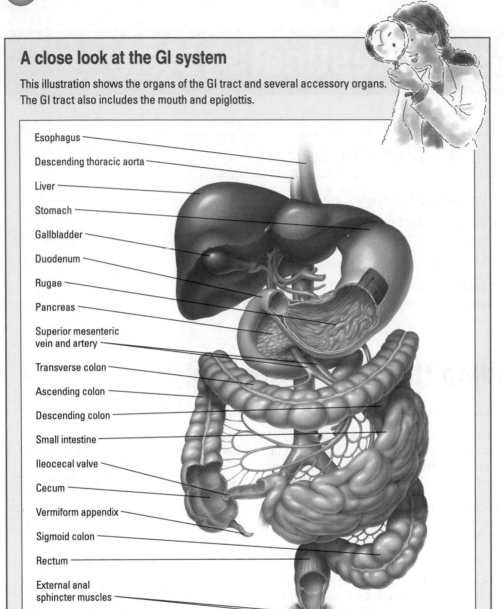

- Esophagus
- Descending thoracic aorta
- Liver
- Stomach
- Gallbladder
- Duodenum
- Rugae
- Pancreas
- Superior mesenteric vein and artery
- Transverse colon
- Ascending colon
- Descending colon
- Small intestine
- Ileocecal valve
- Cecum
- Vermiform appendix
- Sigmoid colon
- Rectum
- External anal sphincter muscles
- Anus

- small intestine
- large intestine.

Mouth and esophagus

When a person smells, tastes, chews, or merely thinks of food, the digestive system gets ready to go to work.

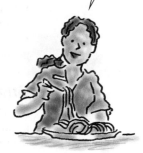

Digestion begins long before food reaches the stomach.

It begins with the first bite

The digestive process begins in the mouth. Chewing and salivation soften food, making it easy to swallow. An enzyme in saliva, called *ptyalin*, begins to convert starches to sugars even before food is swallowed.

Riding the peristaltic wave

When a person swallows, the upper esophageal sphincter relaxes, allowing food to enter the esophagus. In the esophagus, peristaltic waves activated by the glossopharyngeal nerve propel food toward the stomach.

Stomach

Digestion occurs in two phases:

cephalic phase

gastric phase.

Phase 1: Break it down

By the time food is traveling through the esophagus on its way to the stomach, the cephalic phase of digestion has begun. In this phase, the stomach secretes hydrochloric acid and pepsin, digestive juices that help break down food.

Phase 2: Set the stomach on start

The gastric phase of digestion begins when food passes the cardiac sphincter, a circle of muscle at the end of the esophagus. The food exits the esophagus and enters the stomach, causing the stomach wall to distend. This stimulates the mucosal lining of the stomach to release the hormone gastrin. Gastrin serves two purposes:
- stimulation of gastric juice secretion
- stimulation of the stomach's motor functions.

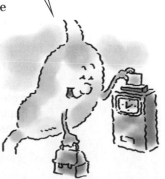

The release of the hormone gastrin means it's time for me to get to work.

Gastric juice, a perfect complement to every meal

Gastric juice secretions are highly acidic, with a pH of 0.9 to 1.5. In addition to hydrochloric acid and pepsin, the gastric juices contain intrinsic factor (which helps the body absorb vitamin B_{12}) and proteolytic enzymes (which help the body use protein). The gastric juices mix with the food, which becomes a thick, gruel-like material called *chyme*.

Hold it, mix it, and empty it out

The stomach has three major motor functions:
- holding food
- mixing food by peristaltic contractions with gastric juices
- slowly emptying chyme into the small intestine for further digestion and absorption.

Small intestine

Nearly all digestion takes place in the small intestine, which is about 20′ (6 m) long. Chyme passes through the small intestine propelled by peristaltic contractions.

The small intestine has three major sections:

 the duodenum

 the jejunum

 the ileum.

Dedicated to the duodenum

The duodenum is a 10″ (25.4-cm) long, C-shaped curve of the small intestine that extends from the stomach. Food passes from the stomach to the duodenum through a narrow opening called the *pylorus*.

The duodenum also has an opening through which bile and pancreatic enzymes enter the intestine to neutralize the acidic chyme and aid digestion. This opening is called the *sphincter of Oddi*.

Just a jejunum? It's the longest part!

The jejunum extends from the duodenum and forms the longest portion of the small intestine. The jejunum leads to the ileum, the narrowest portion of the small intestine.

Let's move these nutrients (and nonnutrients) along

Digestive secretions convert carbohydrates, proteins, and fats into sugars, amino acids, fatty acids, and glycerin. Along with water and electrolytes, these nutrients are absorbed through the intestinal mucosa into the bloodstream for use by the body. Nonnutrients such as vegetable fibers are carried through the intestine.

The small intestine ends at the ileocecal valve, located in the lower right part of the abdomen. The ileocecal valve is a sphincter that empties nutrient-depleted chyme into the large intestine.

Large intestine

After chyme passes through the small intestine, it enters the ascending colon at the cecum, the pouchlike beginning of the large intestine. By this time, the chyme consists of mostly indigestible material. From the ascending colon, chyme passes through the transverse colon, and then down through the descending colon to the rectum and anal canal, where it's finally expelled.

Super-absorbent

The large intestine produces no hormones or digestive enzymes. Rather, it's where absorption takes place. The large intestine absorbs nearly all of the water remaining in the chyme plus large amounts of sodium and chloride.

The large intestine also harbors the bacteria *Escherichia coli, Enterobacter aerogenes, Clostridium welchii,* and *Lactobacillus bifidus,* which help produce vitamin K and break down cellulose into usable carbohydrates.

Joining a mass movement

In the lower part of the descending colon, long, relatively sluggish contractions cause propulsive waves known as mass movements. These movements propel the intestinal contents into the rectum and produce the urge to defecate.

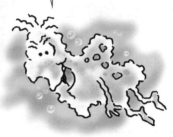

Yeah, it's true. I hang out in the large intestine. I'm real useful, too.

Accessory glands and organs

The liver, gallbladder, and pancreas contribute several substances, such as enzymes, bile, and hormones, that are vital to digestion. These structures deliver their secretions to the duodenum through the ampulla of Vater. (See *Accessory GI organs and vessels,* page 172.)

Liver

A large, highly vascular organ, the liver is enclosed in a fibrous capsule in the upper right area of the abdomen.

No problem with multitasking

The liver performs many complex and important functions, many of which are related to digestion and nutrition:
• It filters and detoxifies blood, removing foreign substances, such as drugs, alcohol, and other toxins.

Accessory GI organs and vessels

Accessory GI organs include the liver, gallbladder, and pancreas, as well as their blood vessels.

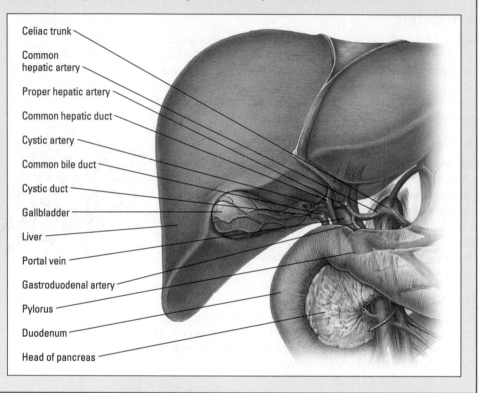

Celiac trunk
Common hepatic artery
Proper hepatic artery
Common hepatic duct
Cystic artery
Common bile duct
Cystic duct
Gallbladder
Liver
Portal vein
Gastroduodenal artery
Pylorus
Duodenum
Head of pancreas

• It removes naturally occurring ammonia from body fluids, converting it to urea for excretion in urine.
• It produces plasma proteins, nonessential amino acids, and vitamin A.
• It stores essential nutrients, such as iron and vitamins K, D, and B_{12}.
• It produces bile to aid digestion.
• It converts glucose to glycogen and stores it as fuel for the muscles.
• It stores fats and converts excess sugars to fats for storage in other parts of the body.

Gallbladder

The gallbladder is a small, pear-shaped organ nestled under the liver and joined to the larger organ by the cystic duct. The gallbladder's job is to store and concentrate bile produced by the liver. Bile is a clear yellowish liquid that helps break down fats and neutralize gastric secretions in the chyme.

You have a delivery

Secretion of the hormone cholecystokinin causes the gallbladder to contract and the ampulla of Vater to relax. This allows the release of bile into the common bile duct for delivery to the duodenum. When the ampulla of Vater closes, bile shunts to the gallbladder for storage.

Pancreas

The pancreas lies behind the stomach, with its head and neck extending into the curve of the duodenum and its tail lying against the spleen.

Between my exocrine and endocrine functions, I sure am busy!

The pancreas is made up of two types of tissue:
• exocrine tissue, from which enzymes are secreted through ducts to the digestive system
• endocrine tissue, from which hormones are secreted into the blood.

An expert analysis...

The pancreas's exocrine function involves small, scattered glands—called *acini*—that secrete more than 1,000 ml of digestive enzymes daily. These lobules of enzyme-producing cells release their secretions into small ducts that merge to form the pancreatic duct. The pancreatic duct runs the length of the pancreas and joins the bile duct from the gallbladder before entering the duodenum. Vagus nerve stimulation and the release of two hormones (secretin and cholecystokinin) control the rate and amount of pancreatic secretion.

...along with an enlightened look

The endocrine function involves the islets of Langerhans, microscopic structures scattered throughout the pancreas. Over 1 million islets house two major cell types:
• alpha cells secrete glucagon, a hormone that stimulates glucose formation in the liver
• beta cells secrete insulin to promote carbohydrate metabolism.

Both hormones flow directly into the blood; their release is mediated by blood glucose levels.

Gastrointestinal disorders

The disorders discussed in this section include:
• appendicitis
• cholecystitis
• cirrhosis
• Crohn's disease
• diverticular disease
• gastroesophageal reflux disease (GERD)
• hiatal hernia
• irritable bowel syndrome
• pancreatitis
• peptic ulcer
• ulcerative colitis
• viral hepatitis.

Appendicitis

Appendicitis occurs when the appendix becomes inflamed. It's the most common major surgical emergency.

Let's get specific

More precisely, this disorder is an inflammation of the vermiform appendix, a small, fingerlike projection attached to the cecum just below the ileocecal valve.

Appendicitis may occur at any age and affects both sexes equally; however, between puberty and age 25, it's more prevalent in men.

How it happens

Until recently, appendicitis was thought to result from an obstruction by a fecal mass, a stricture, barium ingestion, or viral infection. Obstruction does sometimes occur, but mucosal ulceration usually happens first. Although the exact cause of the ulceration is unknown, it may be viral in nature.

Apprehending appendicitis

After ulceration occurs, appendicitis progresses this way:
• Inflammation accompanies the ulceration and temporarily obstructs the appendix.
• Obstruction, if present, is usually caused by stool accumulation around vegetable fibers (*fecalith* is a fancy name for this). (See *Appendix obstruction and inflammation.*)
• Mucus outflow is blocked, which distends the organ.

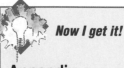

Now I get it!

Appendix obstruction and inflammation

This illustration shows a fecalith obstructing the lumen of the appendix with resulting inflammation.

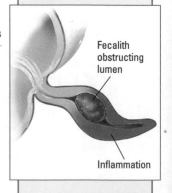

Fecalith obstructing lumen

Inflammation

• Pressure within the appendix increases, and the appendix contracts.
• Bacteria multiply and inflammation and pressure continue to increase, affecting blood flow to the organ and causing severe abdominal pain.

Getting complicated

Inflammation can lead to infection, clotting, tissue decay, and perforation of the appendix. If the appendix ruptures or perforates, the infected contents spill into the abdominal cavity, causing peritonitis, the most common and dangerous complication.

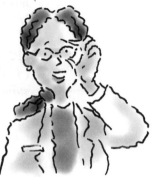

Ulceration and inflammation may cause swelling and rupture.

What to look for

The history and sequence of pain is important in diagnosing appendicitis. The first symptom is almost always vague epigastric pain, sometimes described as a cramping sensation. Over time, the pain becomes more localized and moves to the right lower abdominal area. If the appendix is in back of the cecum or in the pelvis, the patient may have flank tenderness instead of abdominal tenderness.

Other signs and symptoms include:
• anorexia
• nausea or vomiting
• low-grade fever
• rebound tenderness on palpation.

Rupture!

In cases of rupture, spasm will occur, sometimes followed by a brief cessation of abdominal pain.

Untreated appendicitis is invariably fatal. In recent times, the use of antibiotics has reduced the incidence of death from appendicitis. (See *Treating appendicitis*.)

What tests tell you

These tests are sometimes helpful in diagnosis, but normal findings for these don't rule out appendicitis:
• White blood cell (WBC) count is moderately high with an increased number of immature cells.
• X-ray with a radiographic contrast agent aids diagnosis. Failure of the organ to fill with contrast agent indicates appendicitis.

Diagnosis with a difference

Differential diagnosis rules out illnesses with similar symptoms, such as bladder infection, diverticulitis, gastritis, ovarian cyst, pancreatitis, renal colic, and uterine disease.

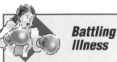

Battling Illness

Treating appendicitis

Appendectomy is the only effective treatment for appendicitis. If peritonitis develops, treatment involves gastric intubation, parenteral replacement of fluids and electrolytes, and antibiotic administration.

Cholecystitis

In cholecystitis, the gallbladder becomes inflamed. Usually, a gallstone becomes lodged in the cystic duct, causing painful gallbladder distention.

Cholecystitis may be acute or chronic. The acute form is most common during middle age; the chronic form, among elderly people.

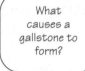

What causes a gallstone to form?

How it happens

Cholecystitis is caused by the formation of calculi called *gallstones*. The exact cause of gallstone formation is unknown. Abnormal metabolism of cholesterol and bile salts play an important role. Acute cholecystitis may also result from poor or absent blood flow to the gallbladder.

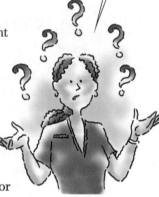

Galling risks

Risk factors that predispose a person to gallstones include:
• obesity and a high-calorie, high-cholesterol diet
• increased estrogen levels from hormonal contraceptives, hormone replacement therapy, or pregnancy
• use of clofibrate, an antilipemic drug
• diabetes mellitus, ileal disease, blood disorders, liver disease, or pancreatitis.

The foundation stone

In acute cholecystitis, inflammation of the gallbladder wall usually develops after a gallstone lodges in the cystic duct. When bile flow is blocked, the gallbladder becomes inflamed and distended. Bacterial growth, usually *E. coli*, may contribute to the inflammation. (See *Understanding gallstone formation.*)

Then this sequence of events takes place:
• Edema of the gallbladder or cystic duct occurs.
• Edema obstructs bile flow, which chemically irritates the gallbladder.
• Cells in the gallbladder wall may become oxygen starved and die as the distended organ presses on vessels and impairs blood flow.
• Dead cells slough off.
• An exudate covers ulcerated areas, causing the gallbladder to adhere to surrounding structures.

Getting complicated

Cholecystitis may lead to complications:
• Pus may accumulate in the gallbladder.
• Fluid may accumulate in the gallbladder (hydrops).

Now I get it!

Understanding gallstone formation

Abnormal metabolism of cholesterol and bile salts plays an important role in gallstone formation. Bile is made continuously by the liver and is concentrated and stored in the gallbladder until the duodenum needs it to help digest fat. Changes in the composition of bile may allow gallstones to form. Changes to the absorptive ability of the gallbladder lining may also contribute to gallstone formation.

Too much cholesterol

Certain conditions, such as age, obesity, and estrogen imbalance, cause the liver to secrete bile that's abnormally high in cholesterol or lacking the proper concentration of bile salts.

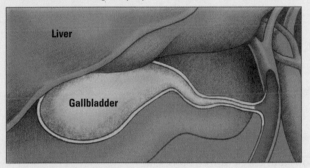

Liver

Gallbladder

Inside the gallbladder

When the gallbladder concentrates this bile, inflammation may occur. Excessive water and bile salts are reabsorbed, making the bile less soluble. Cholesterol, calcium, and bilirubin precipitate into gallstones.

Fat entering the duodenum causes the intestinal mucosa to secrete the hormone cholecystokinin, which stimulates the gallbladder to contract and empty. If a stone lodges in the cystic duct, the gallbladder contracts but can't empty.

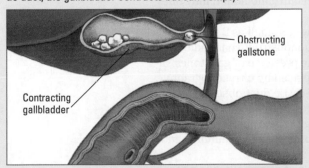

Obstructing gallstone

Contracting gallbladder

Jaundice, irritation, inflammation

If a stone lodges in the common bile duct, the bile flow into the duodenum becomes obstructed. Bilirubin is absorbed into the blood, causing jaundice.

Biliary narrowing and swelling of the tissue around the stone can also cause irritation and inflammation of the common bile duct.

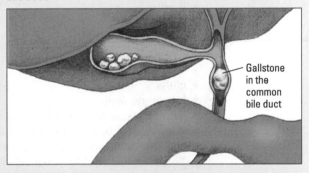

Gallstone in the common bile duct

Up the biliary tree

Inflammation can progress up the biliary tree and cause infection of any of the bile ducts. This causes scar tissue, fluid accumulation, cirrhosis, portal hypertension, and bleeding.

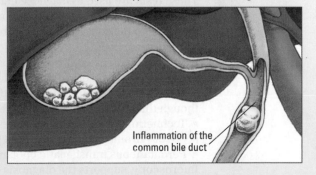

Inflammation of the common bile duct

- The gallbladder may become distended with mucus secretions (mucocele).
- Gangrene may occur, leading to perforation, peritonitis, abnormal passages in the tissues (fistulas), and pancreatitis.
- Chronic cholecystitis may develop.
- Cholangitis (bile duct infection) may develop.

What to look for

Signs and symptoms of acute cholecystitis usually strike after meals that are rich in fats and may occur at night, suddenly awakening the patient. They include:
- acute abdominal pain in the right upper quadrant that may radiate to the back, between the shoulders, or to the front of the chest
- colic due to passage of gallstones along the bile duct (biliary colic)
- pain
- belching
- flatulence
- indigestion
- light-headedness
- nausea
- vomiting
- chills
- low-grade fever
- jaundice (caused by bile in the blood) and clay-colored stools, if a stone obstructs the common bile duct.

Cholecystitis accounts for 10% to 25% of all patients requiring gallbladder surgery. The prognosis is good with treatment. (See *Treating cholecystitis.*)

What tests tell you

These tests are used to diagnose cholecystitis:
- X-rays reveal gallstones if they contain enough calcium to be radiopaque and also help disclose porcelain gallbladder, limy bile, and gallstone ileus.
- Ultrasonography confirms gallstones as small as 2 mm and distinguishes between obstructive and nonobstructive jaundice.
- Oral cholecystography confirms the presence of gallstones, although this test is gradually being replaced by ultrasonography.
- Technetium-labeled scan indicates cystic duct obstruction and acute or chronic cholecystitis if the gallbladder can't be seen.
- Percutaneous transhepatic cholangiography, performed with fluoroscopy, supports the diagnosis of obstructive jaundice and reveals calculi in the ducts.
- Blood studies may reveal high levels of serum alkaline phosphatase, lactate dehydrogenase, aspartate aminotransferase, and

Battling illness

Treating cholecystitis

Surgery is the most common treatment for gallbladder and bile duct disease. Procedures include:
• gallbladder removal (cholecystectomy), with or without X-ray of the bile ducts (operative cholangiography)
• creation of an opening into the common bile duct for drainage (choledochostomy)
• exploration of the common bile duct.

Alternatives to surgery
Other invasive procedures include:
• insertion of a flexible catheter through a sinus tract into the common bile duct and removal of stones using a basket-shaped tool guided by fluoroscopy
• endoscopic retrograde cholangiopancreatography, which removes stones with a balloon or basket-shaped tool passed through an endoscope
• lithotripsy, which breaks up gallstones with ultrasonic waves (contraindicated in patients with pacemakers or implantable defibrillators)
• stone dissolution therapy with oral chenodeoxycholic acid or ursodeoxycholic acid (of limited use).

Diet, drugs, and more
Other treatments include:
• a low-fat diet with replacement of vitamins A, D, E, and K and administration of bile salts to facilitate digestion and vitamin absorption
• opioids to relieve pain during an acute attack
• antispasmodics and anticholinergics to relax smooth muscles and decrease ductal tone and spasm
• antiemetics to reduce nausea and vomiting
• a nasogastric tube connected to intermittent low-pressure suction to relieve vomiting
• cholestyramine if the patient has obstructive jaundice with severe itching from accumulation of bile salts in the skin
• aromatherapy, using a few drops of rosemary oil in a warm bath or inhaled directly, to improve the gallbladder's function.

---

total bilirubin. The icteric index, a measure of bilirubin in the blood, is elevated.
• WBC count is slightly elevated during a cholecystitis attack.

Cirrhosis

Cirrhosis, a chronic liver disease, is characterized by widespread destruction of hepatic cells, which are replaced by fibrous cells. This process is called *fibrotic regeneration*.

Cirrhosis is a common cause of death in the United States and, among people ages 35 to 55, the fourth leading cause of death. It can occur at any age.

How it happens

There are many types of cirrhosis, each with a different cause. The most common include the following:
• Laënnec's cirrhosis, also called *portal, nutritional,* or *alcoholic cirrhosis*, stems from chronic alcoholism and malnutrition. It's most prevalent among malnourished alcoholic men

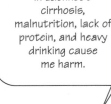

In Laënnec's cirrhosis, malnutrition, lack of protein, and heavy drinking cause me harm.

and accounts for more than one-half of all cirrhosis cases in the United States. Many alcoholics never develop the disease, however, whereas others develop it even with adequate nutrition.

• Postnecrotic cirrhosis is usually a complication of viral hepatitis (inflammation of the liver), but it may also occur after exposure to liver toxins, such as arsenic, carbon tetrachloride, or phosphorus. This form is more common in women and is the most common type of cirrhosis worldwide.

• Biliary cirrhosis results from prolonged bile duct obstruction or inflammation.

• Cardiac cirrhosis is caused by prolonged venous congestion in the liver from right-sided heart failure.

• Idiopathic cirrhosis may develop in some patients with no known cause.

No turning back

Cirrhosis is characterized by irreversible chronic injury of the liver, extensive fibrosis, and nodular tissue growth. These changes result from:

• liver cell death (hepatocyte necrosis)

• collapse of the liver's supporting structure (the reticulin network)

• distortion of the vascular bed (blood vessels throughout the liver)

• nodular regeneration of remaining liver tissue. (See *Cirrhotic changes in the liver.*)

Getting complicated

When the liver begins to malfunction, blood clotting disorders (coagulopathies), jaundice, edema, and various metabolic problems develop.

Fibrosis and the distortion of blood vessels may impede blood flow in the capillary branches of the portal vein and hepatic artery, leading to portal hypertension (elevated pressure in the portal vein). Increased pressure may lead to the development of esophageal varices, enlarged, tortuous veins in the lower part of the esophagus, the area where it meets the stomach. Esophageal varices may easily rupture and leak large amounts of blood into the upper GI tract.

What to look for

Early signs and symptoms of cirrhosis are vague but usually include loss of appetite, indigestion, nausea, vomiting, constipation, diarrhea, dull abdominal ache, and jaundice. The patient may report bruising easily.

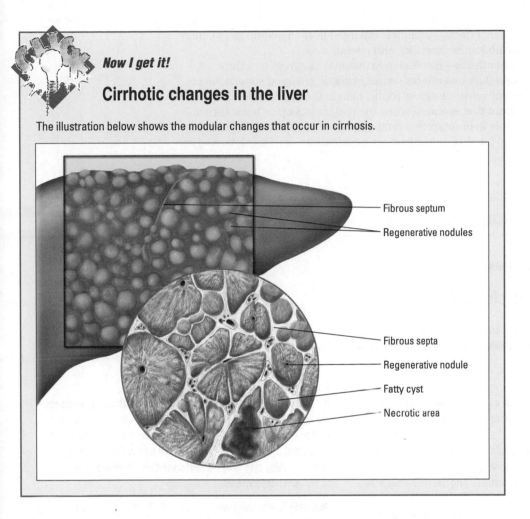

Now I get it!

Cirrhotic changes in the liver

The illustration below shows the modular changes that occur in cirrhosis.

Fibrous septum

Regenerative nodules

Fibrous septa

Regenerative nodule

Fatty cyst

Necrotic area

The final act

Late-stage signs and symptoms affect several body systems and include:
- respiratory effects—fluid in the lungs and weak chest expansion, leading to hypoxia
- central nervous system effects—lethargy, mental changes, slurred speech, asterixis (a motor disturbance marked by intermittent lapses in posture), and peripheral nerve damage
- hematologic effects—nosebleeds, easy bruising, bleeding gums, and anemia
- endocrine effects—testicular atrophy, menstrual irregularities, gynecomastia, and loss of chest and axillary hair
- skin effects—severe itching and dryness, poor tissue turgor, abnormal pigmentation, and spider veins

- hepatic effects—jaundice, enlarged liver (hepatomegaly), fluid in the abdomen (ascites), and edema
- renal effects—insufficiency that may progress to failure
- miscellaneous effects—musty breath, enlarged superficial abdominal veins, muscle atrophy, pain in the upper right abdominal quadrant that worsens when the patient sits up or leans forward, palpable liver or spleen, temperature of 101° to 103° F (38.3° to 39.4° C), and bleeding from esophageal varices. (See *Treating cirrhosis*.)

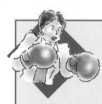

Battling illness

Treating cirrhosis

Therapy for cirrhosis aims to remove or alleviate the underlying cause, prevent further liver damage, and prevent or treat complications.

Drug therapy
Drug therapy requires special caution because the cirrhotic liver can't detoxify harmful substances efficiently. These drugs include:
- vitamins and nutritional supplements to help heal damaged liver cells and improve nutritional status
- antacids to reduce gastric distress and decrease the potential for GI bleeding
- diuretics such as furosemide to reduce fluid accumulation
- vasopressin to treat esophageal varices.

Noninvasive procedures
To control bleeding from esophageal varices or other GI hemorrhage, two measures are attempted first:
- In gastric intubation, the stomach is lavaged until the contents are clear. Antacids and histamine antagonists are then administered if the bleeding is caused by a gastric ulcer.
- In esophageal balloon tamponade, bleeding vessels are compressed to stop blood loss from esophageal varices.

Surgery
In patients with ascites, paracentesis may be used to relieve abdominal pressure. A shunt may be inserted to divert ascites into venous circulation. This treatment causes weight loss, decreased abdominal girth, increased sodium excretion from the kidneys, and improved urine output.

Sclerotherapy
If conservative treatment fails to stop hemorrhaging, a sclerosing agent is injected into the oozing vessels to cause clotting and sclerosis. If bleeding from the varices doesn't stop in 2 to 5 minutes, a second injection is given below the bleeding site. Sclerotherapy also may be performed on nonbleeding varices to prevent hemorrhaging.

Radiologic intervention
A radiologic procedure known as *transjugular intrahepatic portosystemic shunt* may be performed. During this procedure, a shunt is placed between the portal vein and the hepatic vein. The procedure reduces pressure in the varices, preventing them from bleeding.

Last resort
As a last resort, portosystemic shunts may be inserted during surgery to control bleeding from esophageal varices and decrease portal hypertension. These shunts divert a portion of the portal vein blood flow away from the liver. This procedure is seldom performed because it can cause bleeding, infection, and shunt thrombosis. Massive hemorrhage requires blood transfusions to maintain blood pressure.

What tests tell you

These tests help confirm cirrhosis:

• Liver biopsy, the definitive test, reveals tissue destruction (necrosis) and fibrosis.

• Abdominal X-ray shows liver size, cysts or gas within the biliary tract or liver, liver calcification, and massive fluid accumulation (ascites).

• Computed tomography (CT) and liver scans show liver size, abnormal masses, and hepatic blood flow and obstruction.

• Esophagogastroduodenoscopy reveals bleeding esophageal varices, stomach irritation or ulceration, or duodenal bleeding and irritation.

• Blood studies show elevated liver enzymes, total serum bilirubin, and indirect bilirubin levels. Total serum albumin and protein levels decrease; prothrombin time (PT) is prolonged; hemoglobin, hematocrit, and serum electrolyte levels decrease; and vitamins A, C, and K are deficient.

• Urine studies show increased levels of bilirubin and urobilinogen.

• Fecal studies show decreased fecal urobilinogen levels.

Crohn's disease

Crohn's disease is one of the two major types of inflammatory bowel disease. It may affect any part of the GI tract. Inflammation extends through all layers of the intestinal wall and may involve lymph nodes and supporting membranes in the area. Ulcers form as the inflammation extends into the peritoneum.

Crohn's disease is most prevalent in adults ages 20 to 40. It affects men and women equally and tends to run in families—up to 20% of patients have a positive family history.

What's in a name?

When Crohn's disease affects only the small bowel, it's known as *regional enteritis*. When it involves the colon or only affects the colon, it's known as *Crohn's disease of the colon*. Crohn's disease of the colon is sometimes called *granulomatous colitis;* however, not all patients develop granulomas (tumorlike masses of granulation tissue).

How it happens

Although researchers are still studying Crohn's disease, possible causes include:

• lymphatic obstruction

• infection

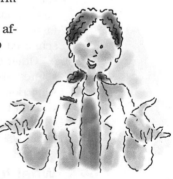

In Crohn's disease, severe inflammation may occur in any part of the GI tract.

- allergies
- immune disorders, such as altered immunoglobulin A production and increased suppressor T-cell activity
- genetic factors. (See *Nod₂ mutation.*)

Comprehending Crohn's

In Crohn's disease, inflammation spreads slowly and progressively. Here's what happens:
- Lymph nodes enlarge and lymph flow in the submucosa is blocked.
- Lymphatic obstruction causes edema, mucosal ulceration, fissures, abscesses and, sometimes, granulomas. Mucosal ulcerations are called skipping lesions because they aren't continuous as in ulcerative colitis.
- Oval, elevated patches of closely packed lymph follicles—called *Peyer's patches*—develop on the lining of the small intestine.
- Fibrosis occurs, thickening the bowel wall and causing stenosis, or narrowing of the lumen. (See *Changes to the bowel in Crohn's disease.*)
- Inflammation of the serous membrane (serositis) develops, inflamed bowel loops adhere to other diseased or normal loops, and diseased bowel segments become interspersed with healthy ones.
- Eventually, diseased parts of the bowel become thicker, narrower, and shorter.

Getting complicated

Severe diarrhea and corrosion of the perineal area by enzymes can cause anal fistula, the most common complication. A perineal abscess may also develop during the active inflammatory state. Fistulas may develop to the bladder, vagina, or even skin in an old scar area. (See *Treating Crohn's disease*, page 186.)
    Other complications include:
- intestinal obstruction
- nutrient deficiencies caused by malabsorption of bile salts and vitamin B_{12} and poor digestion
- fluid imbalances
- rarely, inflammation of abdominal linings (peritonitis).

What to look for

Initially, the patient experiences malaise and diarrhea, usually with pain in the right lower quadrant or generalized abdominal pain and fever.
    Chronic diarrhea results from bile salt malabsorption, loss of healthy intestinal surface area, and bacterial growth. Weight loss, nausea, and vomiting also occur. Stools may be bloody.

The genetic link

Nod₂ mutation

Genetic factors may play a role. Crohn's disease sometimes occurs in identical twins, and 10% to 20% of patients with the disease have one or more affected relatives.

    Researchers recently found a mutation in the gene known as *Nod₂*. The mutation is twice as common in patients with Crohn's disease when compared with the general population. It seems to alter the body's ability to combat bacteria. Currently, there's no practical method to screen for the presence of this genetic mutation.

Now I get it!

Changes to the bowel in Crohn's disease

As Crohn's disease progresses, fibrosis thickens the bowel wall and narrows the lumen. Narrowing—or stenosis—can occur in any part of the intestine and cause varying degrees of intestinal obstruction. At first, the mucosa may appear normal, but as the disease progresses it takes on a "cobblestone" appearance as shown below.

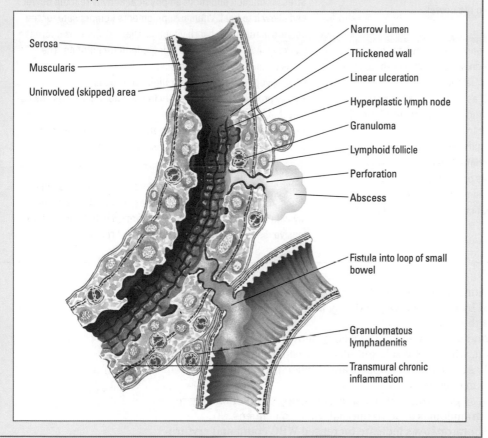

Serosa

Muscularis

Uninvolved (skipped) area

Narrow lumen

Thickened wall

Linear ulceration

Hyperplastic lymph node

Granuloma

Lymphoid follicle

Perforation

Abscess

Fistula into loop of small bowel

Granulomatous lymphadenitis

Transmural chronic inflammation

What tests tell you

These tests and results support a diagnosis of Crohn's disease:
- Fecal occult test shows minute amounts of blood in stools.
- Small-bowel X-ray shows irregular mucosa, ulceration, and stiffening.

Battling illness

Treating Crohn's disease

Treatment for Crohn's disease requires drug therapy, lifestyle changes and, sometimes, surgery. During acute attacks, maintaining fluid and electrolyte balance is the key. Debilitated patients need total parenteral nutrition to provide adequate calories and nutrition while resting the bowel.

Drug therapy
These drugs combat inflammation and relieve symptoms:
• Corticosteroids such as prednisone reduce diarrhea, pain, and bleeding by decreasing inflammation.
• Immunosuppressants, such as azathioprine (Imuran), methotrexate (Rheumatrex), and mercaptopurine (Purinethol), suppress the body's response to antigens.
• Aminosalicylates, such as sulfasalazine (Azulfidine) and mesalamine (Asacol), reduce inflammation.
• Metronidazole (Flagyl) treats perianal complications.
• Antidiarrheals, such as diphenoxylate and atropine, combat diarrhea but aren't used in patients with significant bowel obstruction.
• Opioids control pain and diarrhea.

• Antitumor necrosis factor agent infliximab treats moderate to severe disease that doesn't respond to conventional therapy.

Lifestyle changes
Stress reduction and reduced physical activity rest the bowel and allow it to heal. Vitamin supplements compensate for the bowel's inability to absorb vitamins. Dietary changes decrease bowel activity while still providing adequate nutrition. The foods usually eliminated include:
• fruits, vegetables, and other high-fiber foods
• dairy products, spicy and fatty foods, and other foods and liquids that irritate the mucosa
• carbonated or caffeinated beverages and other foods or liquids that stimulate excessive intestinal activity.

Surgery
Surgery is necessary if bowel perforation, massive hemorrhage, fistulas, or acute intestinal obstruction develop. Colectomy with ileostomy is commonly performed in patients with extensive disease of the large intestine and rectum.

• Barium enema reveals the string sign (segments of stricture separated by normal bowel) and may also show fissures and narrowing of the bowel.
• Sigmoidoscopy and colonoscopy show patchy areas of inflammation, which helps rule out ulcerative colitis. The mucosal surface has a cobblestone appearance. When the colon is involved, ulcers may be seen.
• Biopsy performed during sigmoidoscopy or colonoscopy reveals granulomas in up to one-half of all specimens.

Laboratory tests indicate increased WBC count and erythrocyte sedimentation rate (ESR). Other findings include decreased potassium, calcium, magnesium, and hemoglobin levels in the blood.

Diverticular disease

Diverticular disease is a common problem that affects men and women equally. The risk of disease increases with age. Diverticular disease occurs throughout the world but is more common in developed countries, in which the incidence has increased over time. This suggests that environmental and lifestyle factors may play a role in the development of the disease.

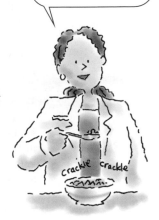

A low-fiber diet seems to be a contributing factor in the development of diverticular disease.

The highs and lows of dietary fiber

One contributing factor may be low intake of dietary fiber. High-fiber diets increase stool bulk, thereby decreasing the wall tension in the colon. High wall tension is thought to increase the risk of developing diverticula.

Diverticula domiciles

In diverticular disease, bulging pouches (diverticula) in the GI wall push the mucosal lining through the surrounding muscle. Although the most common site of diverticula is in the sigmoid colon, they may develop anywhere, from the proximal end of the pharynx to the anus. Other typical sites include the duodenum, near the pancreatic border or the ampulla of Vater, and the jejunum.

Diverticular disease has two clinical forms:
• diverticulosis, in which diverticula are present but don't cause symptoms
• diverticulitis, in which diverticula are inflamed and may cause potentially fatal obstruction, infection, or hemorrhage.

How it happens

Diverticula probably result from high intraluminal pressure on an area of weakness in the GI wall, where blood vessels enter. Diet may be a contributing factor because insufficient fiber reduces fecal residue, narrows the bowel lumen, and leads to high intra-abdominal pressure during defecation.

Diverticular sacs under attack

In diverticulitis, retained undigested food and bacteria accumulate in the diverticular sac. This hard mass cuts off the blood supply to the thin walls of the sac, making them more susceptible to attack by colonic bacteria. Inflammation follows and may lead to perforation, abscess, peritonitis, obstruction, or hemorrhage. Occasionally, the inflamed colon segment may adhere to the bladder or other organs and cause a fistula. (See *Diverticulitis of the colon*, page 188.)

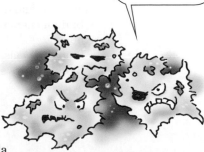

We can cause lots of trouble if we find some undigested food in a diverticular sac.

What to look for

Typically, the patient with diverticulosis is asymptomatic and will remain so unless diverticulitis develops.

Mild diverticulitis

In mild diverticulitis, signs and symptoms include:
• moderate left lower quadrant pain secondary to inflammation of diverticula
• low-grade fever and leukocytosis (from infection) due to trapping of bacteria-rich stool in the diverticula.

Severe diverticulitis

In severe diverticulitis, signs and symptoms include:
• abdominal rigidity from rupture of the diverticula, abscesses, and peritonitis
• left lower quadrant pain secondary to rupture of the diverticula and subsequent inflammation and infection
• high fever, chills, hypotension from sepsis, and shock from the release of fecal material from the rupture site
• microscopic or massive hemorrhage from rupture of diverticulum near a vessel.

Chronic diverticulitis

In chronic diverticulitis, signs and symptoms include:
• constipation, ribbonlike stools, intermittent diarrhea, and abdominal distention resulting from intestinal obstruction (possible when fibrosis and adhesions narrow the bowel's lumen)
• abdominal rigidity and pain, diminishing or absent bowel sounds, nausea, and vomiting secondary to intestinal obstruction. (See *Treating diverticular disease.*)

What tests tell you

These tests help to diagnose and confirm diverticular disease.
• Upper GI series confirms or rules out diverticulosis of the esophagus and upper bowel.
• Barium enema reveals filling of diverticula, which confirms diagnosis.
• Biopsy reveals evidence of benign disease, ruling out cancer.
• Blood studies show an elevated ESR in diverticulitis.

Now I get it!

Diverticulitis of the colon

In diverticulitis retained undigested food and bacteria accumulate in the diverticular sac as shown below.

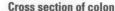

Cross section of colon

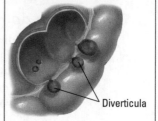

Diverticula

Battling illness

Treating diverticular disease

Treatment for diverticular disease may include:
• liquid or bland diet, stool softeners, and occasional doses of mineral oil to relieve symptoms, minimize irritation, and lessen the risk of progression to diverticulitis
• high-residue diet for treatment of diverticulosis after pain has subsided, to help decrease intra-abdominal pressure during defecation
• exercise, to increase the rate of stool passage
• antibiotics, to treat infection of the diverticula
• analgesics, such as morphine, to control pain and relax smooth muscle

• antispasmodics, to control muscle spasms
• colon resection with removal of involved segment, to correct cases refractory to medical treatment
• temporary colostomy, if necessary, to drain abscesses and rest the colon in diverticulitis accompanied by perforation, peritonitis, obstruction, or fistula
• blood transfusions, if necessary, to treat blood loss from hemorrhage
• fluid replacement as needed.

Gastroesophageal reflux disease

Popularly known as *heartburn*, GERD refers to backflow of gastric or duodenal contents or both into the esophagus and past the lower esophageal sphincter (LES), without associated belching or vomiting. The reflux of gastric contents causes acute epigastric pain, usually after a meal. The pain may radiate to the chest or arms.

Heartburn, yet healthy

Evidence indicates that up to 36% of otherwise healthy Americans experience heartburn at least once per month and about 7% experience heartburn at least once per day. It has been estimated that about 2% of the adult population suffers from GERD. The incidence of GERD increases markedly after age 40. It commonly occurs in pregnant or obese people.

Food or alcohol ingestion or cigarette smoking can lead to GERD.

How it happens

Various factors can lead to GERD, including:
• weakened esophageal sphincter
• increased abdominal pressure, such as with obesity or pregnancy
• hiatal hernia
• medications, such as morphine, diazepam, calcium channel blockers, meperidine, and anticholinergic agents
• food or alcohol ingestion or cigarette smoking that lowers LES pressure

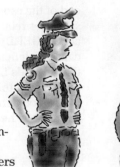
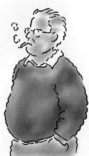

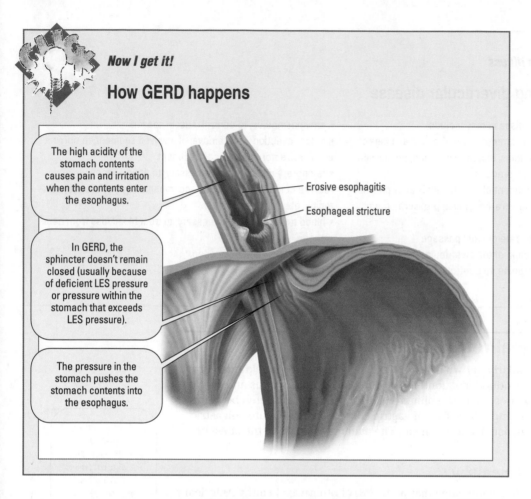

Now I get it!

How GERD happens

The high acidity of the stomach contents causes pain and irritation when the contents enter the esophagus.

In GERD, the sphincter doesn't remain closed (usually because of deficient LES pressure or pressure within the stomach that exceeds LES pressure).

The pressure in the stomach pushes the stomach contents into the esophagus.

Erosive esophagitis

Esophageal stricture

• nasogastric intubation for more than 4 days. (See *How GERD happens.*)

Less LES pressure means more reflux

Normally, the LES maintains enough pressure around the lower end of the esophagus to close it and prevent reflux. Typically the sphincter relaxes after each swallow to allow food into the stomach. In GERD, the sphincter doesn't remain closed (usually because of deficient LES pressure or pressure within the stomach that exceeds LES pressure), and the pressure in the stomach pushes the stomach contents into the esophagus. The high acidity of the stomach contents causes pain and irritation when the contents enter the esophagus.

What to look for

The patient with GERD typically complains of a burning pain in the epigastric area due to the reflux of gastric contents into the esophagus, which causes irritation and esophageal spasm. The pain may radiate to the arms and chest. Pain usually occurs after meals or when the patient lies down because both of these situations cause increased abdominal pressure that leads to reflux.

The patient may also complain of a feeling of fluid accumulating in the throat. The fluid doesn't have a sour or bitter taste because of the hypersecretion of saliva. (See *Treating GERD*.)

What tests tell you

Diagnostic tests are aimed at determining the underlying cause of GERD:
• Esophageal acidity test evaluates the competence of the LES and provides objective measure of reflux.
• Acid perfusion test confirms esophagitis and distinguishes it from cardiac disorders.
• Esophagoscopy allows visual examination of the lining of the esophagus to reveal the extent of the disease and confirm pathologic changes in mucosa.
• Barium swallow identifies hiatal hernia as the cause.
• Upper GI series detects hiatal hernia or motility problems.
• Esophageal manometry evaluates the resting pressure of LES and determines sphincter competence.

Memory jogger

Remember these facts about **GERD**:

Generally known as heartburn.

Epigastric pain and spasm usually follow a meal.

Radiating pain to arms and chest is common.

Diet therapy, antacids and smoking cessation can help alleviate symptoms.

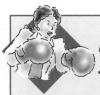

Battling illness

Treating GERD

Treatment of gastroesophageal reflux disease (GERD) is multifaceted and may include:
• diet therapy with frequent, small meals and avoidance of eating before going to bed, to reduce abdominal pressure and incidence of reflux
• positioning—sitting up during and after meals and sleeping with head of bed elevated—to reduce abdominal pressure and prevent reflux
• increased fluid intake, to wash gastric contents out of the esophagus

• antacids, to neutralize acidic content of the stomach and minimize irritation
• histamine-2 receptor antagonists, to inhibit gastric acid secretion
• proton pump inhibitors, to reduce gastric acidity
• cholinergic agents, to increase lower esophageal sphincter (LES) pressure
• smoking cessation, to improve LES pressure (nicotine lowers LES pressure)
• surgery if hiatal hernia is the cause or patient has refractory symptoms.

Hiatal hernia

Hiatal hernia occurs when a defect in the diaphragm permits a portion of the stomach to pass through the diaphragmatic opening (the esophageal hiatus) into the chest cavity. Some people remain asymptomatic whereas others experience reflux, heartburn, and chest pain. It occurs more commonly in women than men.

How it happens

Usually, hiatal hernia results from muscle weakening that's common with aging. It may also be secondary to esophageal cancer, kyphoscoliosis, trauma, and certain surgical procedures. It may also result from certain diaphragmatic malformations that may cause congenital weakness. (See *Stomach herniation.*)

Loosening the collar

In hiatal hernia, the muscular collar around the esophageal and diaphragmatic junction loosens, permitting the lower portion of the esophagus and the stomach to rise into the chest when intra-abdominal pressure increases (possibly causing esophageal reflux). Such increased intra-abdominal pressure may result from ascites, pregnancy, obesity, constrictive clothing, bending, straining, coughing, Valsalva's maneuver, or extreme physical exertion.

Two types of hiatal hernia can occur:
• sliding
• paraesophageal.

A third type may include features of both.

What to look for

Typically a paraesophageal hernia produces no symptoms; it's usually an incidental finding on barium swallow.

A sliding hernia without an incompetent sphincter produces no reflux or symptoms and, consequently, doesn't require treatment. When a sliding hernia does cause symptoms, they're typical of gastric reflux and may include:
• heartburn (pyrosis) occurring 1 to 4 hours after eating, aggravated by reclining and belching and may be accompanied by regurgitation or vomiting
• retrosternal or substernal chest pain, occurring usually after meals or at bedtime, aggravated by reclining, belching, and increased intra-abdominal pressure.

Other signs or symptoms that reflect possible complications include:
• dysphagia (difficulty swallowing)
• bleeding due to esophagitis

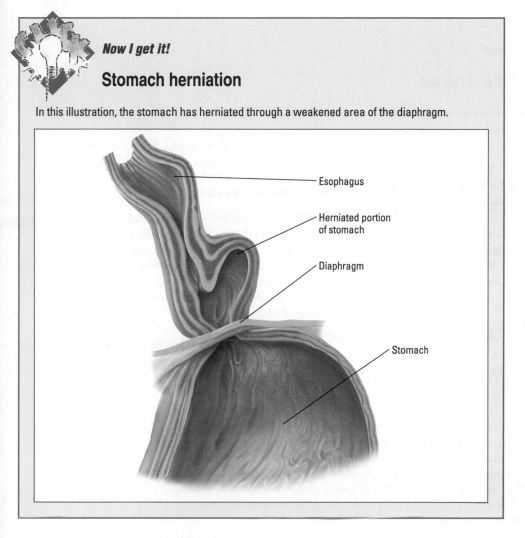

Now I get it!

Stomach herniation

In this illustration, the stomach has herniated through a weakened area of the diaphragm.

Esophagus

Herniated portion
of stomach

Diaphragm

Stomach

• severe pain and shock, which occurs when the hernia becomes strangulated. (See *Treating hiatal hernia*, page 194.)

What tests tell you

A diagnosis of hiatal hernia is based on typical clinical findings as well as the results of these laboratory studies and procedures:

• Chest X-rays occasionally show an air shadow behind the heart with a large hernia and infiltrates in the lower lobes, if the patient has aspirated.

• In a barium study, the hernia may appear as an outpouching that contains barium at the lower end of the esophagus. (Small hernias are difficult to recognize.) This study may also reveal abnormalities in the diaphragm.

Battling illness

Treating hiatal hernia

The primary goal of treatment for hiatal hernia is to relieve symptoms and to prevent or manage complications.

Drug therapy
Anticholinergic agents such as bethanechol are given to strengthen cardiac sphincter tone. Metoclopramide (Reglan) has been used to stimulate smooth-muscle contractions and decrease reflux.

Antiemetics may also be given, if vomiting is an exacerbating factor; antitussives and antidiarrheals may also be given where appropriate. Antacids are also prescribed to decrease the acidity of the gastric contents.

Noninvasive interventions
Activity that increases intra-abdominal pressure (coughing, straining, bending) should be restricted. The patient should be instructed to eat small, frequent, bland meals at least 2 hours before lying down. He should also be instructed to eat slowly and avoid spicy foods, fruit juices, alcoholic beverages, and coffee.

To reduce amount of reflux, the overweight patient should be encouraged to lose weight to help decrease intra-abdominal pressure. Elevating the head of the bed about 6" (15 cm) reduces gastric reflux by gravity.

Surgery
If symptoms can't be controlled medically, or complications, such as bleeding, stricture, pulmonary aspiration, strangulation, or incarceration (constriction) occur, surgical repair is needed. The procedure involves creating an artificial closing mechanism at the gastroesophageal junction to strengthen the function of the esophageal hiatus. A transabdominal fundoplication is performed by wrapping the fundus of the stomach around the lower esophagus to prevent reflux of stomach contents. Although an abdominal or thoracic approach may be used, hiatal hernia is typically repaired via laparoscopy.

- Endoscopy and biopsy differentiate between hiatal hernia, varices, and other small gastroesophageal lesions.
- Esophageal motility studies assess the presence of esophageal motor abnormalities before surgical repair of the hernia.
- pH studies assess for reflux of gastric contents.
- An acid perfusion test indicates that heartburn results from esophageal reflux.

Irritable bowel syndrome

Irritable bowel syndrome is characterized by chronic symptoms of abdominal pain, alternating constipation and diarrhea, and abdominal distention. This disorder is common, although about 20% of patients never seek medical attention. It is twice as common in women as in men.

Is stress to blame?

Irritable bowel syndrome is generally associated with psychological stress; however, it may result from physical factors, such as diverticular disease, ingestion of irritants (coffee, raw vegetables, or fruits), abuse of laxatives, food poisoning, and colon cancer.

How it happens

Typically the patient with irritable bowel syndrome has a normal-appearing GI tract. However, careful examination of the colon may reveal functional irritability—an abnormality in colonic smooth-muscle function marked by excessive peristalsis and spasms, even during remission.

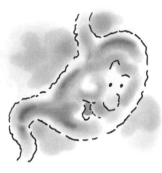

I may appear normal in a patient with irritable bowel syndrome, but you'll soon see I have some problems!

Contract, then relax, contract, then relax...

To understand what happens in irritable bowel syndrome, consider how smooth muscle controls bowel function. Normally, segmental muscle contractions mix intestinal contents while peristalsis propels the contents through the GI tract. Motor activity is most propulsive in the proximal (stomach) and the distal (sigmoid) portions of the intestine. Activity in the rest of the intestines is slower, permitting nutrient and water absorption.

In irritable bowel syndrome, the autonomic nervous system, which innervates the large intestine, doesn't cause the alternating contractions and relaxations that propel stools smoothly toward the rectum. The result is constipation or diarrhea, or both. (See *Effects of irritable bowel syndrome*, page 196.)

A disturbing pattern

Some patients have spasmodic intestinal contractions that set up a partial obstruction by trapping gas and stools. This causes distention, bloating, gas pain, and constipation.

Other patients have dramatically increased intestinal motility. Usually eating or cholinergic stimulation triggers the small intestine's contents to rush into the large intestine, dumping watery stools and irritating the mucosa. The result is diarrhea.

If further spasms trap liquid stools, the intestinal mucosa adsorbs water from the stools, leaving them dry, hard, and difficult to pass. The result is a pattern of alternating diarrhea and constipation.

What to look for

The most commonly reported symptom is intermittent, crampy, lower abdominal pain, usually relieved by defecation or passage of flatus. It usually occurs during the day, and intensifies with stress or 1 to 2 hours after meals. The patient may experience constipation alternating with diarrhea, with one being the dominant problem. Mucus is usually passed through the rectum. Abdominal distention and bloating are common. (See *Treating irritable bowel syndrome*, page 196.)

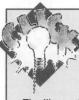

Now I get it!

Effects of irritable bowel syndrome

The illustration below shows partial obstructions in the bowel caused by IBS.

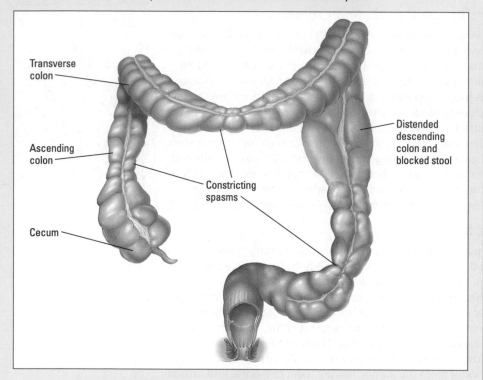

Transverse colon

Ascending colon

Cecum

Constricting spasms

Distended descending colon and blocked stool

Battling illness

Treating irritable bowel syndrome

Treatment for irritable bowel syndrome aims to relieve symptoms.

Medical therapy

Therapy aims to relieve symptoms and includes counseling to help the patient understand the relation between stress and his illness. Dietary restrictions haven't proven to be effective, but the patient is encouraged to be aware of foods that exacerbate symptoms. Rest and heat applied to the abdomen are usually helpful.

In the case of laxative overuse, bowel training is sometimes recommended.

Drug therapy

Antispasmodics, such as diphenoxylate with atropine, are commonly prescribed. A mild barbiturate such as phenobarbital in judicious doses is sometimes helpful as well.

What tests tell you

There are no tests that are specific for diagnosing irritable bowel syndrome. Other disorders, such as diverticulitis, colon cancer, and lactose intolerance, should be ruled out by these tests:
• Stool samples for ova, parasites, bacteria, and blood rule out infection.
• Lactose intolerance test rules out lactose intolerance.
• Barium enema may reveal colon spasm and tubular appearance of descending colon without evidence of cancers and diverticulosis.
• Sigmoidoscopy or colonoscopy may reveal spastic contractions without evidence of colon cancer or inflammatory bowel disease.
• Rectal biopsy rules out malignancy.

Pancreatitis

Pancreatitis is an inflammation of the pancreas. It occurs in acute and chronic forms. In men, the disorder is commonly linked to alcoholism, trauma, or peptic ulcer; in women, to biliary tract disease.

Don't drink and...

The prognosis is good when pancreatitis follows biliary tract disease but poor when it's a complication of alcoholism. Mortality reaches 60% when pancreatitis causes tissue destruction or hemorrhage.

How it happens

The most common causes of pancreatitis are biliary tract disease and alcoholism, but it can also result from:
• abnormal organ structure
• metabolic or endocrine disorders, such as high cholesterol levels or overactive thyroid
• pancreatic cysts or tumors
• penetrating peptic ulcers
• blunt trauma or surgical trauma
• drugs, such as glucocorticoids, sulfonamides, thiazides, and hormonal contraceptives
• kidney failure or transplantation
• endoscopic examination of the bile ducts and pancreas.
    In addition, heredity may predispose a patient to pancreatitis. In some patients, emotional or neurogenic factors play a part.

A permanent change for the pancreas

Chronic pancreatitis is a persistent inflammation that produces irreversible changes in the structure and function of the pancreas. It sometimes follows an episode of acute pancreatitis. Here's what probably happens:
• Protein precipitates block the pancreatic duct and eventually harden or calcify.
• Structural changes lead to fibrosis and atrophy of the glands.
• Growths called *pseudocysts*, containing pancreatic enzymes and tissue debris, form.
• An abscess results if these growths become infected.

Acting prematurely

Acute pancreatitis occurs in two forms:
• edematous (interstitial), causing fluid accumulation and swelling

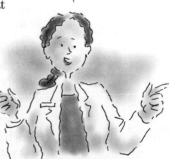

In pancreatitis, the pancreas harms itself.

Now I get it!

Necrotizing pancreatitis

Acute pancreatitis can occur as necrotizing pancreatitis when there is cell death and tissue damage.

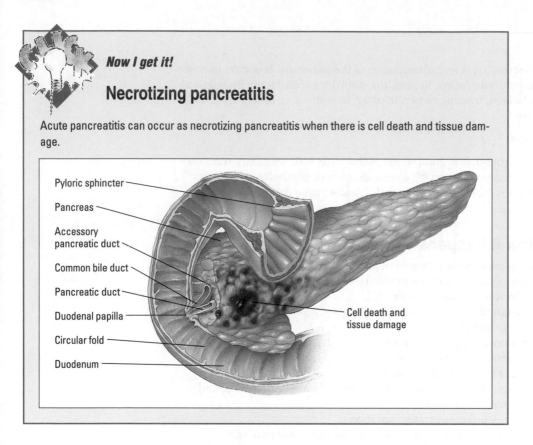

- Pyloric sphincter
- Pancreas
- Accessory pancreatic duct
- Common bile duct
- Pancreatic duct
- Duodenal papilla
- Circular fold
- Duodenum
- Cell death and tissue damage

- necrotizing, causing cell death and tissue damage. (See *Necrotizing pancreatitis*.)

The inflammation that occurs with both types is caused by premature activation of enzymes, which causes tissue damage. Normally, the acini in the pancreas secrete enzymes in an inactive form.

Two theories explain why enzymes become prematurely activated:

A toxic agent, such as alcohol, alters the way the pancreas secretes enzymes. Alcohol probably increases pancreatic secretion, alters the metabolism of the acinar cells, and encourages duct obstruction by causing pancreatic secretory proteins to precipitate.

A reflux of duodenal contents containing activated enzymes enters the pancreatic duct, activating other enzymes and setting up a cycle of more pancreatic damage.

Pain!!! Why? Why?

Pain can be caused by several factors, including:

- escape of inflammatory exudate and enzymes into the back of the peritoneum
- edema and distention of the pancreatic capsule
- obstruction of the biliary tract.

Getting complicated

If pancreatitis damages the islets of Langerhans, diabetes mellitus may result. Sudden, severe pancreatitis causes massive hemorrhage and total destruction of the pancreas. This may lead to diabetic acidosis, shock, or coma.

> Pancreatitis may start with a stomachache and progress to swelling, tissue damage, or bleeding.

What to look for

In many patients, the only symptom of mild pancreatitis is steady epigastric pain centered close to the navel and unrelieved by vomiting.

Acute pancreatitis causes severe, persistent, piercing abdominal pain, usually in the midepigastric region, although it may be generalized or occur in the left upper quadrant radiating to the back.

Eat, drink, and be...in pain

The pain usually begins suddenly after eating a large meal or drinking alcohol. It increases when the patient lies on his back and is relieved when he rests on his knees and upper chest. (See *Treating pancreatitis,* page 200.)

What tests tell you

These tests are used to diagnose pancreatitis:
- Dramatically elevated serum amylase and lipase levels confirm acute pancreatitis. Dramatically elevated amylase levels are also found in urine, ascites, and pleural fluid.
- Blood and urine glucose tests may reveal transient glucose in urine (glycosuria) and hyperglycemia. In chronic pancreatitis, serum glucose levels may be transiently elevated.
- WBC count is elevated.
- Serum bilirubin levels are elevated in both acute and chronic pancreatitis.
- Blood calcium levels may be decreased.
- Stool analysis shows elevated lipid and trypsin levels in chronic pancreatitis.
- Abdominal and chest X-rays detect pleural effusions and differentiate pancreatitis from diseases that cause similar symptoms.
- CT scan and ultrasonography show an enlarged pancreas and pancreatic cysts and pseudocysts.

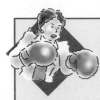

Battling illness

Treating pancreatitis

The goals of treatment for pancreatitis are to maintain circulation and fluid volume, relieve pain, and decrease pancreatic secretions.

Acute pancreatitis
For acute cases, treatment includes the following:
• Shock is the most common cause of death in the early stages, so I.V. replacement of electrolytes and proteins is necessary.
• Metabolic acidosis requires fluid volume replacement.
• Blood transfusions may be needed.
• Food and fluids are withheld to allow the pancreas to rest and to reduce pancreatic enzyme secretion.
• Nasogastric tube suctioning decreases stomach distention and suppresses pancreatic secretions.
• Positioning the patient for comfort in the knee-to-chest position has been helpful in reducing pain.

Drug therapy
Drugs administered for acute pancreatitis include:
• analgesics, such as meperidine (Demerol) to relieve abdominal pain. Demerol is the pain medication of choice for pancreatitis.)
• antacids to neutralize gastric secretions
• histamine antagonists, such as cimetidine (Tagamet), famotidine (Pepcid), or ranitidine (Zantac), to decrease hydrochloric acid production

• antibiotics, such as clindamycin (Cleocin) or gentamicin, to fight bacterial infections
• anticholinergics to reduce vagal stimulation, decrease GI motility, and inhibit pancreatic enzyme secretion
• insulin to correct hyperglycemia.

Surgery
Surgical drainage is necessary for a pancreatic abscess or a pseudocyst. A laparotomy may be needed if biliary tract obstruction causes acute pancreatitis.

Chronic pancreatitis
Pain control measures are similar to those for acute pancreatitis:
• Morphine is the drug of choice.
• Some patients require only over-the-counter pain medications.
• Tricyclic antidepressants may be effective in low doses; they suppress the nervous system's reaction to inflammation.

Other treatment depends on the cause. Surgery relieves abdominal pain, restores pancreatic drainage, and reduces the frequency of attacks. Patients with an abscess or pseudocyst, biliary tract disease, or a fibrotic pancreatic sphincter may undergo surgery. Surgery may also help relieve obstruction and allow drainage of pancreatic secretions.

• Endoscopic retrograde cholangiopancreatography shows the anatomy of the pancreas; identifies ductal system abnormalities, such as calcification or strictures; and differentiates pancreatitis from other disorders such as pancreatic cancer.

Peptic ulcer

A peptic ulcer is a circumscribed lesion in the mucosal membrane of the upper GI tract. Peptic ulcers can develop in the lower esophagus, stomach, duodenum, or jejunum. (See *Common ulcer types and sites.*)

Now I get it!

Common ulcer types and sites

This illustration shows common ulcer types and common sites where they can occur. The illustration also shows how an ulcer can penetrate into and through the muscle layers and muscle wall.

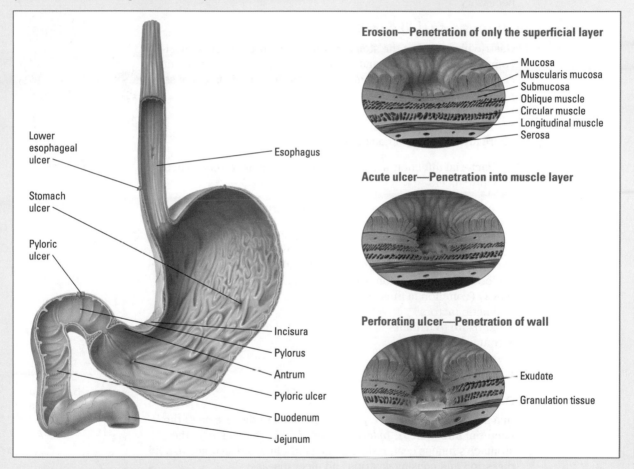

How it happens

The two major forms of peptic ulcer are:
- duodenal
- gastric.

Both of these forms of peptic ulcer are chronic conditions.

Upsetting the upper part

More than 25 million U.S. residents will suffer from an ulcer at some time in their life. Duodenal ulcers affect the upper part of the small intestine. This type of ulcer accounts for about 80% of peptic ulcers, occurs mostly in men between ages 20 and 50, and follows a chronic course of remissions and exacerbations. About 5% to 10% of patients develop complications that make surgery necessary.

> Easy does it. Chronic use of aspirin or alcohol may cause gastric ulcers.

Making the mucosa feel like murder

Gastric ulcers affect the stomach lining (mucosa). They're most common in middle-aged and elderly men, especially poor and undernourished men. They commonly occur in chronic users of aspirin or alcohol.

Peptic promoters

There are three major causes of peptic ulcers:

  bacterial infection with *Helicobacter pylori* is the cause of 90% of peptic ulcers

  use of nonsteroidal anti-inflammatory drugs

  hypersecretory states such as Zollinger-Ellison syndrome.
    Researchers are still discovering the exact mechanisms of ulcer formation. Predisposing factors include:
• blood type A (common in people with gastric ulcers) and blood type O (common in those with duodenal ulcers)
• genetic factors
• exposure to irritants
• trauma
• stress and anxiety
• normal aging.

Aiding and abetting bacterial infection

In a peptic ulcer due to *H. pylori*, acid adds to the effects of the bacterial infection. *H. pylori* releases a toxin that destroys the stomach's mucus coat, reducing the epithelium's resistance to acid digestion and causing gastritis and ulcer disease.

> Bacteria are another major cause of gastric ulcers.

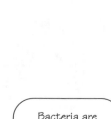

Getting complicated

A possible complication of severe ulceration is erosion of the mucosa. This can cause GI hemorrhage, which can progress to hypovolemic shock, perforation, and obstruction. Obstruction of the pylorus may cause the stomach to distend with food and fluid, block blood flow, and cause tissue damage.

Don't fence me in

The ulcer crater may extend beyond the duodenal wall into nearby structures, such as the pancreas or liver. This phenomenon is called *penetration* and is a fairly common complication of duodenal ulcer.

What to look for

The patient with a gastric ulcer may report:
• recent loss of weight or appetite
• pain, heartburn, or indigestion
• a feeling of abdominal fullness or distention
• pain triggered or aggravated by eating.

The dynamic (if painful) duodenal ulcer

The patient with a duodenal ulcer may describe the pain as sharp, gnawing, burning, boring, aching, or hard to define. He may liken it to hunger, abdominal pressure, or fullness. Typically, pain occurs 90 minutes to 3 hours after eating. However, eating usually reduces the pain, so the patient may report a recent weight gain. The patient may also have pale skin from anemia caused by blood loss. (See *Treating peptic ulcer.*)

What tests tell you

These tests are used to diagnose peptic ulcer:
• Upper GI endoscopy or esophagogastroduodenoscopy confirms an ulcer and permits cytologic studies and biopsy to rule out *H. pylori* or cancer. Endoscopy is the major diagnostic test for peptic ulcers.
• Barium swallow and upper GI or small-bowel series may pinpoint the ulcer in a patient whose symptoms aren't severe.
• Upper GI tract X-ray reveals mucosal abnormalities.
• Stool analysis may detect occult blood in stools.
• WBC count is elevated; other blood tests may also disclose clinical signs of infection.
• Gastric secretory studies show excess hydrochloric acid (hyperchlorhydria).
• Carbon-13 urea breath test reflects activity of *H. pylori*.

Ulcerative colitis

This inflammatory disease causes ulcerations of the mucosa in the colon. It commonly occurs as a chronic condition.

As many as 1 out of 1,000 people may have ulcerative colitis. Peak occurrence is between ages 15 and 30 and between ages 50

Battling illness

Treating peptic ulcer

Drug therapy
Drug therapy for *Helicobacter pylori* infection consists of 1 to 2 weeks of antibiotic therapy using amoxicillin (Amoxil), tetracycline (Sumycin), metronidazole (Flagyl), or clarithromycin (Biaxin). Antibiotics should be used in combination with ranitidine bismuth citrate, bismuth subsalicylate, or a proton pump inhibitor.

According to the Centers for Disease Control and Prevention, duodenal and gastric ulcers recur in up to 80% of patients who receive medications that reduce gastric acid but don't receive antibiotics. In those treated with antibiotics, the recurrence rate is 6%.

More drastic measures
Gastroscopy allows visualization of the bleeding site and coagulation by laser or cautery to control bleeding.

Surgery is indicated if the patient doesn't respond to other treatment or has a perforation, suspected cancer, or other complications.

and 70. The incidence of ulcerative colitis is equal among men and women.

How it happens

Although the cause of ulcerative colitis is unknown, it may be related to an abnormal immune response in the GI tract, possibly associated with genetic factors. Lymphocytes (T cells) in people with ulcerative colitis may have cytotoxic effects on the epithelial cells of the colon.

Stress doesn't cause the disorder, but it can increase the severity of an attack. Although no specific organism has been linked to ulcerative colitis, infection hasn't been ruled out.

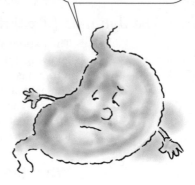

Ulcerative colitis affects the lining of the large intestine. That can't be good!

Surveying the damage

Ulcerative colitis damages the large intestine's mucosal and submucosal layers. Here's how it progresses:
• Usually, the disease originates in the rectum and lower colon and eventually spreads to the entire colon.
• The mucosa develops diffuse ulceration, with hemorrhage, congestion, edema, and exudative inflammation. Unlike Crohn's disease, ulcerations are continuous.
• Abscesses formed in the mucosa drain purulent pus, become necrotic, and ulcerate.
• Sloughing occurs, causing bloody, mucus-filled stools.

Looking closer at the colon

As ulcerative colitis progresses, the colon undergoes changes described below:
• Initially, the colon's mucosal surface becomes dark, red, and velvety.
• Abscesses form and coalesce into ulcers.
• Necrosis of the mucosa occurs.
• As abscesses heal, scarring and thickening may appear in the bowel's inner muscle layer.
• As granulation tissue replaces the muscle layer, the colon narrows, shortens, and loses its characteristic pouches (haustral folds). (See *Mucosal changes in ulcerative colitis.*)

Getting complicated

Progression of ulcerative colitis may lead to intestinal obstruction, dehydration, and major fluid and electrolyte imbalances. Malabsorption is common, and chronic anemia may result from loss of blood in the stools.

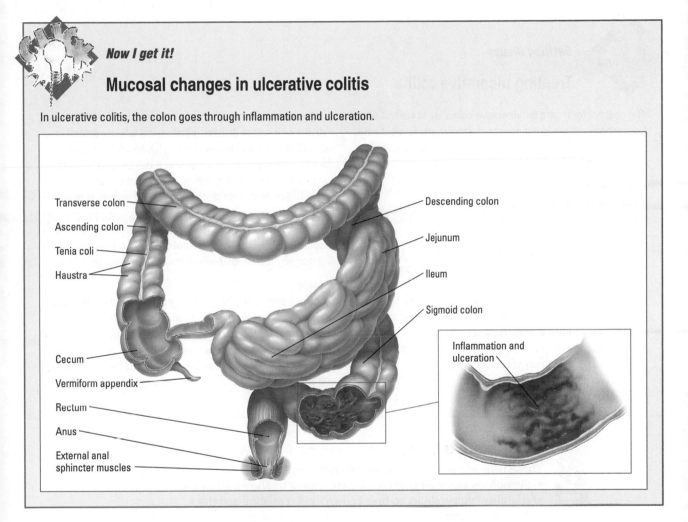

Now I get it!

Mucosal changes in ulcerative colitis

In ulcerative colitis, the colon goes through inflammation and ulceration.

Transverse colon

Ascending colon

Tenia coli

Haustra

Cecum

Vermiform appendix

Rectum

Anus

External anal
sphincter muscles

Descending colon

Jejunum

Ileum

Sigmoid colon

Inflammation and
ulceration

What to look for

The hallmark of ulcerative colitis is recurrent bloody diarrhea—usually containing pus and mucus—alternating with symptom-free remissions. Accumulation of blood and mucus in the bowel causes cramping abdominal pain, rectal urgency, and diarrhea.

Other symptoms include:

- irritability
- weight loss
- weakness
- anorexia
- nausea
- vomiting. (See *Treating ulcerative colitis*, page 206.)

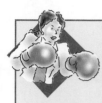

Battling illness

Treating ulcerative colitis

The goals of treatment for ulcerative colitis are to control inflammation, replace lost nutrients and blood, and prevent complications. Supportive measures include bed rest, I.V. fluid replacement, and blood transfusions.

Drug therapy
Medications include:
• corticosteroids, such as prednisone and hydrocortisone, to control inflammation
• aminosalicylates, such as sulfasalazine (Azulfidine), mesalamine (Asacol), and balsalazide (Colazal), to help control inflammation
• antidiarrheals, such as diphenoxylate and atropine, for patients with frequent, troublesome diarrhea and whose ulcerative colitis is otherwise under control
• immunomodulators, such as 6-mercaptopurine (Purinethol) and azathioprine (Imuran), to reduce inflammation by acting on the immune system
• iron supplements to correct anemia.

Diet therapy
Patients with severe disease usually need total parenteral nutrition (TPN) and are allowed nothing by mouth. TPN is also used for patients awaiting surgery or those dehydrated or debilitated from excessive diarrhea. This treatment rests the intestinal tract, decreases stool volume, and restores nitrogen balance.

Patients with moderate signs and symptoms may receive supplemental drinks and elemental feedings. A low-residue diet may be ordered for the patient with mild disease.

Surgery
Surgery is performed if the patient has massive dilation of the colon (toxic megacolon), if he doesn't respond to drugs and supportive measures, or if he finds the symptoms unbearable.

The most common surgical technique is proctocolectomy with ileostomy, although pouch ileostomy and ileoanal reservoir are also done.

What tests tell you

These tests are used to diagnose ulcerative colitis:
• Sigmoidoscopy confirms rectal involvement by showing mucosal friability (vulnerability to breakdown) and flattening and thick, inflammatory exudate.
• Colonoscopy shows the extent of the disease, strictured areas, and pseudopolyps. It isn't performed when the patient has active signs and symptoms.
• Biopsy during colonoscopy can help confirm the diagnosis.
• Barium enema is used to show the extent of the disease, detect complications, and identify cancer. It isn't performed in a patient with active signs and symptoms.
• Stool specimen analysis reveals blood, pus, and mucus but no disease-causing organisms.
• Other laboratory tests show decreased serum potassium, magnesium, and albumin levels; decreased WBC count; decreased hemoglobin levels; and prolonged PT. Increase of the ESR correlates with the severity of the attack.

Viral hepatitis

Viral hepatitis is a common infection of the liver. In most patients, damaged liver cells eventually regenerate with little or no permanent damage. However, old age and serious underlying disorders make complications more likely. More than 70,000 cases are reported annually in the United States.

How it happens

Viral hepatitis is marked by liver cell destruction, tissue death (necrosis), and self-destruction of cells (autolysis). It leads to anorexia, jaundice, and hepatomegaly.

The ABCs of viral hepatitis...

Five types of viral hepatitis are recognized, each caused by a different virus:

Type A is transmitted almost exclusively by the fecal-oral route, and outbreaks are common in areas of overcrowding and poor sanitation. Day-care centers and other institutional settings are common sources of outbreaks. The incidence is also increasing among homosexuals and in people with human immunodeficiency virus (HIV) infection.

Type B, also increasing among HIV-positive people, accounts for 5% to 10% of posttransfusion hepatitis cases in the United States. Vaccinations are available and are now required for health care workers and school children in many states.

Type C accounts for about 20% of all viral hepatitis as well as most cases that follow transfusion.

Type D, in the United States, is confined to people frequently exposed to blood and blood products, such as I.V. drug users and hemophiliacs.

Type E was formerly grouped with type C under the name non-A, non-B hepatitis. In the United States, this type mainly occurs in people who have visited an endemic area, such as India, Africa, Asia, or Central America.

The five major forms of viral hepatitis result from infection with the causative viruses A, B, C, D, or E. (See *Viral hepatitis from A to E*, page 208.)

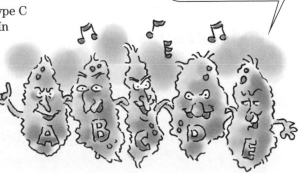

Now you know your ABCs and also how we cause disease.

Viral hepatitis from A to E

The following chart compares the features of each type of viral hepatitis.

Feature	Hepatitis A	Hepatitis B	Hepatitis C	Hepatitis D	Hepatitis E
Incubation	15 to 45 days	30 to 180 days	15 to 160 days	14 to 64 days	14 to 60 days
Onset	Acute	Insidious	Insidious	Acute	Acute
Age-group most affected	Children, young adults	Any age	More common in adults	Any age	Ages 20 to 40
Transmission	Fecal-oral, sexual (especially oral-anal contact), nonpercutaneous (sexual, maternal-neonatal), percutaneous (rare)	Blood-borne; parenteral route, sexual, maternal-neonatal; virus is shed in all body fluids	Blood-borne; parenteral route	Parenteral route; most people infected with hepatitis D are also infected with hepatitis B	Primarily fecal-oral
Severity	Mild	Usually severe	Moderate	Can be severe and lead to fulminant hepatitis	Highly virulent with common progression to fulminant hepatitis and hepatic failure, especially in pregnant patients
Prognosis	Generally good	Worsens with age and debility	Moderate	Fair; worsens in chronic cases; can lead to chronic hepatitis D and chronic liver disease	Good unless pregnant
Progression to chronicity	None	Occasional	10% to 50% of cases	Occasional	None

The result is the same

Despite the different causes, changes to the liver are usually similar in each type of viral hepatitis. Varying degrees of liver cell injury and necrosis occur. These changes in the liver are completely reversible when the acute phase of the disease subsides.

Usually, my cells grow back with little residual damage but old age and other disorders may complicate things.

Getting complicated

A fairly common complication is chronic persistent hepatitis, which prolongs recovery up to 8 months. Some patients also suffer relapses. A few may develop chronic active hepatitis, which destroys part of the liver and causes cirrhosis. In rare cases, severe and sudden (fulminant) hepatic failure and death may result from massive tissue loss. Primary hepatocellular carcinoma is a late complication that can cause death within 5 years, but it's rare in the United States.

What to look for

Signs and symptoms of viral hepatitis progress in three stages:

 prodromal

 clinical

 recovery.

Prodromal stage

In the prodromal stage, the following signs and symptoms may be caused by circulating immune complexes: fatigue, anorexia, mild weight loss, generalized malaise, depression, headache, weakness, joint pain (arthralgia), muscle pain (myalgia), intolerance of light (photophobia), nausea and vomiting, changes in the senses of taste and smell, temperature of 100° to 102° F (37.8° to 38.9° C), right upper quadrant tenderness, and dark-colored urine and clay-colored stools (1 to 5 days before the onset of the clinical jaundice stage).

During this phase, the infection is highly transmissible.

Clinical stage

Also called the *icteric stage*, the clinical stage begins 1 to 2 weeks after the prodromal stage. It's the phase of actual illness.

If the patient progresses to this stage, he may have these signs and symptoms: itching, abdominal pain or tenderness, indigestion, appetite loss (in early clinical stage), and jaundice.

Jaundice lasts for 1 to 2 weeks and indicates that the damaged liver can't remove bilirubin from the blood. However, jaundice doesn't indicate disease severity and, occasionally, hepatitis occurs without jaundice.

Recovery stage

Recovery begins with the resolution of jaundice and lasts 2 to 6 weeks in uncomplicated cases. The prognosis is poor if edema and hepatic encephalopathy develop. (See *Treating viral hepatitis.*)

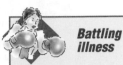

Battling illness

Treating viral hepatitis

Hepatitis C has been treated somewhat successfully with interferon alfa. No specific drug therapy has been developed for other types of viral hepatitis. Instead, the patient is advised to rest in the early stages of the illness and combat anorexia by eating small, high-calorie, high-protein meals.

Protein intake should be reduced if signs of precoma—lethargy, confusion, or mental changes—develop. Large meals are usually better tolerated in the morning because many patients have nausea late in the day.

Acute cases

In acute viral hepatitis, hospitalization is usually required only if severe symptoms or complications occur. Parenteral nutrition may be needed if the patient can't eat because of persistent vomiting.

What tests tell you

These tests are used to diagnose viral hepatitis:
- Hepatitis profile establishes the type of hepatitis.
- Liver function studies show disease stage.
- PT is prolonged.
- WBC count is elevated.
- Liver biopsy may be performed if chronic hepatitis is suspected.

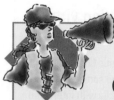

That's a wrap!

Gastrointestinal system review

Understanding the gastrointestinal system

The body's food processing complex supplies essential nutrients that fuel other organs and body systems. The gastrointestinal system's two major components are the:
- GI tract
- accessory glands and organs.

GI tract

Beginning in the mouth and ending at the anus, the GI tract includes the:
- mouth—where chewing and salivation occur to make food soft and easy to swallow
- esophagus—where food enters by peristaltic waves that are activated by the glossopharyngeal nerves
- stomach—where digestion occurs in two phases:
  - the cephalic phase
  - the gastric phase
- small intestine—where digestion takes place in three major sections:
  - the duodenum
  - the jejunum
  - the ileum
- large intestine—where absorption takes place and mostly indigestible material passes through the transverse colon, and then down through the descending colon to the rectum and is expelled through the anal canal.

Accessory glands and organs

Enzymes, bile, and hormones, which are vital to digestion, are produced by the:
- liver—filters and detoxifies blood, removes naturally occurring ammonia from body fluids, produces plasma proteins, stores essential nutrients, produces bile, converts glucose, and stores fat.
- gallbladder—stores and concentrates bile.
- pancreas—secretes more than 1,000 ml of digestive enzymes daily; houses alpha cells, which stimulate glucose formation in the liver, and beta cells, which secrete insulin to promote carbohydrate metabolism.

Digestive disorders

- *Appendicitis*—inflammation of the vermiform appendix
- *Cholecystitis*—inflammation of the gallbladder
- *Cirrhosis*—widespread destruction of hepatic cells in the liver
- *Crohn's disease*—inflammation of any part of the GI tract
- *Diverticular disease*—bulging outpouches in the GI wall push the mucosal lining through surrounding muscle
- *GERD*—backflow of gastric or duodenal contents (or both) into the esophagus and past the lower esophageal sphincter
- *Hiatal hernia*—defect in the diaphragm that permits a portion of the stomach to pass through the diaphragmatic opening into the chest cavity
- *Irritable bowel syndrome*—characterized by chronic symptoms of abdominal pain, alternating constipation and diarrhea, and abdominal distention
- *Pancreatitis*—inflammation of the pancreas; two forms:
  - chronic pancreatitis (persistent inflammation)
  - acute pancreatitis (inflammation causes tissue damage)
- *Peptic ulcer*—circumscribed lesion in the mucosal membrane of the upper GI tract
- *Ulcerative colitis*—inflammation of the mucosa in the colon that causes ulcerations
- *Viral hepatitis*—infection of the liver

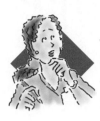

Quick quiz

1. Bleeding from esophageal varices usually stems from:
   A. esophageal perforation.
   B. pulmonary hypertension.
   C. portal hypertension.
   D. systemic hypertension.

Answer: C. Increased pressure within the portal veins causes them to bulge, leading to rupture and bleeding.

2. What are the two phases of digestion?
   A. Gastric and colonic
   B. Salivation and secretion
   C. Esophageal and abdominal
   D. Cephalic and gastric

Answer: D. The cephalic phase begins when the food is on its way to the stomach. Food entering the stomach initiates the gastric phase.

3. Which of the following is usually the initial event in appendicitis?
   A. Lymph node enlargement
   B. Obstruction of the appendiceal lumen
   C. Ulceration of the mucosa
   D. Perforation of the appendix

Answer: C. Although an obstruction can be identified in some cases, ulceration of the mucosa usually occurs first.

4. In women, pancreatitis is usually associated with:
   A. biliary tract disease.
   B. alcoholism.
   C. allergies.
   D. diabetes mellitus.

Answer: A. Biliary tract disease is a leading cause of pancreatitis in women. In men, the leading causes are trauma and peptic ulcer.

Scoring

☆☆☆   If you answered all four items correctly, excellent! When it comes to understanding the GI system, you're on the right tract.

☆☆   If you answered three items correctly, relax and enjoy! Your performance on this test isn't difficult to digest.

☆   If you answered fewer than three items correctly, don't worry. Take your chyme and you'll absorb all the important facts.

6

Musculoskeletal system

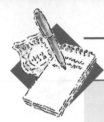

Just the facts

In this chapter, you'll learn:

♦ the function of the musculoskeletal system

♦ essential concepts about bone formation, growth, and re-newal

♦ pathophysiology, diagnostic tests, and treatments for certain musculoskeletal disorders.

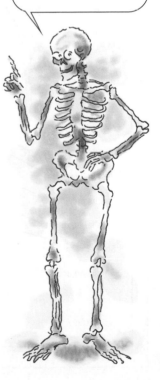

I give the body its shape and ability to move. Let's put on the muscle and go!

Understanding the musculoskeletal system

The structures of the musculoskeletal system work together to provide support and produce movement. This system includes:
• muscles
• bones
• cartilage
• joints, bursae, tendons, and ligaments.

Muscles

There are three major muscle types:

 skeletal (voluntary, striated muscles)

 smooth (involuntary muscles)

 cardiac (involuntary, striated muscles).

A skeletal sketch

This chapter focuses on skeletal muscle, which is attached to bone. Skeletal muscle cells are arranged in long bands or strips, called *striations*. Skeletal muscle is *voluntary*, meaning it can be contracted at will. (See *A close look at skeletal muscles*, page 214, and *Muscle structure*, page 215.)

A close look at skeletal muscles

The human body has about 600 skeletal muscles. Each muscle is classified by the kind of movement for which it's responsible. For example, flexors permit the bending of joints, or flexion. Extensors permit straightening of joints, or extension. These illustrations show some of the major muscles.

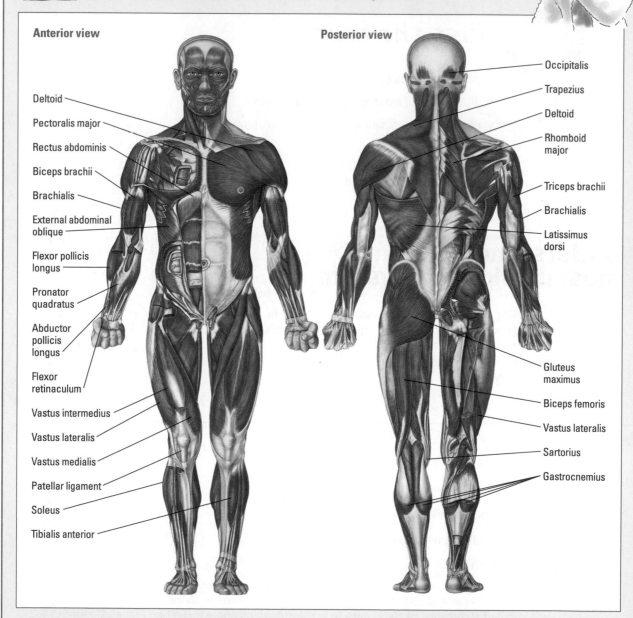

Anterior view

- Deltoid
- Pectoralis major
- Rectus abdominis
- Biceps brachii
- Brachialis
- External abdominal oblique
- Flexor pollicis longus
- Pronator quadratus
- Abductor pollicis longus
- Flexor retinaculum
- Vastus intermedius
- Vastus lateralis
- Vastus medialis
- Patellar ligament
- Soleus
- Tibialis anterior

Posterior view

- Occipitalis
- Trapezius
- Deltoid
- Rhomboid major
- Triceps brachii
- Brachialis
- Latissimus dorsi
- Gluteus maximus
- Biceps femoris
- Vastus lateralis
- Sartorius
- Gastrocnemius

Muscle structure

Each muscle contains cells called *muscle fibers* that extend the length of the muscle. A sheath of connective tissues—called the *perimysium*—binds the fibers into a bundle, or fasciculus. A stronger sheath, the *epimysium*, binds fasciculi together to form the fleshy part of the muscle. Extending beyond the muscle, the epimysium becomes a tendon.

Each muscle fiber is surrounded by a plasma membrane, the sarcolemma. Within the sarcoplasm (or cytoplasm) of the muscle fiber lie tiny myofibrils. Arranged lengthwise, myofibrils contain still finer fibers, called *thick fibers* and *thin fibers*.

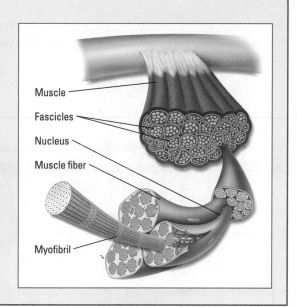

Muscle

Fascicles

Nucleus

Muscle fiber

Myofibril

Smooth muscle, found in the internal organs, such as the gallbladder, lacks striations and is called *involuntary* because it can't be consciously controlled.

Building muscle

Muscle develops when existing muscle fibers grow. Exercise, nutrition, hormones, gender, and genetic factors account for variations in muscle strength and size among individuals.

Bones

There are 206 separate bones in the human body. (See *A close look at the bones*, page 216.)

Sing along! "The leg bone is connected to the..."

Bones are classified by shape and location. They include:
- long, such as arm and leg bones (the humerus, radius, femur, tibia, ulna, and fibula) (see *A typical long bone*, page 217)
- short, such as wrist and ankle bones (the carpals and tarsals)
- flat, such as the shoulder blade (scapula), ribs, and skull
- irregular, such as bones of the vertebrae and jaw (mandible)
- sesamoid such as the kneecap (patella).

A close look at the bones

The human skeleton contains 206 bones; 80 form the axial skeleton and 126 form the appendicular skeleton. This illustration shows some of the major bones and bone groups. The illustration on the next page depicts the interior structure of a bone.

Bone consists of layers of calcified matrix containing spaces occupied by osteocytes (bone cells). Bone layers (lamellae) are arranged concentrically about central canals (haversian canals). Small cavities (lacunae) lying between the lamella contain osteocytes. Tiny canals (canaliculi) connect the lacunae. These canals form the structural units and provide nutrients to bone tissue.

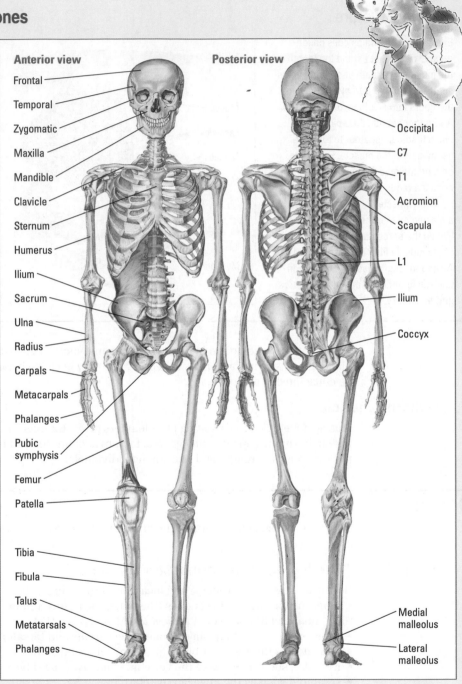

Anterior view

Frontal
Temporal
Zygomatic
Maxilla
Mandible
Clavicle
Sternum
Humerus
Ilium
Sacrum
Ulna
Radius
Carpals
Metacarpals
Phalanges
Pubic symphysis
Femur
Patella
Tibia
Fibula
Talus
Metatarsals
Phalanges

Posterior view

Occipital
C7
T1
Acromion
Scapula
L1
Ilium
Coccyx
Medial malleolus
Lateral malleolus

A typical long bone

A typical long bone has a diaphysis (main shaft) and an epiphysis (end). The epiphyses are separated from the diaphysis with cartilage at the epiphyseal line. Beneath the epiphyseal articular surface lies the articular cartilage, which cushions the joint.

Beneath the bone surface

Each bone consists of an outer layer of dense compact bone containing haversian systems and an inner layer of spongy (cancellous) bone composed of thin plates, called *trabeculae*, that interface to form a latticework. Red marrow fills the spaces between the trabeculae of some bones. Cancellous bone doesn't contain haversian systems.

Compact bone is located in the diaphyses of long bones and the outer layers of short, flat, and irregular bones. Cancellous bone fills central regions of the epiphyses and the inner portions of short, flat, and irregular bones. Periosteum—specialized fibrous connective tissue—consists of an outer fibrous layer and an inner bone-forming layer. Endosteum (a membrane that contains osteoblast producing cells) lines the medullary cavity (inner surface of bone, which contains the marrow).

Blood reaches bone by way of arterioles in haversian canals; vessels in Volkmann's canals, which enter bone matrix from the periosteum; and vessels in the bone ends and within the marrow. In children, the periosteum is thicker than in adults and has an increased blood supply to assist new bone formation around the shaft.

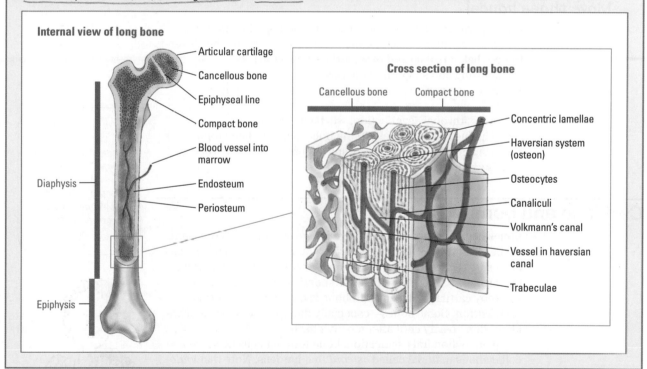

Internal view of long bone

Articular cartilage
Cancellous bone
Epiphyseal line
Compact bone
Blood vessel into marrow
Endosteum
Periosteum
Diaphysis
Epiphysis

Cross section of long bone

Cancellous bone   Compact bone

Concentric lamellae
Haversian system (osteon)
Osteocytes
Canaliculi
Volkmann's canal
Vessel in haversian canal
Trabeculae

Bones of the head and trunk—called the *axial skeleton*—include the:
• facial and cranial bones
• hyoid bone (a U-shaped bone at the base of the tongue, beneath the thyroid cartilage)
• vertebrae

- ribs
- breast bone (sternum).
      Bones of the extremities—called the *appendicular skeleton*—include the:
- collarbone (clavicle)
- scapula
- humerus
- radius
- ulna
- hand bones (metacarpals)
- pelvis
- femur
- patella
- fibula
- tibia
- foot bones (metatarsals).

Move those bones!

Bones perform such mechanical and physiologic functions as:
- protecting internal tissues and organs (for example, the 33 vertebrae that surround and protect the spinal cord)
- stabilizing and supporting the body
- providing a surface for muscle, ligament, and tendon attachment
- moving, through lever action, when contracted
- producing red blood cells in the bone marrow (hematopoiesis)
- storing mineral salts (for example, approximately 99% of the body's calcium).

Cartilage and bone formation

Bones begin as cartilage. Cartilage is a growing fibrous or elastic tissue that hardens to form bone. At 3 months' gestation, cartilage makes up the fetal skeleton. At about 6 months' gestation, the fetal cartilage hardens (ossifies) into bony skeleton. The process whereby cartilage hardens into bone is called *endochondral ossification*. Some bones—especially those of the wrists and ankles—don't ossify until after a baby's birth.

In endochondral ossification, bone-forming cells produce a collagenous material called *osteoid* that hardens. Note that *endochondral* means "occurring within cartilage."

Can you tell an osteoblast from an osteoclast?

Bone-forming cells called *osteoblasts* deposit new bone. In other words, osteoblastic activity results in bone formation.

Large cells called *osteoclasts* reabsorb material from previously formed bones, tearing down old or excess bone structure and

The fontanels of the skull are incomplete at birth. These "soft spots" allow for compression during birth and brain growth during infancy.

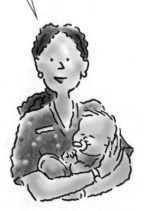

allowing osteoblasts to rebuild new bone (a process called *resorption*). Osteoblastic and osteoclastic activity promotes longitudinal bone growth. This growth continues until adolescence, when bones stop lengthening. During adolescence, the epiphyseal growth plates located at bone ends close.

Interior decorating

Osteoblasts and osteoclasts are responsible for remodeling—the continuous creation and destruction of bone within the body. When osteoblasts complete their bone-forming function and are located within the mineralized bone matrix, they transform themselves into osteocytes (mature bone cells). Bone renewal continues throughout life, although it slows down with age.

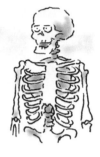

Are you ready to remodel? Osteoblasts and osteoclasts work at remodeling your bones throughout your whole life.

The estrogen connection

Researchers have found that estrogen secretion plays a role in calcium uptake and release and helps regulate osteoblastic activity (bone formation). Decreased estrogen levels have been linked to decreased osteoblastic activity, which contributes to osteoporosis.

Bones of contention

A patient's sex, race, and age also influence bone. They affect:
• bone mass
• bone's structural ability to withstand stress
• bone loss.

Men commonly have denser bones than women; Blacks commonly have denser bones than Whites. Bone density and structural integrity decrease after age 30 in women and age 45 in men. Thereafter, bone density and strength tend to continually decline at a more or less steady rate.

Cartilage cushions and absorbs shock, preventing direct transmission to the bone.

Making connections

Cartilage is dense connective tissue made up of fibers embedded in a strong, gel-like substance that supports, cushions, and shapes body structures. It's avascular (bloodless) and isn't innervated (supplied with nerves), and it may be fibrous, hyaline, or elastic:
• Fibrous cartilage forms the symphysis pubis and the intervertebral disks. This type of cartilage provides good cushioning and strength.
• Hyaline cartilage covers the articular bone surfaces (where one or more bones meet at a joint). It also appears in the trachea, bronchi, and nasal septum and covers the entire skeleton of the fetus. This type of cartilage cushions against shock.
• Elastic cartilage is located in the auditory canal, external ear, and epiglottis. It provides support with flexibility.

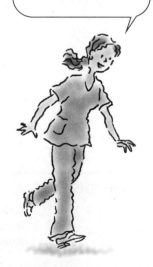

Joints

The union of two or more bones is called a *joint*.

Is the joint jumpin'?

The body contains three major types of joints, classified by how much movement they allow:

☝ Synarthrosis joints permit no movement; for example, joints between bones in the skull.

✌ Amphidiarthrosis joints allow slight movement; for example, joints between the vertebrae.

✌ Diarthrosis joints permit free movement; for example, the ankle, wrist, knee, hip, and shoulder.

Joints are further classified by shape and by connective structure, such as fibrous, cartilaginous, and synovial.

A joint venture

In a free-moving joint, a fluid-filled space known as the *joint space* exists between the bones. The synovial membrane, which lines this cavity, secretes a viscous lubricating substance called *synovial fluid*, which allows two bones to move against one another without friction. Ligaments, tendons, and muscles help to stabilize the joint.

Easing the blow

Bursae (small sacs of synovial fluid) are located at friction points around joints and between tendons, ligaments, and bones. In joints, such as the shoulder and knee, they act as cushions, easing stress on adjacent structures.

Tendons are bands of fibrous connective tissue that attach muscles to the fibrous membrane that covers the bones (the *periosteum*). Tendons enable bones to move when skeletal muscles contract.

Ligaments are dense, strong, flexible bands of fibrous connective tissue that tie bones to other bones. Ligaments that connect the joint ends of bones either limit or facilitate movement. They also provide stability.

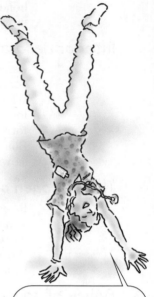

Joints get additional support from bursae, tendons, and ligaments!

Movement

Skeletal movement results primarily from muscle contractions, although other musculoskeletal structures also play a role. Here's a general description of how body movement takes place:

- Skeletal muscle is loaded with blood vessels and nerves. To contract, it needs an impulse from the nervous system and oxygen and nutrients from the blood.
- When a skeletal muscle contracts, force is applied to the tendon.
- The force pulls one bone toward, away from, or around a second bone, depending on the type of muscle contracted and the type of joint involved.

A bone's origin...more or less

Usually, one bone moves less than the other. The muscle tendon attachment to the more stationary bone is called the *origin;* the attachment to the more movable bone is the insertion site.

13 ways to shake your bones

The 13 angular and circular musculoskeletal movements are:

- circumduction—moving in a circular manner
- flexion—bending, decreasing the joint angle
- extension—straightening, increasing the joint angle
- internal rotation—turning toward midline
- external rotation—turning away from midline
- abduction—moving away from midline
- adduction—moving toward midline
- supination—turning upward
- pronation—turning downward
- eversion—turning outward
- inversion—turning inward
- retraction—moving backward
- protraction—moving forward.

Most movement involves groups of muscles rather than one muscle. Most skeletal movement is mechanical; the bones act as levers and the joints act as fulcrums (points of support for movement of the bones).

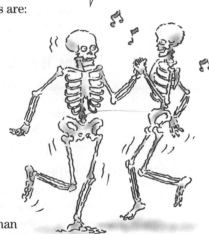

Look at all my moves!

Musculoskeletal disorders

The musculoskeletal disorders discussed in this chapter include:
- carpal tunnel syndrome
- gout
- osteoarthritis
- osteomyelitis
- osteoporosis
- rhabdomyolysis.

Carpal tunnel syndrome

Compression of median Nerve

The most common of the nerve entrapment syndromes, carpal tunnel syndrome (CTS), results from compression of the median nerve at the wrist within the carpal tunnel. This nerve passes through the carpal tunnel, along with blood vessels and flexor tendons, to the fingers and thumb. The compression neuropathy causes sensory and motor changes in the hand, especially the palm and middle finger.

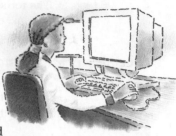

CTS is commonly the result of repetitive movements at work.

An occupational hazard

CTS usually occurs between ages 30 and 60 and poses a serious occupational health problem. Those who use a computer frequently, assembly-line workers and packers, and persons who repeatedly use poorly designed tools are most likely to develop this disorder. Any strenuous use of the hands—sustained grasping, twisting, or flexing—aggravates this condition.

How it happens

The carpal tunnel is formed by the carpal bones and the transverse carpal ligament. Inflammation or fibrosis of the tendon sheaths that pass through the carpal tunnel typically causes edema and compression of the median nerve. (See *Cross section of the wrist with CTS.*)

Carpal tunnel vision

Many conditions can cause the contents or structure of the carpal tunnel to swell and press the median nerve against the transverse carpal ligament, including:
- rheumatoid arthritis
- pregnancy
- renal failure
- menopause
- diabetes mellitus
- acromegaly
- edema following Colles' fracture of the wrist
- hypothyroidism
- amyloidosis
- myxedema
- benign tumors
- tuberculosis.

Another source of damage to the median nerve is dislocation or acute sprain of the wrist.

Now I get it!

Cross section of the wrist with CTS

Increased pressure on the median nerve decreases blood flow. If compression persists, the nerve begins to swell. The myelin sheath begins to thin and degenerate.

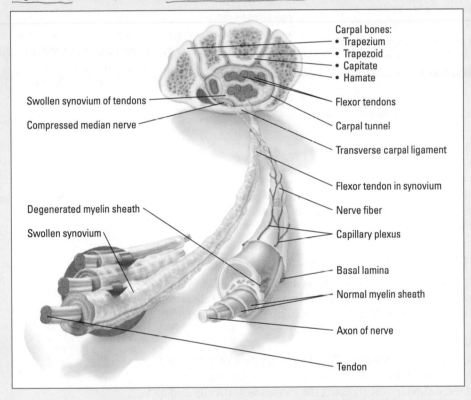

Carpal bones:
• Trapezium
• Trapezoid
• Capitate
• Hamate

Swollen synovium of tendons

Compressed median nerve

Flexor tendons

Carpal tunnel

Transverse carpal ligament

Flexor tendon in synovium

Nerve fiber

Degenerated myelin sheath

Swollen synovium

Capillary plexus

Basal lamina

Normal myelin sheath

Axon of nerve

Tendon

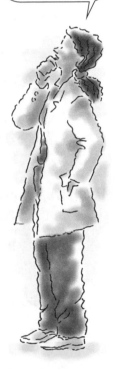

For such a small area, the carpal tunnel can sure cause severe pain.

What to look for

The patient with carpal tunnel syndrome usually complains of weakness, pain, burning, numbness, or tingling in one or both hands. This paresthesia affects the thumb, forefinger, middle finger, and half of the fourth finger. The patient can't clench his hand into a fist. The nails may be atrophic; the skin, dry and shiny.

Shaking it off

Symptoms are usually worse at night and in the morning. The pain may spread to the forearm and, in severe cases, as far as the shoulder. The patient can usually relieve such pain by shaking his

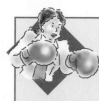

Battling illness

Treating carpal tunnel syndrome

Conservative treatment should be tried first, including resting the hands by splinting the wrist in neutral extension for 1 to 2 weeks. If a definite link has been established between the patient's occupation and the development of carpal tunnel syndrome, he should alter his work environment, if possible—or seek other work, when necessary. Effective treatment may also require correction of an underlying disorder.

Drug therapy
These drugs may be used in the treatment of carpal tunnel syndrome:
NSAIDs
• nonsteroidal anti-inflammatory drugs to decrease inflammation around the nerve and relieve symptoms

• steroids injected directly into the carpal tunnel to decrease swelling and inflammation around the median nerve.

Surgical intervention
When conservative treatment fails, the only alternative is surgical decompression of nerve by resecting the entire transverse carpal tunnel ligament or by using endoscopic surgical techniques. Neurolysis (freeing of the nerve fibers) may also be necessary.

hands vigorously or dangling his arms at his side. (See *Treating carpal tunnel syndrome.*)

What tests tell you
Physical examination reveals decreased sensation to light touch or pinpricks in the affected fingers. Thenar (palm) muscle atrophy occurs in about half of all cases of carpal tunnel syndrome.

Positive signs
The patient exhibits a positive Tinel's sign (tingling over the median nerve on light percussion). He also responds positively to Phalen's wrist-flexion test (holding the forearms vertically and allowing both hands to drop into complete flexion at the wrists for 1 minute reproduces symptoms of carpal tunnel syndrome).

Put the pressure on
These tests aid in the diagnosis of carpal tunnel syndrome:
• A compression test supports the diagnosis. A blood pressure cuff inflated above systolic pressure on the forearm for 1 to 2 minutes provokes pain and paresthesia along the distribution of the median nerve.
• Electromyography detects a median nerve motor conduction delay of more than 5 milliseconds.
• Other laboratory tests may identify underlying disease.

Gout

A metabolic disease, gout is marked by red, swollen, and acutely painful joints. Gout may affect any joint but is found mostly in joints of the feet, especially the great toe, ankle, and midfoot.

How it happens

Primary gout usually occurs in men older than age 30 and in postmenopausal women who take diuretics. It follows an intermittent course. Between attacks, patients may be symptom-free for years.

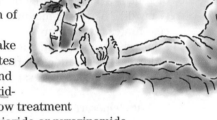

Uric acid salt deposits cause painfully arthritic joints.

About gout

The underlying cause of primary gout is unknown. In many patients it results from decreased excretion of uric acid by the kidneys. In a few patients, gout is linked to a genetic defect that causes overproduction of uric acid. This is called *hyperuricemia*.

Secondary gout may develop in the wake of another disease, such as obesity, diabetes mellitus, high blood pressure, leukemia and other blood disorders, bone cancer, and kidney disease. Secondary gout can also follow treatment with certain drugs, such as hydrochlorothiazide or pyrazinamide.

They call this progress?

Left untreated, gout progresses in four stages:

☝ During the first stage, the patient develops hyperuricemia (urate levels rise but don't produce symptoms).

✌ The second stage is marked by acute gouty arthritis. During this time, the patient experiences painful swelling and tenderness. Symptoms usually lead the patient to seek medical attention.

🖖 The third stage, the interictal stage, may last for months to years. The patient may be asymptomatic or experience exacerbations.

🖐 The fourth stage is the chronic stage. Without treatment, urate pooling may continue for years. Tophi (clusters of urate crystals) may develop in cartilage, synovial membranes, tendons, and soft tissues. This final unremitting stage of the disease is also known as *tophaceous gout*.

The tale of the tophi

Tophi are clusters of urate crystals generally surrounded by inflamed tissue. This can cause deformity and destruction of hard and soft tissues. In joints, tophi lead to destruction of cartilage and bone as well as other degeneration. (See *A close look at gout tophi*.)

Tophi form in diverse areas, including:
• hands
• knees
• feet
• outer sides of the forearms
• pinna of the ear
• Achilles tendon.

Rarely, internal organs, such as the kidneys and heart, may be affected. Kidney involvement may cause kidney dysfunction.

Hyperuricemia: The hallmark of gout

Urates are uric acid salts. They predominate in the plasma, fluid around the cells, and synovial fluid. Hyperuricemia, the hallmark of gout, is a plasma urate concentration greater than 420 μmol/L (7 mg/dl). Hyperuricemia indicates increased total-body urate. Excess urates result from:
• increased urate production
• decreased excretion of uric acid
• a combination of increased production and decreased excretion.

With hyperuricemia, plasma and extracellular fluids are supersaturated with urate. This leads to urate crystal formation. When crystals are deposited in other tissues, a gout attack strikes.

These things get your gout

Many different factors may provoke an acute attack of gout, including:
• stress
• trauma
• infection
• hospitalization
• surgery
• starvation
• excessive intake of foods containing purine
• use of alcohol
• some medications.

A sudden increase in serum urate may cause new crystals to form. However, a drop in serum and extracellular urate concentrations may cause previously formed crystals to partially dissolve and be excreted.

A close look at gout tophi

In advanced gout, urate crystal deposits develop into hard, irregular, yellow-white nodules called *tophi*. These bumps commonly protrude from the finger and the pinna, as shown below.

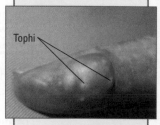

Tophi

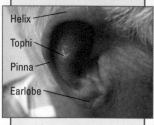

Helix
Tophi
Pinna
Earlobe

Stress? I know all about stress! I know it's one of many factors that can provoke an acute attack of gout!

What to look for

In some patients, serum urate levels increase but produce no symptoms. In symptom-producing gout, the first acute attack strikes suddenly and peaks quickly.

First strike

Although it may involve only one or a few joints, the first acute attack causes extreme pain. Untreated gout attacks usually resolve in 10 to 14 days. Mild acute attacks usually subside quickly but tend to recur at irregular intervals. Severe attacks may last for days or weeks.

Ahhh, a respite...

Patients with gout usually enjoy symptom-free intervals between attacks. Most patients have a second attack between 6 months and 2 years after the first; in some patients, however, the second attack is delayed for 5 to 10 years. Delayed attacks, which may involve several joints, are more common in untreated patients. These attacks tend to last longer and produce more symptoms than initial episodes.

A persistent plight

Chronic gout is marked by numerous, persistently painful joints. With tophi development, joints are typically swollen and dusky red or purple, with limited movement. The actual tophi—hard, irregular, yellow-white nodules—may be seen, especially on the ears, hands, and feet.

Late in the chronic stage of gout, the skin over the tophi may ulcerate and release a chalky white exudate or pus. Chronic inflammation and tophi lead to joint degeneration; deformity and disability may develop.

Warmth and extreme tenderness may be felt over the joint. The patient may have a sedentary lifestyle and a history of hypertension and renal calculi. The patient may wake during the night with pain in the great toe or other part of the foot.

Initially moderate pain may grow so intense that eventually the patient can't bear the weight of bed linens or the vibrations of a person walking across the room. He may report chills and a mild fever.

Getting complicated

Potential complications include kidney disorders, such as renal calculi, infection that develops with tophi rupture and nerve damage, and circulatory problems, such as atherosclerotic disease, cardiovascular lesions, stroke, coronary thrombosis, and hypertension.

Patients who receive treatment for gout have a good prognosis. (See *Treating gout*, page 228.)

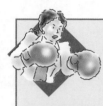

Battling illness

Treating gout

Treatment for gout varies, depending on whether gout is acute or chronic. Dietary restrictions and weight loss may also be a part of care.

Treatment goals

 terminate the acute attack

 reduce uric acid levels

 prevent recurrent gout and renal calculi.

Acute attacks

Treatment of an acute attack includes:
• elevation of the extremity, when possible
• immobilization and protection of the inflamed, painful joints
• local application of cold.

A bed cradle can be used to keep bed linens off sensitive, inflamed joints. Analgesics, such as acetaminophen, relieve the pain of mild attacks. Acute inflammation, however, requires nonsteroidal anti-inflammatory drugs or I.V. corticosteroids if the patient is hospitalized.

Colchicine or oral corticosteroids are occasionally used to treat acute attacks, although they don't affect uric acid levels. The patient should also drink plenty of fluids (at least 2 qt [2 L]/day) to help prevent renal calculi.

Acute gout can attack 24 to 96 hours after surgery; even minor surgery can trigger an attack. Colchicine may be administered before and after surgery to help prevent gout attacks.

Chronic gout

To treat chronic gout, serum uric acid levels are reduced to less than 6.5 mg/dl using various medications, depending on whether the patient over- or underproduces uric acid. If he overproduces uric acid, he may be given allopurinol. If he underproduces uric acid, he may be treated with probenecid or sulfinpyrazone. Serum uric acid levels are monitored regularly, and sodium bicarbonate or other agents may be given to alkalinize the patient's urine.

Adjunctive therapy

Adjunctive therapy emphasizes:
• avoiding alcohol (especially beer and wine)
• avoiding purine-rich foods (which raise urate levels), such as anchovies, liver, sardines, kidneys, sweetbreads, and lentils.

Weight loss

Obese patients should begin a weight-loss program because weight reduction decreases uric acid levels and stress on painful joints as well. To diffuse anxiety and promote coping, the patient should be encouraged to express his concerns about his condition.

What tests tell you

These tests aid in the diagnosis of gout:
• Needle aspiration of synovial fluid (called *arthrocentesis*) or of tophi for microscopic examination reveals needlelike crystals of sodium urate in the cells and establishes the diagnosis. If test results identify calcium pyrophosphate crystals, the patient probably has pseudogout, a disease similar to gout.
• Blood and urine analysis are used to determine serum and urine uric acid levels.
• X-ray studies initially produce normal results. However, in chronic gout, X-rays show damage to cartilage and bone. Outward displacement of the overhanging margin from the bone contour characterizes gout.

Osteoarthritis

Osteoarthritis, the most common form of arthritis, is widespread, occurring equally in both sexes. Incidence occurs after age 40; its earliest symptoms generally begin in middle age and may progress with advancing age.

The degree of disability depends on the site and severity of involvement; it can range from minor limitation of the fingers to severe disability in a person with hip or knee involvement. The rate of progression varies, and joints may remain stable for years in an early stage of deterioration.

As a result of...

Primary osteoarthritis, a normal part of aging, results from many things, including:
- metabolic factors
- genetics
- chemical factors
- mechanical factors.

The wear and tear

Secondary osteoarthritis usually follows an identifiable predisposing event—most commonly trauma, congenital deformity, or obesity—and leads to degenerative changes.

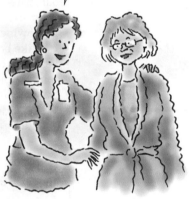

The normal aging process commonly leads to primary osteoarthritis.

How it happens

Osteoarthritis is chronic, causing deterioration of the joint cartilage and formation of reactive new bone at the margins and subchondral (below the cartilage) areas of the joints. This degeneration results from a breakdown of chondrocytes (cartilage cells), most commonly in the hips and knees.

What to look for

The most common symptom of osteoarthritis is a deep, aching joint pain, particularly after exercise or weight bearing, that's usually relieved by rest. Other signs and symptoms of osteoarthritis include:
- stiffness in the morning and after exercise (relieved by rest)
- aching during changes in weather
- "grating" of the joint during motion
- altered gait contractures
- limited movement.

These signs and symptoms increase with poor posture, obesity, and occupational stress.

The nodes know

Osteoarthritis involving the joints of the fingers produces irreversible changes in the distal joints (Heberden's nodes) and proximal joints (Bouchard's nodes). These nodes may be painless at first but eventually become red, swollen, and tender, causing numbness and loss of dexterity. (See *A close look at the effects of osteoarthritis* and *Treating osteoarthritis*.)

What tests tell you

A thorough physical examination confirms typical symptoms, and the absence of systemic symptoms rules out an inflammatory joint disorder. X-rays of the affected joint help confirm diagnosis of osteoarthritis but may be normal in the early stages.

X-rays may require many views and typically show:
- narrowing of the joint space or margins
- cystlike bony deposits in joint space and margins
- sclerosis of the subchondral space
- joint deformity due to degeneration or articular damage
- bony growths at weight-bearing areas
- fusion of joints.

No laboratory test is specific for osteoarthritis.

A close look at the effects of osteoarthritis

Involvement of the interphalangeal (finger bone) joints produces irreversible changes in the distal joints (Heberden's nodes) and the proximal joints (Bouchard's nodes), as shown below. These nodes can be painless initially, with gradual progression to or sudden flare-ups of redness, swelling, tenderness, and impaired sensation and dexterity.

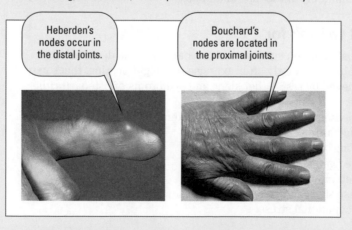

Heberden's nodes occur in the distal joints.

Bouchard's nodes are located in the proximal joints.

Battling illness

Treating osteoarthritis

The goal of osteoarthritis treatment is to:
- relieve pain
- maintain or improve mobility
- minimize disability.

Drug therapy

Drugs used to treat osteoarthritis include:
- acetaminophen (Tylenol)
- aspirin (or other nonopioid analgesics)
- celecoxib (Celebrex)
- meloxicam (Mobic)
- ibuprofen (Advil)
- naproxen (Aleve).

In some cases, intra-articular injections of corticosteroids given every 4 to 6 months may delay the development of nodes in the hands.

Noninvasive interventions

Weight loss helps decrease stress on joints.

Strengthening exercises for muscles around the knee and hip help stabilize these joints and improve alignment of the articular surfaces, preventing further cartilage deterioration. Exercise may also help with weight management.

Effective treatment also reduces stress by supporting or stabilizing the joint with crutches, braces, a cane, a walker, a cervical collar, or traction.

Surgical interventions

Surgical treatment, reserved for patients who have severe disability or uncontrollable pain, may include:
- arthroplasty—replacement of the deteriorated part of joint with prosthetic appliance
- arthrodesis—surgical fusion of bones; used primarily in the spine (laminectomy)
- osteoplasty—scraping and lavage of deteriorated bone from joint
- osteotomy—change in alignment of bone to relieve stress by excision of bone wedge or cutting of bone.

Osteomyelitis

Osteomyelitis is a bone infection characterized by progressive inflammatory bone destruction after formation of new bone. It may be acute or chronic and commonly results from a combination of local trauma—usually trivial but causing a hematoma—and an acute infection originating elsewhere in the body. It can also occur from severe open fractures with contamination from dirt or paving material. Although osteomyelitis typically remains localized, it can spread through the bone to the marrow, cortex, and periosteum.

Common in children

Acute osteomyelitis is usually a blood-borne disease and most commonly affects rapidly growing children. Chronic osteomyelitis, which is rare, is characterized by draining sinus tracts and widespread lesions.

Typical sites in tykes

Osteomyelitis occurs more commonly in children (particularly boys) than in adults—usually as a complication of an acute localized infection. Typical sites of osteomyelitis in children are the lower end of the femur and the upper ends of the tibia, humerus, and radius. The most common sites in adults are the pelvis and vertebrae, generally after surgery or trauma. (See *Stages of osteomyelitis*.)

How it happens

The most common causative organism in osteomyelitis is *Staphylococcus aureus*. Other organisms that can cause osteomyelitis include:

- *Streptococcus pyogenes*
- pneumococcus
- *Pseudomonas aeruginosa*
- *Escherichia coli*
- *Proteus vulgaris*
- *Pasteurella multocida* (part of the normal mouth flora of cats and dogs).

> No bones about it! We move into an area weakened by trauma or infection and travel through the bloodstream to the metaphysis.

Now I get it!

Stages of osteomyelitis

The illustrations show the progression of osteomyelitis.

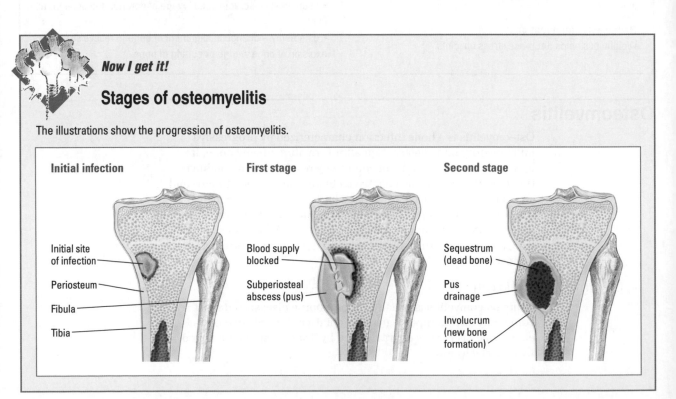

Initial infection

- Initial site of infection
- Periosteum
- Fibula
- Tibia

First stage

- Blood supply blocked
- Subperiosteal abscess (pus)

Second stage

- Sequestrum (dead bone)
- Pus drainage
- Involucrum (new bone formation)

Typically, these organisms find a culture site in a hematoma (from recent trauma) or in a weakened area (such as the site of local infection) and travel through the bloodstream to the metaphysis, the section of a long bone that's continuous with the epiphysis plates, where blood flows into sinusoids.

What to look for

Signs and symptoms of acute and chronic osteomyelitis are generally the same and may include:
• rapid onset (acute osteomyelitis), with sudden pain in the affected bone accompanied by tenderness, heat, swelling, erythema, guarding of the affected region of the limb, and restricted movement
• chronic infection persisting intermittently for years, flaring after minor trauma or persisting as drainage of pus from an old pocket in a sinus tract; occurs in chronic osteomyelitis, yet acute osteomyelitis may progress to this
• fever
• dehydration (in children)
• irritability and poor feeding in infants. (See *Treating osteomyelitis.*)

Battling illness

Treating osteomyelitis

Treatment for osteomyelitis should be initiated as soon as osteomyelitis is suspected.

Acute osteomyelitis
Therapy for acute osteomyelitis includes drug therapy and other interventions.

Drug therapy
Drugs used to treat acute osteomyelitis include:
• I.V. antibiotics, such as nafcillin or oxacillin, after blood cultures are obtained
• Analgesics to relieve pain
• Intracavity instillation of antibiotics through closed-system continuous irrigation with low intermittent suction.

Other interventions
• Surgical drainage to relieve pressure and abscess formation
• I.V. fluids to maintain hydration
• Immobilization of the affected body part

Chronic osteomyelitis
Treatment of chronic osteomyelitis may include:
• surgery to remove dead bone and promote drainage
• hyperbaric oxygen therapy to stimulate healing
• skin, bone, and muscle grafts to increase blood supply
• placement of antibiotic beads directly into the affected bone.

What tests tell you

These test results help diagnose osteomyelitis:
• White blood cell count shows leukocytosis.
• Erythrocyte sedimentation rate is elevated.
• Blood cultures reveal the causative organism.
• Bone cultures reveal the causative organism.
• Magnetic resonance imaging (MRI) delineates bone marrow from soft tissue to show the extent of the infection.
• X-rays show bone involvement after the disease has been active for 2 to 3 weeks.
• Bone scan detects early infection.

Osteoporosis

Osteoporosis is a metabolic bone disorder in which the rate of bone resorption accelerates and the rate of bone formation decelerates. The result is decreased bone mass. Bones affected by this disease lose calcium and phosphate and become porous, brittle, and abnormally prone to fracture.

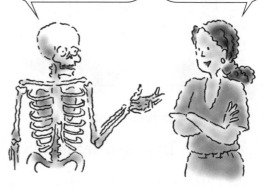

With osteoporosis, bone resorption accelerates while bone formation decelerates.

That means decreased bone mass, leaving bones very prone to fracture.

By the numbers

Osteoporosis is four times more common in women than men. White and Asian women are more likely to develop the disease than Black or Hispanic women.

How it happens

Osteoporosis may be a primary disorder or occur secondary to an underlying disease. (See *What is osteoporosis?*)

Boning up on osteoporosis

The cause of primary osteoporosis is unknown. However, contributing factors include:
• mild but prolonged lack of calcium due to poor dietary intake or poor absorption by the intestine secondary to age
• hormonal imbalance due to endocrine dysfunction
• faulty metabolism of protein due to estrogen deficiency
• a sedentary lifestyle.
   Primary osteoporosis is classified as one of three types:

Postmenopausal osteoporosis (type I) usually affects women ages 51 to 75. It's related to the loss of estrogen and its protective effect on bone and characterized by vertebral and wrist fractures

Now I get it!

What is osteoporosis?

Osteoporosis is a metabolic disease of the skeleton that reduces the amount of bone tissue. Bones weaken as local cells resorb, or take up, bone tissue. Trabecular bone at the core becomes less dense, and cortical bone on the perimeter loses thickness.

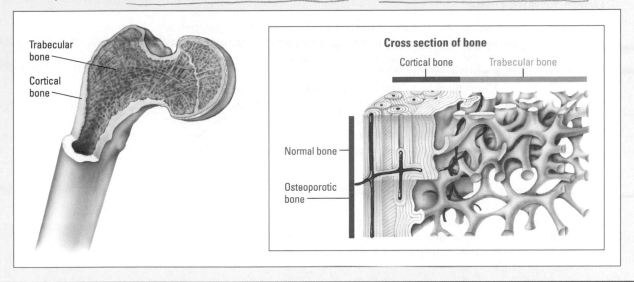

Senile osteoporosis (type II) occurs mostly between ages 70 and 85. It's related to osteoblast or osteoclast shrinkage or decreased physical activity and characterized by fractures of the humerus, tibia, femur, and pelvis.

Premenopausal osteoporosis (type III) involves higher estrogen levels that may increase bone resorption by affecting the sensitivity of osteoclasts to parathyroid hormone.

Other factors take their toll

Secondary osteoporosis may result from:
- prolonged therapy with steroids or heparin
- bone immobilization or disuse (such as paralysis)
- alcoholism
- malnutrition
- rheumatoid arthritis
- liver disease
- malabsorption of calcium
- scurvy (vitamin C deficiency)

- lactose intolerance
- hyperthyroidism
- osteogenesis imperfecta (an inherited condition that causes brittle bones)
- trauma leading to atrophy in the hands and feet, with recurring attacks (Sudeck's disease)
- smoking.

Down to the bone

Osteoporosis is characterized by a reduction in the bone matrix and in remineralization, resulting in soft bones that fracture easily. Bone mass is lost because of an imbalance between bone resorption and formation.

Cancellous bone, the inner layer of spongy bone, is composed of trabeculae, sharp, needlelike structures forming a meshwork of interconnecting spaces. Trabeculae have a larger surface volume than compact bone (the outer layer of dense bone) and therefore are lost more rapidly as bone mass decreases. This loss leads to fractures.

What to look for

Bone fractures are the major complication of osteoporosis. Fractures occur mostly in the vertebrae, femur, and distal radius. Signs of redness, warmth, and new sites of pain may indicate new fractures.

Patient profile

The patient is typically postmenopausal or has one of the conditions that cause secondary osteoporosis. She may report that she heard a snapping sound and felt a sudden pain in her lower back when she bent down to lift something. Alternatively, she may say that the pain developed slowly over several years. If the patient has vertebral collapse, she may describe a backache and pain radiating around the trunk. Movement or jarring aggravates the pain.

Don't get bent out of shape

The patient may have a humped back (dowager's hump); the curvature worsens as repeated vertebral fractures increase spinal curvature. The abdomen eventually protrudes to compensate for the changed center of gravity. The patient commonly reports a gradual loss of height, decreased exercise tolerance, and trouble breathing. Palpation may reveal muscle spasm. The patient may also have decreased spinal movement, with flexion more limited than extension. (See *Height loss in osteoporosis* and *Treating osteoporosis*, page 238.)

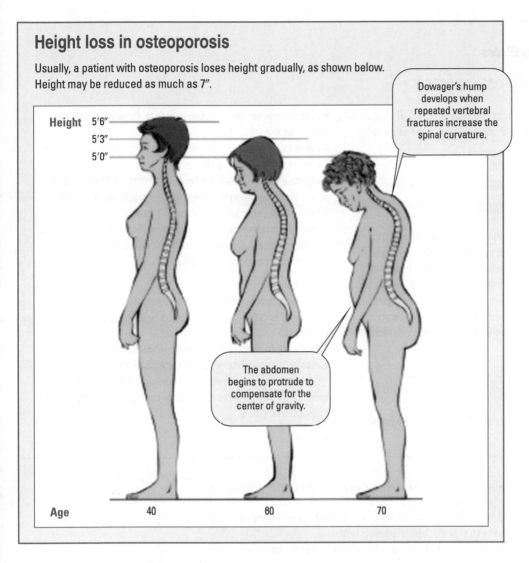

Height loss in osteoporosis

Usually, a patient with osteoporosis loses height gradually, as shown below. Height may be reduced as much as 7".

Dowager's hump develops when repeated vertebral fractures increase the spinal curvature.

The abdomen begins to protrude to compensate for the center of gravity.

Height   5'6"   5'3"   5'0"

Age   40   60   70

What tests tell you

A diagnosis excludes other causes of bone disease, especially those that affect the spine, such as cancer or tumors. These tests help confirm a diagnosis of osteoporosis:
- <u>X-ray studies</u> show characteristic degeneration in the lower vertebrae. Loss of bone mineral appears in later disease.
- Serum calcium, phosphorus, and alkaline phosphatase levels remain within normal limits; parathyroid hormone levels may be elevated.
- Bone biopsy allows direct examination of changes in bone cells.
- Computed tomography scan allows accurate assessment of spinal bone loss.

Battling illness

Treating osteoporosis

Treatment focuses on a physical therapy program of gentle exercise and activity and drug therapy to slow the disease's progress. Care seeks to:
- control bone loss
- prevent fractures
- control pain.

How goals are achieved

Measures may include supportive devices such as a back brace and, possibly, surgery to correct fractures. Estrogen may be prescribed within 3 years after menopause to decrease the rate of bone resorption. A balanced diet should be rich in nutrients, such as vitamin D, calcium, and protein, that support skeletal metabolism. Low-impact weight bearing exercises can help stimulate osteoblast formation. Heat may be applied to relieve pain.

Drug therapy

Drugs used to treat osteoporosis include:
- analgesics to relieve pain
- alendronate, risedronate, or raloxifene to treat and prevent osteoporosis

- calcium and vitamin D supplements to support normal bone metabolism
- calcitonin to reduce bone resorption and slow the decline in bone mass and relieve pain
- etidronate is the first agent proved to increase bone density and restore lost bone by inhibiting osteoblast activity
- teriparatide, an injectable form of human parathyroid hormone, for postmenopausal women and men with osteoporosis who are at high risk for developing fractures; the drug stimulates bone formation in the spine and hips.

Keep it safe

Preventing falls is the top priority. Safety precautions include keeping side rails up on the patient's bed and moving the patient gently and carefully at all times.

Be sure to discuss with ancillary hospital personnel how easily an osteoporotic patient's bones can fracture.

Instruct the patient and family members about home safety measures such as removing scatter rugs and installing tub and shower safety bars.

- Radionuclide bone scans display injured or diseased areas as darker portions.
- Dual photon or dual energy X-ray absorptiometry can detect bone loss in a safe, noninvasive test.
- Bone density measurements confirm the diagnosis.

Rhabdomyolysis

Rhabdomyolysis, a disease involving the breakdown of muscle tissue, may cause myoglobinuria, in which varying amounts of muscle protein (myoglobin) appear in the urine. Approximately 26,000 cases of rhabdomyolysis are reported annually in the United States.

Major muscle trauma means major problems

The term *rhabdomyolysis* was first used to describe crush injuries seen in the victims of London bombing raids during World War II.

Rhabdomyolysis usually follows major muscle trauma, especially a muscle crush injury. Long-distance running, certain severe infections, and exposure to electric shock can cause extensive muscle damage and excessive release of myoglobin.

A drug connection

Most recently, a connection has been noted between the combined use of cerivastatin and gemfibrozil and the development of rhabdomyolysis.

Prognosis for rhabdomyolysis is good if contributing causes are discovered and eliminated or if the disease is checked before damage has progressed to an irreversible stage. Unchecked, rhabdomyolysis can cause renal failure and death.

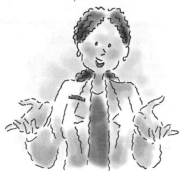

Prognosis for rhabdomyolysis is good if contributing causes are eliminated or if the disease is checked before it reaches an irreversible stage.

How it happens

Possible causes of rhabdomyolysis include:
• alcohol abuse and use of illicit drugs
• familial tendency
• strenuous exertion
• infection and inflammatory processes
• anesthetic agents such as halothane that can cause intraoperative rigidity
• heatstroke
• electrolyte disturbances
• cardiac arrhythmias
• excessive muscular activity associated with status epilepticus, electroconvulsive therapy, or high-voltage electric shock
• medications, including HMG-CoA reductase inhibitors (especially in conjunction with nicotinic acid), cyclosporine, itraconazole, erythromycin, colchicine, zidovudine, and corticosteroids.

Getting complicated

Muscle trauma that compresses tissue causes ischemia and necrosis. The ensuing local edema further increases compartment pressure and tamponade; pressure from severe swelling causes blood vessels to collapse, leading to tissue hypoxia, muscle infarction, and neural damage in the area of the fracture. Myoglobin, potassium, creatine kinase, and urate are released from the necrotic muscle fibers into the circulation.

What to look for

Patients with rhabdomyolysis may experience local and systemic symptoms, including:
• local—muscle pain, tenderness, swelling, and muscle weakness caused by muscle trauma and pressure

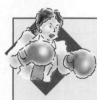

Battling illness

Treating rhabdomyolysis

Therapy for rhabdomyolysis typically includes treating the underlying disorder and taking measures to prevent renal failure. These measures may be used for treatment:
• I.V. hydration initiated as early as possible (Infuse normal saline solution at a rate of 1.5 L/hour to maintain urine output of at least 300 ml/hour. Continue the infusion until the creatine kinase level falls below 1,000 units/L. Then, change I.V. fluids to half normal saline solution with 40 mEq of sodium bicarbonate and 10 g/L of mannitol.)

• Bed rest
• Anti-inflammatory agents
• Corticosteroids in extreme cases
• Analgesics to relieve pain
• Immediate fasciotomy and debridement to relieve pressure and promote circulation (if compartment venous pressure is greater that 25 mm Hg).

• systemic—urine that darkens and becomes reddish brown as myoglobin enters the urine, fever, malaise, nausea, vomiting, confusion, agitation, delirium, and anuria. (See *Treating rhabdomyolysis.*)

What tests tell you

These diagnostic tests help confirm the diagnosis of rhabdomyolysis:
• Urine myoglobin level is greater than 0.5 mg/dl.
• Creatine kinase level is severely elevated.
• Serum potassium, phosphate, and creatinine levels are elevated.
• Calcium levels are decreased in early stages and elevated in later stages.
• CT scans, MRI, and bone scintigraphy reveal muscle necrosis.
• Intracompartmental venous pressure measurements are elevated
• Electrocardiogram will show changes resulting from elevated potassium levels.

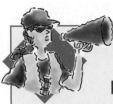

That's a wrap!

Musculoskeletal system review

Understanding the structures

Working together to provide support and produce movement, the structures of the musculoskeletal system include:
• muscles
• bones
• cartilage
• joints, bursae, tendons, and ligaments.

Muscles

Three major muscle types:
• Skeletal muscles (voluntary, striated muscles)
• Smooth (involuntary muscles)
• Cardiac (involuntary, striated muscles)

Bones

• 206 in the human body
• Classified by shape and location
• Perform mechanical and physiologic functions
• Begin as cartilage
• Formed by process called *endochondral ossification*
• Continuously torn down and rebuilt by osteoclasts and osteoblasts

Cartilage

• Dense connective tissue consisting of fibers embedded in a strong, gel-like substance
• Avascular and not innervated
• Supports, cushions, and shapes body structures
• May be fibrous, hyaline, or elastic

Joints

• The union of two or more bones
• Classified by how much movement they allow; synarthrosis, no movement; amphiarthrosis, slight movement; diarthrosis, free movement
• Supporting the joints:
  – Bursae—cushions located at friction points around joints and between tendons, ligaments, and bones
  – Tendons— bands of fibrous connective tissue that attach muscle to bone to stabilize joints
  – Ligaments—bands of fibrous connective tissue that tie bones to other bones to stabilize joints

Musculoskeletal disorders

• *Carpal tunnel syndrome*—caused by inflammation or fibrosis of tendon sheath that results in median nerve compressed by edema
• *Gout*—caused by decreased uric acid excretion by the kidneys resulting in painful swelling and tenderness caused by rising urate levels
• *Osteoarthritis*—caused by deterioration of joint cartilage that results in reactive new bone forming in the joints
• *Osteomyelitis*—bone infection characterized by progressive inflammatory destruction after formation of new bone
• *Osteoporosis*—caused by reduction in bone matrix and bone remineralization that results in bones becoming soft and easily fractured
• *Rhabdomyolysis*—breakdown of muscle tissue that may cause myoglobinuria, in which varying amounts of muscle protein appear in the urine

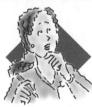

Quick quiz

1. Which types of muscles make up most of the musculoskeletal system?

    A. Striated and involuntary
    B. Smooth and voluntary
    C. Striated and voluntary
    D. Smooth and involuntary

Answer: C. The musculoskeletal system consists mostly of skeletal muscle, which is striated and can be moved at will.

2. Which of the following is a positive sign of carpal tunnel syndrome?
 A. Trousseau's sign
 B. Tinel's sign
 C. Tzanck test
 D. Ortolani's sign

Answer: B. Tinel's sign, a complaint of tingling over the median nerve on light percussion, is a positive sign of carpal tunnel syndrome.

3. Irreversible changes in the distal joints of the fingers caused by osteoarthritis are known as:
 A. Bouchard's nodes.
 B. lymph nodes.
 C. Haygarth's nodes.
 D. Heberden's nodes.

Answer: D. Heberden's nodes are the result of changes in the distal joints of the fingers.

4. Osteoporosis is characterized by:
 A. porosity and brittleness.
 B. brittleness and swelling of the joints.
 C. crystal deposition and brittleness.
 D. progressive inflammatory destruction after new bone formation.

Answer: A. Osteoporosis is a metabolic bone disorder in which bone loses calcium and phosphate and becomes porous, brittle, and abnormally vulnerable to fractures.

Scoring

☆☆☆ If you answered all four items correctly, take a bow! You're great—no bones about it.

☆☆ If you answered three items correctly, right on! Jump up and dance a victory jig using any of the 13 angular and circular musculoskeletal movements.

☆ If you answered fewer than three items correctly, there's only one thing we can say: You're going to have to bone up.

7

Endocrine system

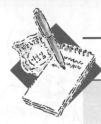

Just the facts

In this chapter, you'll learn:

♦ the role of the hypothalamus in regulating hormones

♦ the function of the adrenal glands, pancreas, pituitary gland, and thyroid gland

♦ the pathophysiology, signs and symptoms, diagnostic tests, and treatments for several endocrine disorders.

Understanding the endocrine system

The endocrine system consists of glands, specialized cell clusters, and hormones, which are chemical transmitters secreted by the glands in response to stimulation.

Together with the central nervous system (CNS), the endocrine system regulates and integrates the body's metabolic activities and maintains homeostasis.

Hypothalamus: The heart of the system

The hypothalamus is the integrative center for the endocrine and autonomic (involuntary) nervous systems. It helps control some endocrine glands by neural and hormonal pathways.

On the path to the posterior pituitary gland

Neural pathways connect the hypothalamus to the posterior pituitary gland. Neural stimulation of the posterior pituitary gland in turn causes the secretion of two effector hormones—antidiuretic hormone (ADH) and oxytocin. When ADH is secreted, the body retains water. Oxytocin stimulates uterine contractions during labor and milk secretion in lactating women.

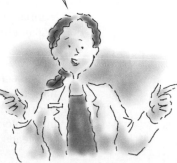

The functions of the endocrine and nervous systems are interrelated.

Please release me

The hypothalamus also exerts hormonal control at the anterior pituitary gland by releasing or inhibiting hormones. Hypothalamic hormones stimulate the anterior pituitary gland to release four types of trophic (gland-stimulating) hormones:

- adrenocorticotropic hormone (ACTH), also called *corticotropin*

- thyroid-stimulating hormone (TSH)

- luteinizing hormone (LH)

- follicle-stimulating hormone (FSH).

The secretion of trophic hormones stimulates their respective target glands, such as the adrenal cortex, the thyroid gland, and the gonads.

Hypothalamic hormones also control the release of effector hormones from the pituitary gland. Examples are growth hormone (GH) and prolactin.

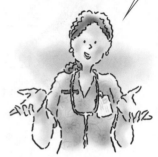

Why are ADH and oxytocin called effector hormones?

Getting feedback

A negative feedback system regulates the endocrine system by inhibiting hormone overproduction. This system may be simple or complex. (See *The feedback loop.*)

A patient with a possible endocrine disorder needs careful assessment to identify the cause of the dysfunction. Dysfunction may result from defects:

- in the gland
- in the release of trophic or effector hormones
- in hormone transport
- of the target tissue.

How do you end up with an endocrine disorder?

Endocrine disorders may be caused by:

- hypersecretion or hyposecretion of hormones
- hyporesponsiveness of hormone receptors
- inflammation of glands
- gland tumors.

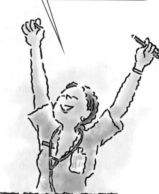

Because they produce an effect when secreted.

Dysfunctional

Hypersecretion or hyposecretion may originate in the hypothalamus, the pituitary effector glands, or the target gland. Regardless of origin, however, the result is abnormal hormone concentrations in the blood. Hypersecretion leads to elevated levels; hyposecretion leads to deficient levels.

Now I get it!

The feedback loop

This diagram shows the negative feedback mechanism that helps regulate the endocrine system.

From simple . . .

Simple feedback occurs when the level of one substance regulates secretion of hormones (simple loop). For example, a low serum calcium level stimulates the parathyroid gland to release parathyroid hormone (PTH). PTH, in turn, promotes resorption of calcium. A high serum calcium level inhibits PTH secretion.

. . . to complex

When the hypothalamus receives feedback from target glands, the mechanism is more complicated (complex loop). Complex feedback occurs through an axis established between the hypothalamus, pituitary gland, and target organ. For example, secretion of the hypothalamic corticotropin-releasing hormone stimulates release of pituitary corticotropin, which in turn stimulates cortisol secretion by the adrenal gland (the target organ). A rise in serum cortisol levels inhibits corticotropin secretion by decreasing corticotropin-releasing hormone.

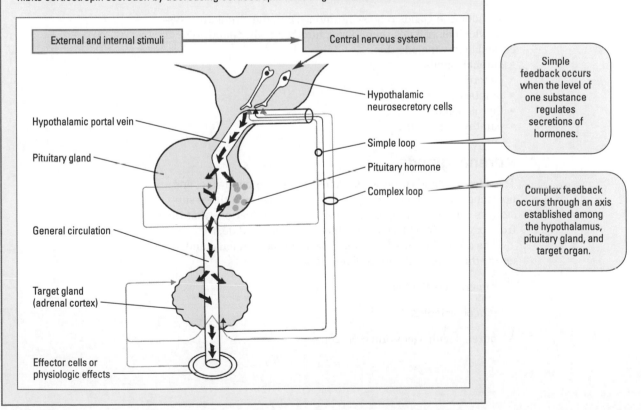

Turn it off! What? Turn it off!!!

In hyporesponsiveness, the cells of the target organ don't have appropriate receptors for a hormone. This means the effects of the hormone aren't detected. Because the receptors don't detect the hormone, there's no feedback mechanism to turn the hormone off. Blood levels of the hormone are normal or high. Hyporesponsiveness causes the same clinical symptoms as hyposecretion.

> Hey, there are hormones there! The receptors aren't detecting it...turn it off!

An inflamed discussion (and tumor talk)

Inflammation is usually chronic, commonly resulting in glandular secretion of hormones. However, it may be acute or subacute, as in thyroiditis.

Tumors can occur within a gland, as in thyroid carcinoma. In addition, tumors occurring in other areas of the body can cause abnormal hormone production (ectopic hormone production). For example, certain lung tumors secrete ADH or parathyroid hormone (PTH).

Glands

The endocrine glands release hormones into the circulatory system, which distributes them throughout the body. Glands discussed below include the:
- adrenal glands
- pancreas
- pituitary gland
- thyroid gland
- parathyroid glands.

Adrenal glands

The adrenal glands produce steroids, amines, epinephrine, and norepinephrine. Hyposecretion or hypersecretion of these substances causes a variety of disorders and complications that range from psychiatric and sexual problems to coma and death.

The adrenal cortex is the outer layer of the adrenal gland. It secretes three types of steroidal hormones:

 mineralocorticoids

 glucocorticoids

 adrenal androgens and estrogens.

Aldosterone in action

Aldosterone is a mineralocorticoid. It regulates the reabsorption of sodium and the excretion of potassium by the kidneys. Aldosterone may be involved with other hormones in the development of hypertension.

Cue cortisol

Cortisol, a glucocorticoid, carries out these five important functions:

☝ stimulation of gluconeogenesis (formation of glycogen from noncarbohydrate sources), which occurs in the liver in response to low carbohydrate intake or starvation

✌ breakdown of increased protein and mobilization of free fatty acid

🖖 suppression of immune response

🖐 assistance with stress response

🖐 assistance with maintenance of blood pressure and cardiovascular function.

Androgens (male sex hormones) promote male traits, especially secondary sex characteristics. Examples of such characteristics are facial hair and a low-pitched voice. Estrogens promote female traits. They are also thought to be responsible for sex drive.

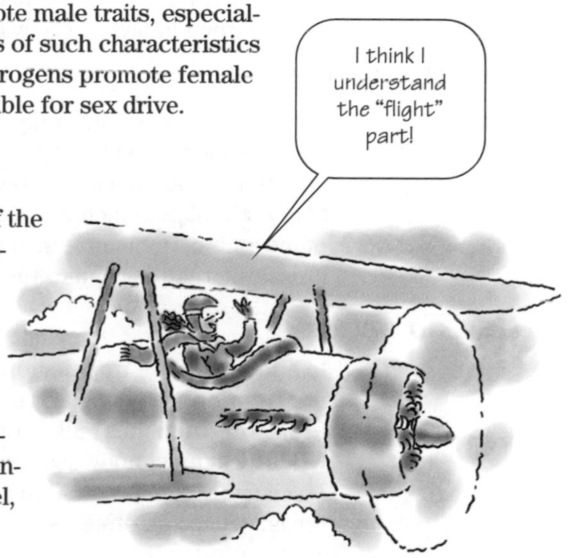

A gland with a lot of nerve

The adrenal medulla is the inner portion of the adrenal gland. It's an aggregate of nerve tissue that produces the catecholamine hormones epinephrine and norepinephrine that cause vasoconstriction.

Epinephrine causes the response to physical or emotional stress called the *fight-or-flight response.* This response produces marked dilation of bronchioles and increased blood pressure, blood glucose level, and heart rate.

I think I understand the "flight" part!

Pancreas

The pancreas produces glucagon and insulin.

Fasting? You'll need glucose fast . . .

Glucagon is a hormone released when a person is in a fasting state. It stimulates the release of stored glucose from the liver to raise blood glucose levels.

Multiple roles of insulin

Insulin is a hormone released during the postprandial (nourished) state. It aids glucose transport into the cells and promotes glucose storage. It also stimulates protein synthesis and enhances free fatty acid uptake and storage. Insulin deficiency or resistance causes diabetes mellitus.

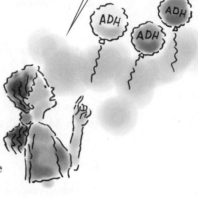

Low blood pressure and low blood volume stimulate the release of ADH.

Pituitary gland

The posterior pituitary gland, located at the base of the brain, secretes two effector hormones:

☞ oxytocin, which stimulates uterine contractions during labor and causes the milk let-down reflex in lactating women

✌ ADH, which controls the concentration of body fluids by altering the permeability of the distal renal tubules and collecting ducts in the kidneys, thereby conserving water.

The ABCs of ADH

ADH secretion depends on plasma osmolality (concentration), which is monitored by hypothalamic neurons. Hypovolemia and hypotension are the most powerful stimulators of ADH release. Other stimulators include pain, stress, trauma, nausea, and the use of morphine, tranquilizers, certain anesthetics, and a positive-pressure breathing apparatus.

The thyroid secretes hormones that a person needs to grow and develop normally.

It's no secret

In addition to the trophic hormones—ACTH, TSH, LH, and FSH—the anterior pituitary gland secretes prolactin and GH. Prolactin stimulates milk secretion in lactating females. GH affects most body tissues. It triggers growth by increasing protein production and fat mobilization and decreasing carbohydrate use.

Thyroid gland

The thyroid gland, located in the anterior neck, secretes the iodine-containing hormones thyroxine (T_4) and triiodothyronine (T_3). Thyroid hormones are necessary for normal growth and development. They also act on many tissues by increasing metabolic activity and protein synthesis.

A good prognosis with treatment

Diseases of the thyroid are caused by thyroid hormone overproduction or deficiency and gland inflammation and enlargement. Most patients have a good prognosis with treatment. Untreated, thyroid disease may progress to an emergency, as in thyroid crisis or storm. It can also cause irreversible disabilities such as vision loss.

Parathyroid glands

There are four parathyroid glands located behind the thyroid gland. These glands secrete PTH, which helps regulate calcium levels and control bone formation.

Disorderly conduct

Disorders of the parathyroid gland involve hyposecretion of PTH resulting in a reduction of serum calcium that can lead to tetany and seizures, or hypersecretion of PTH, which results in elevated serum calcium levels that can lead to cardiac arrhythmias, muscle and bone weakness, and renal calculi.

Endocrine disorders

The endocrine disorders discussed in this chapter include:
• two adrenal disorders (Addison's disease and Cushing's syndrome)
• a pituitary disorder of water metabolism (diabetes insipidus) and a pancreatic disorder (diabetes mellitus)
• three thyroid gland disorders (simple goiter, hyperthyroidism, and hypothyroidism).

Addison's disease

Addison's disease, also called *adrenal hypofunction* or *adrenal insufficiency*, occurs in two forms: primary and secondary. It's a relatively uncommon disorder that occurs in people of all ages and in both sexes. Either primary or secondary Addison's disease can progress into adrenal crisis.

Primary report

The primary form of Addison's disease originates within the adrenal glands. It's characterized by decreased mineralocorticoid, glucocorticoid, and androgen secretion.

Outside influence

The secondary form of Addison's disease is caused by a disorder outside the gland, such as a pituitary tumor with corticotropin deficiency. In secondary forms of the disorder, aldosterone secretion may be unaffected.

Crisis!

Also called *addisonian crisis*, adrenal crisis is a critical deficiency of mineralocorticoids and glucocorticoids. It's a medical emergency that requires immediate, vigorous treatment. (See *Understanding adrenal crisis*.)

How it happens

In primary Addison's disease, more than 90% of both adrenal glands are destroyed. Massive destruction usually results from an autoimmune process whereby circulating antibodies attack adrenal tissue. Destruction of the gland may also be idiopathic (no known cause).

Other causes of primary Addison's disease include:
• tuberculosis
• removal of both adrenal glands
• hemorrhage into the adrenal gland
• neoplasms
• infections, such as human immunodeficiency virus infection, histoplasmosis, meningococcal pneumonia, and cytomegalovirus (CMV).

In rare cases, a familial tendency toward autoimmune disease predisposes a patient to Addison's disease and other endocrine disorders.

The signs and symptoms of primary adrenal insufficiency result from decreased glucocorticoid production. Signs and symptoms may develop slowly and stay unrecognized if production is adequate for the normal demands of life. It may progress to adrenal crisis when trauma, surgery, or other severe physical stress completely exhausts the body's store of glucocorticoids.

Secondary disease

Secondary Addison's disease may result from:
• hypopituitarism, which may lead to decreased corticotropin secretion (Usually it occurs when long-term corticosteroid therapy is abruptly stopped, because such therapy suppresses pituitary corticotropin secretion and causes adrenal gland atrophy.)
• removal of a nonendocrine corticotropin-secreting tumor
• disorders in hypothalamic-pituitary function that diminish the production of corticotropin.

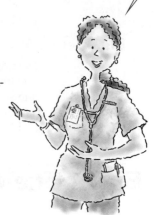

In primary disease, destruction of the adrenal glands usually results from an autoimmune process.

Now I get it!

Understanding adrenal crisis

Adrenal crisis (acute adrenal insufficiency) is the most serious complication of Addison's disease. It may occur gradually or suddenly.

Who's at risk

This potentially lethal condition usually develops in patients who:

- don't respond to hormone replacement therapy
- undergo extreme stress without adequate glucocorticoid replacement
- abruptly stop hormone therapy

- undergo trauma
- undergo bilateral adrenalectomy
- develop adrenal gland thrombosis after a severe infection (Waterhouse-Friderichsen syndrome).

What happens

In adrenal crisis, destruction of the adrenal cortex leads to a rapid decline in the steroid hormones cortisol and aldosterone. This directly affects the liver, stomach, and kidneys. The flowchart below illustrates what happens in adrenal crisis.

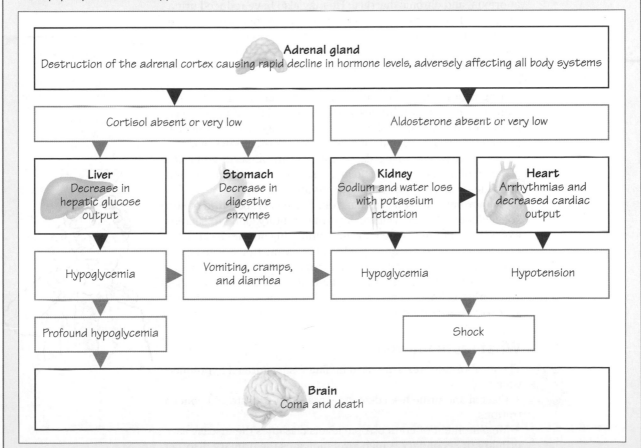

What to look for

These signs and symptoms may indicate Addison's disease:
- confusion
- fatigue
- GI disturbances and weight loss
- hyperkalemia
- hyperpigmentation
- hypoglycemia
- hyponatremia
- hypotension
- muscle weakness.

Patient history may reveal synthetic steroid use, adrenal surgery, or recent infection. The patient may complain of fatigue, light-headedness when rising from a chair or bed, cravings for salty food, decreased tolerance for even minor stress, anxiety, irritability, and various GI disturbances, such as nausea, vomiting, anorexia, and chronic diarrhea. He may also have reduced urine output and other symptoms of dehydration. Women may have decreased libido from reduced androgen production and amenorrhea.

Getting physical

During your examination, you may detect poor coordination, dry skin and mucous membranes, and sparse axillary and pubic hair in women. The patient's skin is typically a deep bronze, especially in the creases of the hands and on the knuckles, elbows, and knees. He may also have a darkening of scars, areas of vitiligo (an absence of pigmentation), and increased pigmentation of the mucous membranes, especially in the mouth.

Abnormal coloration results from decreased secretion of cortisol, a glucocorticoid, which causes the pituitary gland to secrete excessive amounts of melanocyte-stimulating hormone (MSH) and corticotropin. Secondary adrenal hypofunction doesn't cause hyperpigmentation because corticotropin and MSH levels are low.

With early diagnosis and treatment, the prognosis for a patient with either primary or secondary Addison's disease is good. (See *Treating Addison's disease.*)

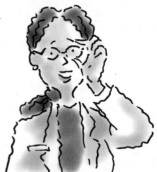

If your patient has a change in skin color, you may think it's jaundice. But if he has Addison's disease, discoloration is caused by a lack of cortisol.

What tests tell you

These laboratory tests are used in diagnosing adrenal hypofunction:
- Plasma and urine tests detect decreased corticosteroid concentrations.
- Measurement of corticotropin levels classifies the disease as primary or secondary. A high level indicates the primary disorder, and a low level points to the secondary disorder.

Battling illness

Treating Addison's disease

Lifelong corticosteroid replacement is the main treatment for patients with primary or secondary Addison's disease. In general, cortisone or hydrocortisone is given because they have a mineralocorticoid effect. Fludrocortisone, a synthetic drug that acts as a mineralocorticoid, may also be given to prevent dehydration and hypotension. Women with muscle weakness and decreased libido may benefit from testosterone injections, but they risk masculinizing effects.

In stressful situations, the patient may need to double or triple his usual corticosteroid dose. These situations include acute illness (because a fever increases the basal metabolic rate), injury, or psychologically stressful episodes.

Crisis control

Treatment for adrenal crisis is prompt I.V. bolus administration of 100 mg of hydrocortisone, followed by hydrocortisone diluted with dextrose in normal saline solution and given I.V. until the patient's condition stabilizes. Up to 300 mg/day of hydrocortisone and 3 to 5 L of I.V. normal saline solution may be required during the acute stage.

With proper treatment, the crisis usually subsides quickly, with blood pressure stabilizing and water and sodium levels returning to normal. Afterward, maintenance doses of hydrocortisone keep the patient's condition stable.

• Rapid corticotropin test (ACTH stimulation test) demonstrates plasma cortisol response to corticotropin. After obtaining plasma cortisol samples, an I.V. infusion of cosyntropin is administered. Plasma samples are taken 30 and 60 minutes later. If the plasma cortisol level doesn't increase, adrenal insufficiency is suspected.

Is it a crisis?

In a patient with typical symptoms of Addison's disease, these laboratory findings strongly suggest adrenal crisis:
• reduced serum sodium levels
• increased serum potassium, serum calcium, and blood urea nitrogen levels
• elevated hematocrit and elevated lymphocyte and eosinophil counts
• X-rays showing a small heart and adrenal calcification
• decreased plasma cortisol levels—less than 10 mcg/dl in the morning, with lower levels at night. (Because this test is time-consuming, crisis therapy shouldn't be delayed while waiting for results.)

Cushing's syndrome

Cushing's syndrome is a cluster of physical abnormalities that occur when the adrenal glands secrete excess glucocorticoids. It may also be caused by excessive androgen secretion. When glucocorticoid excess is caused by pituitary-dependent conditions, it's called *Cushing's syndrome*.

How it happens

Cushing's syndrome appears in three forms:
- primary, caused by a disease of the adrenal cortex
- secondary, caused by hyperfunction of corticotropin-secreting cells of the anterior pituitary gland
- tertiary, caused by hypothalamic dysfunction or injury.

Cancel the corticotropin

In about 70% of patients, Cushing's syndrome results from an excess of corticotropin. This leads to hyperplasia (excessive cell proliferation) of the adrenal cortex. Corticotropin overproduction may stem from:
- pituitary hypersecretion (Cushing's disease)
- a corticotropin-producing tumor in another organ, especially a malignant tumor of the pancreas or bronchus
- administration of synthetic glucocorticoids.

In the remaining 30% of patients, Cushing's syndrome results from a cortisol-secreting adrenal tumor, which is usually benign. In infants, the usual cause is adrenal carcinoma.

Administration of steroids during treatment can also lead to Cushing's syndrome.

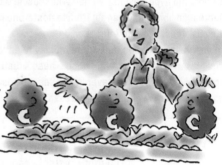

In most patients, Cushing's syndrome results from overproduction of the hormone corticotropin.

It's getting complicated

Complications associated with Cushing's syndrome are caused by the effects of cortisol, the principal glucocorticoid. These complications may include:
- osteoporosis and pathologic fractures, caused by increased calcium resorption from bone
- peptic ulcer, caused by increased gastric secretions, pepsin production, and decreased gastric mucus
- lipidosis (a disorder of fat metabolism)
- impaired glucose tolerance, caused by increased hepatic gluconeogenesis and insulin resistance.

Compromised

Frequent infections or slow wound healing due to decreased lymphocyte production and suppressed antibody formation may occur. Suppressed inflammatory response may mask infection.

Taking it to heart

Hypertension due to sodium and water retention is common in Cushing's syndrome. It may lead to ischemic heart disease and heart failure.

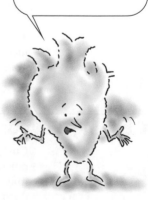

Hypertension is common in Cushing's syndrome and can cause ischemic heart disease and heart failure. Yikes!

Sexual and psychological complications

Menstrual disturbances and sexual dysfunction also occur because of increased adrenal androgen secretion. Decreased ability to handle stress may result in psychiatric problems, ranging from mood swings to psychosis.

What to look for

If your patient has some or all of these signs, he might have Cushing's syndrome:
- weight gain
- muscle weakness
- fatigue
- buffalo hump
- thinning extremities with muscle wasting and fat mobilization
- thin, fragile skin
- thinning scalp hair
- moon face and ruddy complexion
- hirsutism
- truncal obesity
- broad purple striae
- bruising
- impaired wound healing.

The prognosis depends on early diagnosis, identification of the underlying cause, and effective treatment. (See *Treating Cushing's syndrome*, page 256.)

What tests tell you

Diagnosis of Cushing's syndrome depends on a demonstrated increase in cortisol production and the failure to suppress endogenous cortisol secretion after dexamethasone is given. These tests may be performed:
- ACTH level determines whether Cushing's syndrome is ACTH dependent.
- Low-dose dexamethasone suppression test or 24-hour urine test determines the free cortisol excretion rate. Failure to suppress plasma and urine cortisol levels confirms the diagnosis.
- High-dose dexamethasone suppression test determines whether Cushing's syndrome results from pituitary dysfunction. If dexamethasone suppresses plasma cortisol levels, the test result is positive. Failure to suppress plasma cortisol levels indicates an adrenal tumor or a nonendocrine, corticotropin-secreting tumor. This test can produce false-positive results.
- Radiologic evaluation locates a causative tumor in the pituitary or adrenal glands. Tests include ultrasonography, computed tomography (CT) scan, and magnetic resonance imaging (MRI) enhanced with gadolinium.

Battling illness

Treating Cushing's syndrome

Restoring hormone balance and reversing Cushing's syndrome may require radiation, drug therapy, or surgery. Treatment depends on the cause of the disease.

A patient with pituitary-dependent Cushing's disease and adrenal hyperplasia may require hypophysectomy (removal of the pituitary gland) or pituitary irradiation. If these treatments are unsuccessful or impractical, bilateral adrenalectomy may be performed.

Diverse drugs

A patient with a nonendocrine corticotropin-producing tumor requires excision of the tumor, followed by drug therapy with mitotane, metyrapone, or aminoglutethimide. A combination of aminoglutethimide, cyproheptadine, and ketoconazole decreases cortisol levels and helps some patients. Aminog-

lutethimide, alone or with metyrapone, may also be useful in metastatic adrenal carcinoma.

An ounce of prevention

Before surgery, the patient needs to control edema, diabetes, hypertension, and other cardiovascular manifestations and prevent infection. Glucocorticoids given before surgery can help prevent acute adrenal insufficiency during surgery. Cortisol therapy is essential during and after surgery to combat the physiologic stress imposed by the removal of the pituitary or adrenal glands.

If normal cortisol production resumes, steroid therapy may gradually be tapered and eventually discontinued. However, the patient who has a bilateral adrenalectomy or a total hypophysectomy requires lifelong steroid replacement.

• Petrosal sinus sampling is the most accurate way to determine whether Cushing's syndrome is due to a pituitary tumor or some other cause. ACTH levels higher in the petrosal sinuses than in a forearm vein indicate the presence of a pituitary adenoma.

Diabetes insipidus

Diabetes insipidus is a disorder of water metabolism caused by a deficiency of ADH, also called *vasopressin*. The absence of ADH allows filtered water to be excreted in the urine instead of reabsorbed. The disease causes excessive urination and excessive thirst and fluid intake. It may first appear in childhood or early adulthood and is more common in men than in women.

How it happens

Some drugs as well as injury to the posterior pituitary gland can cause abnormalities in ADH secretion. A less common cause is a failure of the kidneys to respond to ADH. Lesions of the hypothalamus, infundibular stem, and posterior pituitary gland can also interfere with ADH synthesis, transport, or release. Lesions may be caused by brain tumor, removal of the pituitary gland (hypophysectomy), aneurysm, thrombus, immunologic disorder, or infection.

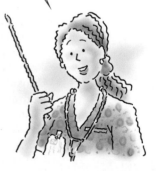

Without ADH, the kidneys are unable to reabsorb fluid, which causes excretion of large quantities of dilute urine and excessive thirst.

When ADH is absent

Normally, ADH is synthesized in the hypothalamus and then stored by the posterior pituitary gland. When it's released into the general circulation, ADH increases the water permeability of the distal and collecting tubules of the kidneys, causing water reabsorption. If ADH is absent, the filtered water is excreted in the urine instead of being reabsorbed, and the patient excretes large quantities of dilute urine. (See *Understanding ADH*.)

What to look for

The patient's history shows:
• abrupt onset of extreme polyuria (usually 4 to 16 L/day of dilute urine, but sometimes as much as 30 L/day)
• polydipsia (extreme thirst) and consumption of extraordinarily large volumes of fluid.

Now I get it!

Understanding ADH

In response to increased serum osmolality and reduced circulating volume, the posterior pituitary gland releases antidiuretic hormone (ADH). Circulating ADH alters permeability of the distal renal tubules and collecting ducts in the kidney, resulting in increased reabsorption of water. This decreases serum osmolality and increases circulating volume. Through a negative feedback mechanism, decreased osmolality and increased volume halt the release of ADH.

ADH release	Negative feedback halting release of ADH
Hemoconcentration or hypovolemia occurs.	Hemodilution or hypervolemia occurs.
Stimulation of receptors in posterior pituitary releases more ADH.	Stimulation of receptors in posterior pituitary decreases amount of ADH released.
Kidneys become more permeable to water.	Kidneys become less permeable to water.
Water is conserved and reabsorbed.	Water isn't reabsorbed and diuresis occurs.
Serum osmolality and urine output decrease and urine osmolality increases.	Serum osmolality and urine output increase and urine osmolality decreases.

In severe cases, fatigue occurs because sleep is interrupted by the need to void and drink fluids. Children often have enuresis (involuntary urination), sleep disturbances, irritability, anorexia, and decreased weight gain and linear growth.

Additional signs and symptoms may include:
- weight loss
- dizziness
- weakness
- constipation
- increased serum sodium and osmolality.

What lies underneath?

The prognosis is good for uncomplicated diabetes insipidus with adequate water replacement, and patients usually lead normal lives. However, when the disease is complicated by an underlying disorder such as cancer, the prognosis varies. (See *Treating diabetes insipidus.*)

One thing leads to another

Untreated diabetes insipidus can produce hypovolemia, hyperosmolality, circulatory collapse, loss of consciousness, and CNS damage. These complications are most likely to occur if the patient has an impaired or absent thirst mechanism.

A prolonged urine flow may produce chronic complications, such as bladder distention, enlarged calyces, hydroureter (distention of the ureter with fluid), and hydronephrosis (collection of urine in the kidney). Complications may also result from underlying conditions, such as metastatic brain lesions, head trauma, and infections.

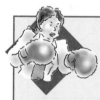

Battling illness

Treating diabetes insipidus

Until the cause of diabetes insipidus is identified and eliminated, patients are given various forms of vasopressin to control fluid balance and prevent dehydration. The following may be administered:
- Aqueous vasopressin is a replacement agent administered by subcutaneous injection. It's used in the initial management of diabetes insipidus after head trauma or a neurosurgical procedure.
- Desmopressin acetate, a synthetic vasopressin analogue, affects prolonged antidiuretic activ-ity and has no pressor ef-

fects. A long-acting drug, desmopressin acetate is administered intra-nasally.
- Lypressin is a synthetic vasopressin replacement given as a short-acting nasal spray. It has significant disadvantages, including a variable absorption rate, nasal congestion and irritation, nasal passage ulceration with repeated use, substernal chest tightness, coughing, and dyspnea after accidental inhalation of large doses.

What tests tell you

These tests distinguish diabetes insipidus from other disorders causing polyuria:

• Urinalysis reveals almost colorless urine of low osmolality (50 to 200 mOsm/kg of water, less than that of plasma) and low specific gravity (less than 1.005).

• Dehydration test differentiates ADH deficiency from other forms of polyuria by comparing urine osmolality after dehydration and after ADH administration. Diabetes insipidus is diagnosed if the increase in urine osmolality after ADH administration exceeds 9%. Patients with pituitary diabetes insipidus have decreased urine output and increased urine specific gravity. Those with nephrogenic diabetes insipidus show no response to ADH.

• Plasma or urinary ADH evaluation may be performed after fluid restriction or hypertonic saline infusion to determine whether diabetes insipidus originated from damage to the posterior pituitary gland (neurogenic) or failure of the kidneys to respond to ADH (nephrogenic). ADH levels are decreased in neurogenic diabetes insipidus and elevated in the nephrogenic type.

If the patient is critically ill, diagnosis may be based on these laboratory values alone:

• urine osmolality of 200 mOsm/kg
• urine specific gravity of 1.005
• serum osmolality of 300 mOsm/kg
• serum sodium of 147 mEq/L.

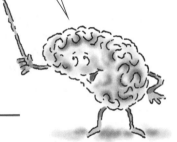

Diabetes insipidus is a pituitary disorder...

Diabetes mellitus

Diabetes mellitus is a disease in which the body doesn't produce or properly use insulin, leading to hyperglycemia.

The disease occurs in two primary forms:

type 1 (formerly referred to as *insulin-dependent diabetes mellitus*)

type 2 (formerly referred to as *non–insulin-dependent diabetes mellitus*), the more prevalent form.

Several secondary forms also exist, caused by such conditions as pancreatic disease, pregnancy (gestational diabetes mellitus), hormonal or genetic problems, and certain drugs or chemicals.

Diabetes mellitus affects about 6.3% of the U.S. population (18.2 million people); 5.2 million people are unaware that they have the disease. The incidence increases with age. Diabetes is the fifth leading cause of death in the United States.

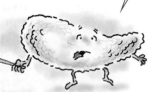

...while diabetes mellitus is a pancreatic disorder.

How it happens

Normally, insulin allows glucose to travel into cells. There, it's used for energy and stored as glycogen. It also stimulates protein synthesis and free fatty acid storage in adipose tissue. Insulin deficiency blocks tissues' access to essential nutrients for fuel and storage. The pathophysiology behind each type of diabetes differs.

Type 1 diabetes

In type 1 diabetes, the beta cells in the pancreas are destroyed or suppressed. Type 1 diabetes is subdivided into idiopathic and immune-mediated types. With the idiopathic type, patients have a permanent insulin deficiency with no evidence of autoimmunity.

In the immune-mediated type, a local or organ-specific deficit may induce an autoimmune attack on beta cells. This attack, in turn, causes an inflammatory response in the pancreas called *insulitis*.

Islet cell antibodies may be present long before symptoms become apparent. These immune markers also precede evidence of beta cell deficiency. Autoantibodies against insulin have also been noted.

By the time the disease becomes apparent, 80% of the beta cells are gone. Some experts believe that the beta cells aren't destroyed by the antibodies but that they're disabled and might later be reactivated.

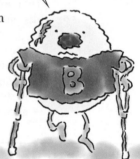

It looks like my days of producing insulin are over!

Type 2 diabetes

Type 2 diabetes may be caused by:
• resistance to insulin action in target tissues
• abnormal insulin secretion
• inappropriate hepatic gluconeogenesis (overproduction of glucose).

Type 2 diabetes may also develop as a consequence of obesity. (See *Understanding type 2 diabetes* and *Screening guidelines*, page 262.)

Secondary diabetes

Three common causes of secondary diabetes are:
• physical or emotional stress, which may cause prolonged elevation in levels of the stress hormones cortisol, epinephrine, glucagon, and GH (this, in turn, raises the blood glucose level and increases demands on the pancreas)
• pregnancy, which causes weight gain and high levels of estrogen and placental hormones
• use of adrenal corticosteroids, hormonal contraceptives, and other drugs that antagonize the effects of insulin.

Some viral infections have been implicated, such as CMV, adenovirus, rubella, and mumps.

Now I get it!

Understanding type 2 diabetes

Normally, in response to blood glucose levels, the pancreatic islets of Langerhans release insulin. In type 2 diabetes, problems arise when insufficient insulin is produced or when the body's cells resist insulin.

Normal body cell

Normally, insulin molecules bind to the preceptors on the body's cells. When activated by insulin, portals open to allow glucose to enter the cell, where it's converted to energy.

Diabetic body cell

In type 2 diabetes, the body's cells develop a resistance to insulin, making it more difficult for glucose to enter the cell.

As a result, cells don't get enough energy. This lack of energy causes glucose to build up in the blood vessels, resulting in damage to all body organs.

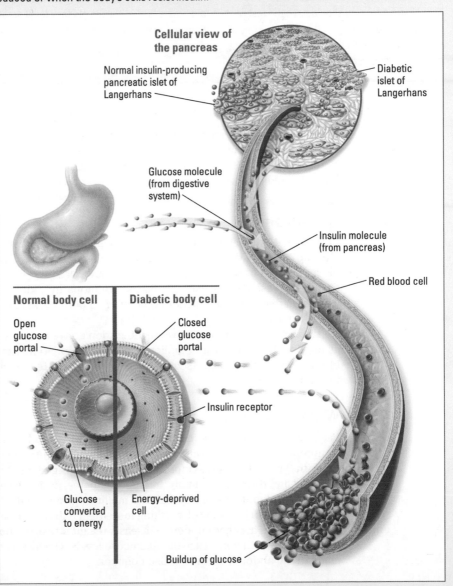

Cellular view of the pancreas

Normal insulin-producing pancreatic islet of Langerhans

Diabetic islet of Langerhans

Glucose molecule (from digestive system)

Insulin molecule (from pancreas)

Red blood cell

Normal body cell

Diabetic body cell

Open glucose portal

Closed glucose portal

Insulin receptor

Glucose converted to energy

Energy-deprived cell

Buildup of glucose

Screening guidelines

The guidelines below, from the American Diabetes Association, are also endorsed by the National Institutes of Health.

• Adults should be tested for diabetes every 3 years starting at age 45. Those who get a high glucose reading should have the test repeated on another day.

• People at increased risk may need to be tested earlier or more often. Higher-risk groups include Native Americans, Blacks, Asians, Hispanics, and anyone who is overweight or has high blood pressure, high cholesterol, or a strong family history of diabetes.

• The cutoff used for declaring someone as diabetic is a fasting plasma glucose level greater than or equal to 126 mg/dl on at least two occasions.

Acute danger

Two acute metabolic complications of diabetes are diabetic ketoacidosis (DKA) and hyperosmolar hyperglycemic nonketotic syndrome (HHNS). These life-threatening conditions require immediate medical intervention. (See *Understanding DKA and HHNS*.)

Chronic complications

Patients with diabetes mellitus also have a higher risk of various chronic complications affecting virtually all body systems. The most common chronic complications are cardiovascular disease, peripheral vascular disease, eye disease (retinopathy), kidney disease, skin disease (diabetic dermopathy), and peripheral and autonomic neuropathy.

Research shows that glucose readings don't have to be as high as previously thought for complications to develop. So meticulous blood glucose control is essential to help prevent acute and chronic complications.

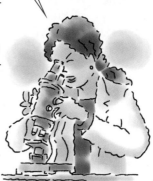

Research shows that glucose readings don't have to be as high as previously thought for complications to develop.

What to look for

Patients with type 1 diabetes usually report rapidly developing symptoms, including muscle wasting and loss of subcutaneous fat.

With type 2 diabetes, symptoms are generally vague and long-standing and develop gradually. In type 2 diabetes, patients generally report a family history of diabetes mellitus, gestational diabetes, delivery of a baby weighing more than 9 lb (4 kg), severe viral infection, another endocrine disease, recent stress or trauma, or use of drugs that increase blood glucose levels. Obesity, especially in the abdominal area, is also common.

Understanding DKA and HHNS

Diabetic ketoacidosis (DKA) and hyperosmolar hyperglycemic nonketotic syndrome (HHNS) are acute complications of hyperglycemic crisis that may occur with diabetes. If not treated properly, either may result in coma or death.

DKA occurs most often in patients with type 1 diabetes and may be the first evidence of the disease. HHNS occurs most often in patients with type 2 diabetes, but it also occurs in anyone whose insulin tolerance is stressed and in patients who have undergone certain therapeutic procedures, such as peritoneal dialysis, hemodialysis, tube feedings, or total parenteral nutrition.

Acute insulin deficiency (absolute in DKA; relative in HHNS) precipitates both conditions. Causes include illness, stress, infection and, in patients with DKA, failure to take insulin.

Buildup of glucose

Inadequate insulin hinders glucose uptake by fat and muscle cells. Because the cells can't take in glucose to convert to energy, glucose accumulates in the blood. At the same time, the liver responds to the demands of the energy-starved cells by converting glycogen to glucose and releasing glucose into the blood, further increasing the blood glucose level. When this level exceeds the renal threshold, excess glucose is excreted in urine.

Still, the insulin-deprived cells can't utilize glucose. Their response is rapid metabolism of protein, which results in loss of intracellular potassium and phosphorus and excessive liberation of amino acids. The liver converts these amino acids into urea and glucose.

As a result of these processes, blood glucose levels are grossly elevated. The aftermath is increased serum osmolarity and glycosuria (high amounts of glucose in the urine), leading to osmotic diuresis. Glycosuria is higher in HHNS than in DKA because blood glucose levels are higher in HHNS.

A deadly cycle

The massive fluid loss from osmotic diuresis causes fluid and electrolyte imbalances and dehydration. Water loss exceeds glucose and electrolyte loss, contributing to hyperosmolarity. This, in turn, perpetuates dehydration, decreasing the glomerular filtration rate and reducing the amount of glucose excreted in the urine. This leads to a deadly cycle: Diminished glucose excretion further raises blood glucose levels, producing hyperosmolarity and dehydration and finally causing shock, coma, and death.

DKA complication

All of these steps hold true for DKA and HHNS, but DKA involves an additional, simultaneous process that leads to metabolic acidosis. The absolute insulin deficiency causes cells to convert fats into glycerol and fatty acids for energy. The fatty acids can't be metabolized as quickly as they're released, so they accumulate in the liver, where they're converted into ketones (ketoacids). These ketones accumulate in the blood and urine and cause acidosis. Acidosis leads to more tissue breakdown, more ketosis, more acidosis, and eventually shock, coma, and death.

It takes both types

Patients with type 1 or type 2 diabetes may report symptoms related to hyperglycemia, such as:

- excessive urination (polyuria)
- excessive thirst (polydipsia)

- excessive eating (polyphagia)
- weight loss
- fatigue
- weakness
- vision changes
- frequent skin infections
- dry, itchy skin
- vaginal discomfort.

Patients with either type of diabetes may have poor skin turgor, dry mucous membranes related to dehydration, decreased peripheral pulses, cool skin temperature, and decreased reflexes. Patients in crisis with DKA may have a fruity breath odor because of increased acetone production. (See *Treating diabetes mellitus.*)

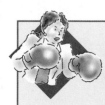

Battling illness

Treating diabetes mellitus

Effective treatment for diabetes optimizes blood glucose levels and decreases complications. In type 1 diabetes, treatment includes insulin replacement, meal planning, and exercise. Current forms of insulin replacement include single-dose, mixed-dose, split-mixed-dose, and multiple-dose regimens. The multiple-dose regimens may use an insulin pump.

Insulin action
Insulin may be rapid-acting (Humalog), fast-acting (Regular), intermediate-acting (NPH and Lente), or a premixed combination of fast-acting and intermediate-acting. Purified human insulin is used commonly today. Patients may inject insulin subcutaneously throughout the day or receive insulin through an insulin pump.

Inhaled insulin in patients with type 1 and type 2 diabetes is proving to be a viable alternative for patients who can't or don't want to take insulin injections before meals.

Personalized meal plan
Treatment for both types of diabetes also requires a meal plan to meet nutritional needs, to control blood glucose levels, and to help the patient reach and maintain his ideal body weight. A dietitian estimates the total amount of energy a patient needs per day based on his ideal body weight. Then she plans meals with the appropriate carbohydrate, fat, and protein content. For the diet to work, the patient must follow it consistently and eat at regular times.

In type 1 diabetes, the calorie allotment may be high, depending on the patient's growth stage and activity level. Weight reduction is a goal for the obese patient with type 2 diabetes.

Other treatments
Exercise is also useful in managing type 2 diabetes because it increases insulin sensitivity, improves glucose tolerance, and promotes weight loss. In addition, patients with type 2 diabetes may need oral antidiabetic drugs to stimulate endogenous insulin production and increase insulin sensitivity at the cellular level.

Treatment for long-term complications may include dialysis or kidney transplantation for renal failure, photocoagulation for retinopathy, and vascular surgery for large vessel disease. Pancreas transplantation is also an option.

What tests tell you

In nonpregnant adults, a diagnosis of diabetes mellitus may be confirmed by:
• symptoms of diabetes and a random blood glucose level equal to or above 200 mg/dl
• a fasting plasma glucose level equal to or greater than 126 mg/dl on at least two occasions
• a blood glucose level above 200 mg/dl on the second hour of the glucose tolerance test and on at least one other occasion during a glucose tolerance test.

Three other tests may be done:
• An ophthalmologic examination may show diabetic retinopathy.
• Urinalysis shows the presence of acetone.
• Blood tests for glycosylated hemoglobin monitor the long-term effectiveness of diabetes therapy. These tests show variants in hemoglobin levels that reflect average blood glucose levels during the preceding 2 to 3 months. The goal is to achieve a glycosylated hemoglobin of 7%.

Goiter

A goiter is an enlargement of the thyroid gland. It isn't caused by inflammation or neoplasm and isn't initially associated with hyperthyroidism or hypothyroidism. This condition is commonly referred to as nontoxic goiter. It's classified two ways:

☝ endemic, caused by lack of iodine in the diet

✌ sporadic, related to ingestion of certain drugs or food and occurring randomly.

Nontoxic goiter is most common in females, especially during adolescence, pregnancy, and menopause. At these times, the demand for thyroid hormone increases.

A toxic topic

Toxic goiter arises from long-standing nontoxic goiter and occurs in elderly people. The enlarged thyroid gland develops small rounded masses and secretes excess thyroid hormone.

How it happens

Nontoxic goiter occurs when the thyroid gland can't secrete enough thyroid hormone to meet metabolic needs. As a result, the thyroid mass increases to compensate. This usually overcomes mild to moderate hormonal impairment. (See *Simple, nontoxic goiter*, page 266.)

TSH levels in nontoxic goiter are generally normal. Enlargement of the gland probably results from impaired hormone pro-

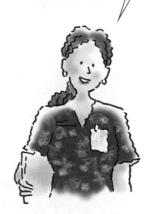

A goiter is an enlargement of the thyroid gland and can be either nontoxic or toxic.

duction in the thyroid and depleted iodine, which increases the thyroid gland's reaction to TSH.

Pass the iodine, please

Endemic goiter usually results from inadequate dietary intake of iodine, which leads to inadequate synthesis of thyroid hormone. In Japan, goiter resulting from iodine excess from excessive ingestion of seaweed has been found.

Some areas, called *goiter belts*, have a high incidence of endemic goiter. This is caused by iodine-deficient soil and water. Goiter belts include areas in the Midwest, Northwest, and Great Lakes region.

Too much of a good thing

Sporadic goiter commonly results from ingestion of large amounts of goitrogenic foods or use of goitrogenic drugs. These foods and drugs contain agents that decrease T_4 production. Such foods include rutabagas, cabbage, soybeans, peanuts, peaches, peas, strawberries, spinach, and radishes.

Goitrogenic drugs include:
• propylthiouracil
• iodides
• aminosalicylic acid
• cobalt
• lithium (Eskalith).

A closer look

Here's a more detailed account of what happens in goiter:
• Depletion of glandular organic iodine along with impaired hormone synthesis increases the thyroid's responsiveness to normal TSH levels.
• Resulting increases in both thyroid mass and cellular activity overcome mild impairment of hormone synthesis. Although the patient has a goiter, his metabolic function is normal.
• When the underlying disorder is severe, compensatory responses may cause both a goiter and hypothyroidism. (See *Treating nontoxic goiter.*)

What to look for

A nontoxic goiter causes these signs and symptoms:
• single or multinodular, firm, irregular enlargement of the thyroid gland
• stridor
• respiratory distress and dysphagia from compression of the trachea and esophagus

Simple, nontoxic goiter

A simple or nontoxic goiter involves thyroid gland enlargement that isn't caused by inflammation or a neoplasm. It's commonly classified as endemic or sporadic. Thyroid enlargement may range from a mildly enlarged gland to massive multinodular goiter.

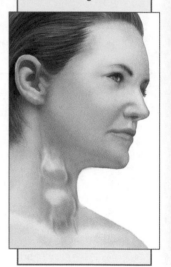

Battling illness

Treating nontoxic goiter

The goal of treatment for nontoxic goiter is to reduce thyroid hyperplasia.

Hormone replacement

Thyroid hormone replacement with levothyroxine, dessicated thyroid, or liothyronine is the treatment of choice because it inhibits thyroid-stimulating hormone secretion and allows the gland to rest. Small doses of iodide (Lugol's solution or potassium iodide solution) often relieve goiters caused by iodine deficiency.

Diet

Patients with sporadic goiters must avoid known goitrogenic drugs or food.

Radiation

Radioiodine ablation therapy to the thyroid gland is used to destroy the cells that concentrate iodine to make thyroxine.

Surgery

In rare cases of a large goiter unresponsive to treatment, partial removal of the thyroid gland may relieve pressure on surrounding structures.

• dizziness or syncope when arms are raised above the head due to obstructed venous return.

Bigger isn't always better

The enlarged thyroid gland frequently undergoes exacerbations and remissions, with areas of hypervolution and involution. Fibrosis may alternate with hyperplasia, and nodules containing thyroid follicles may develop. Production of excessive amounts of thyroid hormone may lead to thyrotoxicosis.

Complications from a large retrosternal goiter mainly result from the compression and displacement of the trachea or esophagus. Thyroid cysts and hemorrhage into the cysts may increase the pressure on and compression of the surrounding tissues and structures. Large goiters may obstruct venous return, produce venous engorgement and, rarely, cause collateral circulation of the chest.

With treatment, the prognosis is good for patients with either endemic or sporadic goiter.

Pressure from a goiter can displace or obstruct surrounding tissues and structures, such as the trachea and veins.

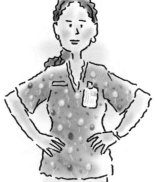

What tests tell you

These tests are used to diagnose nontoxic goiter and rule out other diseases with similar clinical effects:
• Serum thyroid hormone levels are usually normal. Abnormalities in T_3, T_4, and TSH levels rule out this diagnosis. Transient increased levels of TSH, which occur infrequently, may be missed by diagnostic tests.

- Thyroid antibody titers are usually normal. Increases indicate chronic thyroiditis.
- Radioactive iodine (^{131}I) uptake is usually normal but may increase in the presence of iodine deficiency or a biosynthetic defect.
- Urinalysis may show low urinary excretion of iodine.
- Radioisotope scanning identifies thyroid neoplasms.

Hyperthyroidism

When thyroid hormone is overproduced, it creates a metabolic imbalance called *hyperthyroidism* or *thyrotoxicosis*. Excess thyroid hormone can cause various thyroid disorders; Graves' disease is the most common. (See *Types of hyperthyroidism*.)

How grave is Graves' disease?

Graves' disease is an autoimmune disorder that causes goiter and multiple systemic changes. It occurs mostly in people ages 30 to 60, especially when their family histories include thyroid abnormalities. Only 5% of patients are younger than age 15.

Types of hyperthyroidism

In addition to Graves' disease, other forms of hyperthyroidism include toxic adenoma, thyrotoxicosis factitia, functioning metastatic thyroid carcinoma, thyroid-stimulating hormone (TSH)–secreting pituitary tumor, and subacute thyroiditis.

Toxic adenoma

The second most common cause of hyperthyroidism, toxic adenoma is a small, benign nodule in the thyroid gland that secretes thyroid hormone. The cause of toxic adenoma is unknown; its incidence is highest in elderly people. Clinical effects are similar to those of Graves' disease except that toxic adenoma doesn't induce ophthalmopathy, pretibial myxedema, or acropachy (clubbing of fingers or toes). A radioactive iodine (^{131}I) uptake and a thyroid scan show a single hyperfunctioning nodule suppressing the rest of the gland. Treatment includes ^{131}I therapy or surgery to remove the adenoma after antithyroid drugs restore normal gland function.

Thyrotoxicosis factitia

Thyrotoxicosis factitia results from chronic ingestion of thyroid hormone for TSH suppression in patients with thyroid carcinoma. It may also result from thyroid hormone abuse by people trying to lose weight.

Functioning metastatic thyroid carcinoma

This rare disease causes excess production of thyroid hormone.

TSH-secreting pituitary tumor

This form of hyperthyroidism causes excess production of thyroid hormone.

Subacute thyroiditis

A virus-induced granulomatous inflammation of the thyroid, subacute thyroiditis produces transient hyperthyroidism associated with fever, pain, pharyngitis, and tenderness of the thyroid gland.

Understanding thyroid storm

Thyrotoxic crisis—also known as *thyroid storm*—usually occurs in patients with preexisting, though often unrecognized, thyrotoxicosis. Left untreated, it's usually fatal.

Pathophysiology
The thyroid gland secretes the thyroid hormones triiodothyronine (T_3) and thyroxine (T_4). When T_3 and T_4 are overproduced, systemic adrenergic activity increases. The result is epinephrine overproduction and severe hypermetabolism, leading rapidly to cardiac, GI, and sympathetic nervous system decompensation.

Assessment findings
Initially, the patient may have marked tachycardia, vomiting, and stupor. If left untreated, he may experience vascular collapse, hypotension, coma, and death. Other findings may include a combination of irritability and restlessness, visual disturbance (such as diplopia), tremor and weakness, angina, shortness of breath, cough, and swollen extremities. Palpation may disclose warm, moist, flushed skin and a high fever that begins insidiously and rises rapidly to a lethal level.

Precipitating factors
Onset is almost always abrupt and evoked by a stressful event, such as trauma, surgery, or infection. Other less common precipitating factors include:
- insulin-induced ketoacidosis
- hypoglycemia or diabetic ketoacidosis
- stroke
- myocardial infarction
- pulmonary embolism
- sudden discontinuation of antithyroid drug therapy
- initiation of radioactive iodine therapy
- preeclampsia
- subtotal thyroidectomy with accompanying excessive intake of synthetic thyroid hormone.

Taken by storm

Thyrotoxic crisis, also known as *thyroid storm*, is an acute exacerbation of hyperthyroidism. It's a medical emergency that may lead to life-threatening cardiac, hepatic, or renal failure. Inadequately treated hyperthyroidism and stressful conditions, such as surgery, infection, toxemia of pregnancy, and DKA, can lead to thyrotoxic crisis. (See *Understanding thyroid storm*.)

How it happens

In Graves' disease, thyroid-stimulating antibodies bind to and stimulate the TSH receptors of the thyroid gland.

The trigger for this autoimmune response is unclear; it may have several causes. Genetic factors may play a part; the disease tends to occur in identical twins. Immunologic factors may also be the culprit; the disease occasionally coexists with other autoimmune endocrine abnormalities, such as type 1 diabetes mellitus, thyroiditis, and hyperparathyroidism.

Graves' disease is also associated with the production of several autoantibodies formed because of a defect in suppressor T-lymphocyte function.

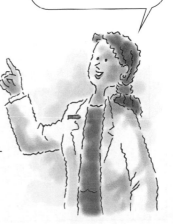

Graves' disease may result from genetic and immunologic influences.

Hyperthyroidism in hiding

In a person with latent hyperthyroidism, excessive iodine intake and, possibly, stress can cause active hyperthyroidism.

What to look for

The onset of signs and symptoms commonly follows a period of acute physical or emotional stress. The classic features of Graves' disease are:
- an enlarged thyroid gland
- exophthalmos (abnormal protrusion of the eye)
- nervousness
- heat intolerance
- weight loss despite increased appetite
- excessive sweating
- diarrhea
- tremors
- palpitations. (See *Recognizing hyperthyroidism.*)

Because thyroid hormones have widespread effects on almost all body systems, many other signs and symptoms are common with hyperthyroidism:
• CNS (most common in younger patients)—difficulty concentrating, anxiety, excitability or nervousness, fine tremor, shaky hand-

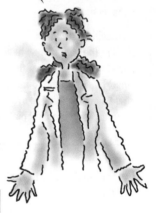

Signs and symptoms of Graves' disease commonly follow a period of acute physical or emotional stress.

Recognizing hyperthyroidism

Below illustrates the common signs of an overactive thyroid.

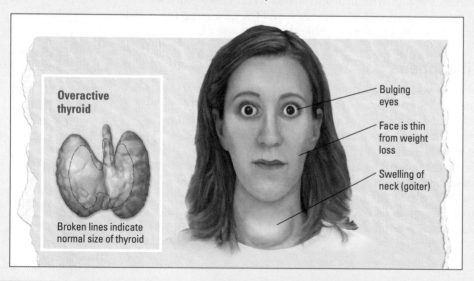

Overactive thyroid

Broken lines indicate normal size of thyroid

Bulging eyes

Face is thin from weight loss

Swelling of neck (goiter)

writing, clumsiness, emotional instability, and mood swings ranging from occasional outbursts to overt psychosis
• cardiovascular system (most common in elderly patients)—arrhythmias, especially atrial fibrillation; cardiac insufficiency; cardiac decompensation; and resistance to the usual therapeutic dose of digoxin
• integumentary system—vitiligo and skin hyperpigmentation; warm, moist, flushed skin with a velvety texture; fine, soft hair; premature graying; hair loss in both sexes; fragile nails; onycholysis (separation of distal nail from nail bed); and pretibial myxedema producing raised, thickened skin and plaquelike or nodular lesions
• respiratory system—dyspnea on exertion and, possibly, at rest and breathlessness when climbing stairs
• GI system—anorexia, nausea, and vomiting
• musculoskeletal system—muscle weakness, generalized or localized muscle atrophy, acropachy (soft-tissue swelling with underlying bone changes where new bone formation occurs), and osteoporosis
• reproductive system—menstrual abnormalities, impaired fertility, decreased libido, and gynecomastia (abnormal development of mammary glands in men)
• eyes—infrequent blinking, lid lag, reddened conjunctiva and cornea, corneal ulcers, impaired upward gaze, convergence, strabismus (eye deviation), and exophthalmos, which causes the characteristic staring gaze. (See *Treating hyperthyroidism*, page 272.)

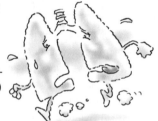

Breathlessness when taking a slow jog or climbing stairs could mean Graves' disease is affecting the respiratory system.

Touch tells you

On palpation, the thyroid gland may feel asymmetrical, lobular, and enlarged to three or four times its normal size. The liver may also be enlarged. Hyperthyroidism may cause tachycardia, commonly accompanied by a full, bounding, palpable pulse. Hyperreflexia is also present.

Listen and learn

Auscultation of the heart may detect an accelerated heart rate, which may prove to be paroxysmal supraventricular tachycardia or atrial fibrillation when verified by electrocardiogram, especially in elderly patients. Occasionally, a systolic murmur occurs at the left sternal border. Wide pulse pressures may be audible when blood pressure readings are taken. In Graves' disease, an audible bruit over the thyroid gland indicates thyrotoxicity but, occasionally, it may also be present in other hyperthyroid disorders. With treatment, most patients can lead normal lives.

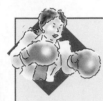

Battling illness

Treating hyperthyroidism

In Graves' disease, the most common hyperthyroid disorder, treatment consists of drug therapy, including radioactive iodine (^{131}I) therapy, and surgery.

Drug therapy

Antithyroid drugs, such as propylthiouracil and methimazole, are used for children, young adults, pregnant women, and patients who refuse other treatments.

Radioactive iodine therapy

A single oral dose of ^{131}I is the treatment of choice. This form of therapy is contraindicated during pregnancy; therefore, pregnancy should be ruled out before the initiation of treatment. Women should be cautioned to avoid pregnancy for 3 months after treatment. Radioactive iodine should be used cautiously in patients younger than age 20.

During treatment, the thyroid gland picks up the radioactive element as it would regular iodine. Subsequently, the radioactivity destroys some of the cells that normally concentrate iodine and produce thyroxine (T_4), thus decreasing thyroid hormone production and normalizing thyroid size and function.

In most patients, hypermetabolic symptoms diminish within 6 to 8 weeks. However, some patients may require a second dose.

Surgery

Partial thyroidectomy is indicated for patients younger than age 40 who have a very large goiter and whose hyperthyroidism has repeatedly relapsed after drug therapy, for pregnant patients, and for patients allergic to ^{131}I and other antithyroid drugs. The surgery involves removal of part of the thyroid gland, decreasing its size and capacity for hormone production.

Preoperative preparations

Preoperatively, the patient may receive iodide (Lugol's solution or potassium iodide solution), antithyroid drugs, or high doses of propranolol to help prevent thyroid storm. If normal thyroid function isn't achieved, surgery should be delayed and propranolol administered to decrease the risk of cardiac arrhythmias.

Other treatments

Therapy for hyperthyroid ophthalmopathy includes local applications of topical drugs but may require high doses of corticosteroids. A patient with severe exophthalmos that causes pressure on the optic nerve may require surgical decompression to reduce pressure on the orbital contents.

Treatment for thyrotoxic crisis includes giving an antithyroid drug, I.V. propranolol to block sympathetic effects, a corticosteroid to inhibit the conversion of triiodothyronine to T_4 and replace depleted cortisol, and an iodide to block the release of thyroid hormones. Supportive measures include the administration of nutrients, vitamins, fluids, and sedatives.

What tests tell you

These laboratory tests confirm Graves' disease:
- Radioimmunoassay shows increased serum T_3 and T_4 concentrations.
- TSH level is low in primary hyperthyroidism and elevated when excessive TSH secretion is the cause.
- Thyroid scan reveals increased uptake of ^{131}I.

Other tests show increased serum protein-bound iodine and decreased serum cholesterol and total lipid levels.

Hypothyroidism

In thyroid hormone deficiency (hypothyroidism) in adults, metabolic processes slow down. That's because of a deficit in T_3 or T_4, both of which regulate metabolism. The disorder is most prevalent in women and in people with Down syndrome. Its incidence in the United States is increasing in people ages 40 to 50.

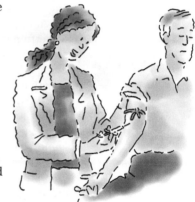

Low thyroid hormone levels in the blood may result from a problem in the pituitary gland, thyroid gland, or hypothalamus.

Primary or secondary

Hypothyroidism is classified as primary or secondary. The primary form stems from a disorder of the thyroid gland itself. The secondary form stems from a failure to stimulate normal thyroid function. This form may progress to myxedema coma, a medical emergency. (See *Understanding myxedema coma.*)

How it happens

Primary hypothyroidism has several possible causes:
- thyroidectomy
- inflammation from radiation therapy
- other inflammatory conditions, such as amyloidosis and sarcoidosis
- chronic autoimmune thyroiditis (Hashimoto's disease).

Secondary hypothyroidism is caused by a failure to stimulate normal thyroid function. For example, the pituitary may fail to produce TSH (thyrotropin) or the hypothalamus may fail to produce thyrotropin-releasing hormone.

Secondary hypothyroidism may also be caused by an inability to synthesize thyroid hormones because of iodine deficiency (usually dietary) or the use of antithyroid medications.

Understanding myxedema coma

A medical emergency, myxedema coma commonly has a fatal outcome. Progression is usually gradual but when stress, such as infection, exposure to cold, or trauma, aggravates severe or prolonged hypothyroidism, coma may develop abruptly. Other precipitating factors are thyroid medication withdrawal and the use of sedatives, opioids, or anesthetics.

What happens
Patients in myxedema coma have significantly depressed respirations, so their partial pressure of carbon dioxide in arterial blood may rise. Decreased cardiac output and worsening cerebral hypoxia may also occur. The patient becomes stuporous and hypothermic. Vital signs reflect bradycardia and hypotension. Lifesaving interventions are needed.

Throughout the organ-ization

Because insufficient synthesis of thyroid hormones affects almost every organ system in the body, signs and symptoms vary according to the organs involved as well as the duration and severity of the condition.

What to look for

The signs and symptoms of hypothyroidism may be vague and varied. Early ones include:

- energy loss
- fatigue
- forgetfulness
- sensitivity to cold
- unexplained weight gain
- constipation.

As the disease progresses, the patient may have:

- anorexia
- decreased libido
- menorrhagia (painful menstruation)
- paresthesia (numbness, prickling, or tingling)
- joint stiffness
- muscle cramping.

Other signs and symptoms include:

- CNS—psychiatric disturbances, ataxia (loss of coordination), intention tremor (tremor during voluntary motion), carpal tunnel syndrome, benign intracranial hypertension, and behavioral changes ranging from slight mental slowing to severe impairment
- integumentary system—dry, flaky, inelastic skin; puffy face, hands, and feet; dry, sparse hair with patchy hair loss and loss of the outer third of the eyebrow; thick, brittle nails with transverse and longitudinal grooves; and a thick, dry tongue, causing hoarseness and slow, slurred speech (see *Recognizing hypothyroidism*)
- cardiovascular system—hypercholesterolemia (high cholesterol) with associated arteriosclerosis and ischemic heart disease, poor peripheral circulation, heart enlargement, heart failure, and pleural and pericardial effusions
- GI system—achlorhydria (absence of free hydrochloric acid in the stomach), pernicious anemia, and adynamic (weak) colon, resulting in megacolon (extremely dilated colon) and intestinal obstruction
- reproductive system—impaired fertility
- eyes and ears—conductive or sensorineural deafness and nystagmus
- hematologic system—anemia, which may result in bleeding tendencies and iron deficiency anemia.

Recognizing hypothyroidism

Below illustrates the common signs of an underactive thyroid.

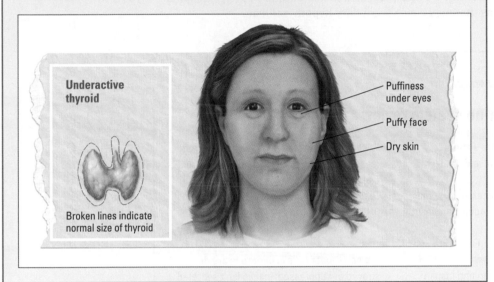

Underactive thyroid

Broken lines indicate normal size of thyroid

Puffiness under eyes

Puffy face

Dry skin

Going to extremes

Severe hypothyroidism, or myxedema, is characterized by thickening of the facial features and induration of the skin. The skin may feel rough, doughy, and cool. Other signs and symptoms are weak pulse, bradycardia, muscle weakness, sacral or peripheral edema, and delayed reflex relaxation time (especially in the Achilles tendon). Unless a goiter is present, the thyroid tissue itself may not be easily palpable.

Hyponatremia (low blood sodium) may result from impaired water excretion and from poor regulation of ADH secretion. (See *Treating hypothyroidism*.)

What tests tell you

Primary hypothyroidism is confirmed by an elevated TSH level and low serum free T_4 level. Additional tests may be performed:
• Serum TSH levels determine whether the disorder is primary or secondary. An increased serum TSH level is due to thyroid insufficiency; a decreased or normal level is due to hypothalamic or pituitary insufficiency.
• Serum antithyroid antibodies show elevated levels in autoimmune thyroiditis.

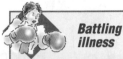

Battling illness

Treating hypothyroidism

Treatment consists of gradual thyroid hormone replacement with the synthetic hormone levothyroxine. Treatment begins slowly, particularly in elderly patients, to avoid adverse cardiovascular effects. The dosage is increased every 2 to 3 weeks until the desired response is obtained.

In underdeveloped areas, prophylactic iodine supplements have successfully decreased the incidence of iodine-deficient goiter.

No time to waste
Rapid treatment is necessary for patients with myxedema coma and those having emergency surgery. These patients need both I.V. administration of levothyroxine and hydrocortisone therapy.

- Perchlorate discharge tests identify enzyme deficiency within the thyroid gland. A deficiency will affect the uptake of iodine.
- Radioisotope scanning identifies ectopic thyroid tissue.
- Skull X-ray, CT scan, and MRI locate pituitary or hypothalamic lesions that may cause secondary hypothyroidism.

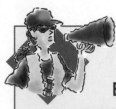

That's a wrap!

Endocrine system review

Understanding the endocrine system
- Hypothalamus helps control endocrine glands
- Adrenal cortex secretes mineralocorticoids, glucocorticoids, adrenal androgens, and estrogen
- Adrenal medulla produces epinephrine and norepinephrine
- Pancreas produces glucagon and insulin
- Pituitary gland secretes oxytocin and antidiuretic hormone
- Thyroid gland secretes thyroxine and triiodothyronine
- Parathyroid glands secrete parathyroid hormone

Causes of endocrine disorders
- Hypersecretion or hyposecretion of hormones
- Hyporesponsiveness of receptors of hormones
- Inflammation of gland
- Tumor of gland

Endocrine disorders
- *Addison's disease*—autoimmune disease (primary) that causes massive destruction of both adrenal glands

- *Cushing's syndrome*—typically results from excess corticotropin, which leads to hyperplasia of the adrenal cortex
- *Diabetes insipidus*—caused by deficiency of ADH
- *Diabetes mellitus*—occurs in two primary forms:
  - *type 1*—beta cells in pancreas are destroyed or suppressed; insulin isn't secreted
  - *type 2*—may be insulin resistance, overproduction of glucose, or abnormal insulin secretion
- *Goiter*—enlargement of the thyroid gland; occurs in two forms:
  - *nontoxic goiter*—thyroid gland is enlarged because it's unable to secrete enough thyroid hormone to meet metabolic needs
  - *toxic goiter*—occurs after long-standing nontoxic goiter
- *Hyperthyroidism*—autoimmune disorder that overproduces thyroid hormone
- *Hypothyroidism*—a thyroid deficiency that causes metabolic processes to slow down

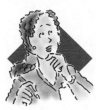

Quick quiz

1. A patient with weight loss, GI disturbances, dehydration, fatigue, and a craving for salty food probably has which disorder?

    A.   Cushing's syndrome
    B.   Addison's disease
    C.   Hypothyroidism
    D.   Diabetes insipidus

Answer: B. Other classic symptoms of Addison's disease are muscle weakness, anxiety, light-headedness, and amenorrhea.

2. Cushing's syndrome may be caused by which of the following?

    A.   Destruction of more than 90% of the adrenal gland
    B.   Thyroid hormone overproduction
    C.   Glucocorticoid excess
    D.   Insufficient antidiuretic hormone production

Answer: C. Cushing's syndrome is also caused by excess androgen secretion.

3. Which treatment is commonly indicated for type 2 diabetes mellitus?

    A.   High-fiber, low-fat diet
    B.   Fluid restriction
    C.   Insulin
    D.   Oral antidiabetic agent

Answer: D. Oral antidiabetic agents are commonly indicated for treatment of type 2 diabetes mellitus.

4. Nontoxic goiter is more common in:

    A.   females.
    B.   blacks.
    C.   older adults.
    D.   children.

Answer: A. The disorder occurs more commonly in females, especially during adolescence, pregnancy, and menopause, when the demand on the body for thyroid hormone increases.

Scoring

☆☆☆   If you answered all four items correctly, hooray! You're hyper-informed about hormones.

☆☆   If you answered three items correctly, exceptional! Your endocrine expertise is indeed endearing.

☆   If you answered fewer than three items correctly, just remember, never give up. Let's hope your glands will release test-taking hormones that will stimulate you to stick with it.

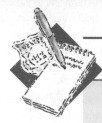

8

Renal system

Just the facts

In this chapter, you'll learn:

♦ the structures of the renal system

♦ how the renal system functions

♦ pathophysiology, signs and symptoms, diagnostic tests, and treatments for several common renal system disorders.

Understanding the renal system

The renal system, which consists of the kidneys, ureters, bladder, and urethra, serves as the body's water treatment plant by collecting the body's waste products and expelling them as urine. It also filters electrolytes.

The kidneys are located on each side of the vertebral column in the upper abdomen outside the peritoneal cavity. These compact organs contain an amazingly efficient filtration system—they filter about 45 gallons of fluid each day. The by-product of this filtration is urine, which contains water, electrolytes, and waste products. (See *A close look at the kidney*, page 280.)

It's all downhill from here

After it's produced by the kidneys, urine passes through the urinary system and is expelled from the body. Other structures of the renal system, extending downward from the kidneys, include:
• ureters—16″ to 18″ (40.5- to 45.5-cm) muscular tubes that contract rhythmically (peristaltic action) to transport urine from each kidney to the bladder
• urinary bladder—a sac with muscular walls that collects and holds urine (300 to 500 ml) that's expelled from the ureters every few seconds

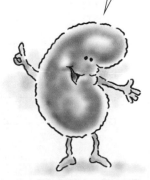

I filter about 45 gallons of fluid per day!

A close look at the kidney

Illustrated below is a kidney along with an enlargement of a nephron, the kidney's functional unit. Major structures of the kidney include:

• medulla—inner portion of the kidney, made up of renal pyramids and tubular structures
• renal artery—supplies blood to the kidney
• renal pyramid—channels output to renal pelvis for excretion
• renal calyx—channels formed urine from the renal pyramids to the renal pelvis
• renal vein—about 99% of filtered blood is reabsorbed and circulated through the renal vein back to the general circulation; the remaining 1%, which contains waste products, undergoes further processing in the kidney
• renal pelvis—after blood that contains waste products is processed in the kidney, formed urine is channeled to the renal pelvis
• ureter—tube that terminates in the urethra; urine enters the urethra for excretion
• cortex—outer layer of the kidney.

Note the nephron

The nephron is the functional and structural unit of the kidney. Each kidney contains about 1 million nephrons. Its two main activities are selective reabsorption and secretion of ions and mechanical filtration of fluids, wastes, electrolytes, and acids and bases.

Components of the nephron include:

• glomerulus—a network of twisted capillaries which acts as a filter for the passage of protein-free and red blood cell–free filtrate to Bowman's capsule
• Bowman's capsule—contains the glomerulus and acts as a reservoir for glomerular filtrate
• proximal convoluted tubule—site of reabsorption of glucose, amino acids, metabolites, and electrolytes from filtrate; reabsorbed substances return to circulation
• loop of Henle—a U-shaped nephron tubule located in the medulla and extending from the proximal convoluted tubule to the distal convoluted tubule; site for further concentration of filtrate through reabsorption
• distal convoluted tubule—site from which filtrate enters the collecting tubule
• collecting tubule—releases urine.

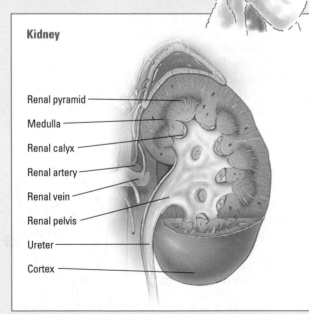

Kidney

- Renal pyramid
- Medulla
- Renal calyx
- Renal artery
- Renal vein
- Renal pelvis
- Ureter
- Cortex

Nephron

- Glomerulus
- Bowman's capsule
- Efferent arteriole
- Afferent arteriole
- Proximal convoluted tubule
- Renal artery
- Renal vein
- Peritubular capillaries
- Loop of Henle
- Collecting tubule

- urethra—a narrow passageway, surrounded by the prostate gland in men, from the bladder to the outside of the body through which urine is excreted.

Renal labor

Vital functions that the kidneys perform include:
- maintaining fluid and acid-base balance as well as regulating electrolyte concentration
- detoxifying the blood and eliminating wastes
- regulating blood pressure
- aiding red blood cell (RBC) production (erythropoiesis)
- regulating vitamin D and calcium formation.

Maintaining fluid and acid-base balance

Two important kidney functions are maintaining fluid and acid-base balance.

Fluid balance

The kidneys maintain fluid balance in the body by regulating the amount and makeup of the fluids inside and around the cells.

At the exchange

The kidneys maintain the volume and composition of extracellular and, to a lesser extent, intracellular fluid by continuously exchanging water and solutes, such as hydrogen, sodium, potassium, chloride, bicarbonate, sulfate, and phosphate ions, across their cell membranes.

Hormones...sometimes a help...

Hormones partially control the kidneys' role in fluid balance. This control depends on the response of specialized sensory nerve endings (osmoreceptors) to changes in osmolality (the ionic, or solute, concentration of a solution).

The two hormones involved are:
- antidiuretic hormone (ADH), produced by the pituitary gland
- aldosterone, produced by the adrenal cortex.

...sometimes a hindrance

Problems in hormone concentration may cause fluctuations in sodium and potassium concentrations that, in turn, may lead to hypertension.

The ABC's of ADH

ADH alters the collecting tubules' permeability to water. When ADH concentration in plasma is high, the tubules are most perme-

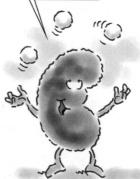

Regulating, balancing, detoxifying— no wonder the body finds me vital.

able to water. This causes more water to be absorbed, creating a highly concentrated but small volume of urine that has a high specific gravity. If ADH concentration is low, the tubules are less permeable to water. This causes more water to be excreted, creating a larger volume of less concentrated urine with a low specific gravity.

All that's known about aldosterone

Aldosterone is produced and released by the adrenal cortex. Aldosterone regulates water reabsorption by the distal tubules and changes urine concentration by increasing sodium reabsorption. A high plasma aldosterone concentration increases sodium and water reabsorption by the tubules and decreases sodium and water excretion in the urine. A low plasma aldosterone concentration promotes sodium and water excretion.

Aldosterone helps control the secretion of potassium by the distal tubules. A high aldosterone concentration increases the excretion of potassium. Other factors that affect potassium secretion include:
• the amount of potassium ingested
• the number of hydrogen ions secreted
• potassium levels in the cells
• the amount of sodium in the distal tubule
• the glomerular filtration rate (GFR), the rate at which plasma is filtered as it flows through the glomerular capillary filtration membrane.

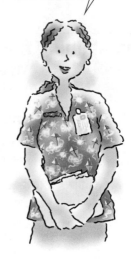

Aldosterone regulates sodium and water retention.

Going against the current

The kidneys concentrate urine through the countercurrent exchange system. In this system, fluid flows in opposite directions through parallel tubes, up and down parallel sides of the loops of Henle. A concentration gradient causes fluid exchange; the longer the loop, the greater the concentration gradient.

Acid-base balance

To regulate acid-base balance, the kidneys:
• secrete hydrogen ions
• reabsorb sodium and bicarbonate ions
• acidify phosphate salts
• produce ammonia.

Earning a PhD in pH balance

All of these regulating activities keep the blood at its normal pH of 7.35 to 7.45. Acidosis occurs when the pH falls below 7.35, and alkalosis occurs when the pH rises above 7.45.

Waste collection

The kidneys collect and eliminate wastes from the body in a three-step process:

☝ *Glomerular filtration*—The *glomeruli*, a collection of nephron capillaries, filter blood flowing through them to form filtrate.

✌ *Tubular reabsorption*—Next, the tubules (minute canals that make up the nephron) re-absorb the filtered fluid in surrounding blood vessels.

🖐 *Tubular secretion*—The filtered substance, known as *glomerular filtrate*, passes through the tubules to the collecting tubules and ducts.

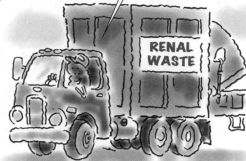

How do I go about waste collection? Easy. First, I get to work by filtering the blood.

RENAL WASTE

Clear the way

Clearance is the complete removal of a substance from the blood—commonly described in terms of the amount of blood that can be cleared in a specific amount of time. For example, creatinine clearance is the volume of blood in milliliters that the kidneys can clear of creatinine in 1 minute.

Some substances are filtered out of the blood by the glomeruli. Dissolved substances that remain in the fluid may be reabsorbed by the renal tubular cells. (See *Understanding the glomerular filtration rate.*)

Understanding the glomerular filtration rate

The glomerular filtration rate (GFR) is the rate at which the glomeruli filter blood. The normal GFR is about 120 ml/minute. GFR depends on:
• permeability of capillary walls
• vascular pressure
• filtration pressure.

GFR and clearance
Clearance is the complete removal of a substance from the blood. The most accurate measure of glomerular filtration is creatinine clearance, because creatinine is filtered by the glomeruli but not reabsorbed by the tubules. Creatinine is a waste product of skeletal muscles.

Equal to, greater than, or less than
Here's more about how the GFR affects clearance measurements for a substance in the blood:
• If the tubules neither reabsorb nor secrete the substance—as happens with creatinine—clearance equals the GFR.
• If the tubules reabsorb the substance, clearance is less than the GFR.
• If the tubules secrete the substance, clearance exceeds the GFR.
• If the tubules reabsorb and secrete the substance, clearance may be less than, equal to, or greater than the GFR.

Too little, too late

In a patient whose kidneys have shrunk from disease, healthy nephrons (the filtering units of the kidney) enlarge to compensate. However, as nephron damage progresses, the enlargement can no longer adequately compensate, and the GFR slows.

Don't saturate the system

The amount of a substance that's reabsorbed or secreted depends on the substance's maximum tubular transport capacity—the maximum amount of a substance that can be reabsorbed or secreted in 1 minute without saturating the renal system.

For example, in diabetes mellitus, excess glucose in the blood overwhelms the renal tubules and causes glucose to appear in the urine (glycosuria). In other cases, when glomeruli are damaged, protein appears in the urine (proteinuria) because the large protein molecules pass into the urine instead of being reabsorbed.

Blood pressure regulation

The kidneys help regulate blood pressure by producing and secreting the enzyme renin in response to an actual or perceived decline in extracellular fluid volume. Renin, in turn, forms angiotensin I, which is converted to the more potent vasopressor, angiotensin II.

Angiotensin II raises low arterial blood pressure levels by:
• increasing peripheral vasoconstriction
• stimulating aldosterone secretion.

The increase in aldosterone promotes the reabsorption of sodium and water to correct the fluid deficit and inadequate blood flow (renal ischemia).

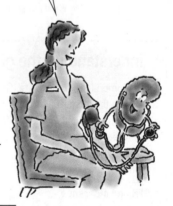

I do my part in blood pressure regulation, too. If I see it getting low, I give it some renin.

Hypertension: A serious threat

Hypertension can stem from a fluid and electrolyte imbalance as well as renin-angiotensin hyperactivity. High blood pressure can damage blood vessels as well as cause hardening of the kidneys (nephrosclerosis), one of the leading causes of chronic renal failure.

RBC production

Erythropoietin is a hormone that prompts the bone marrow to increase RBC production.

"Eryth"-ing you need to know about erythropoietin

The kidneys secrete erythropoietin when the oxygen supply in blood circulating through the tissues drops. Loss of renal function results in chronic anemia and insufficient calcium levels (hypocalcemia) because of a decrease in erythropoietin.

Vitamin D regulation and calcium formation

The kidneys help convert vitamin D to its active form. Active vitamin D helps regulate calcium and phosphorus balance and bone metabolism. When the kidneys fail, hypocalcemia and hypophosphatemia occur.

Renal disorders

The renal disorders discussed in this chapter include:
- acute tubular necrosis
- benign prostatic hyperplasia
- glomerulonephritis
- hydronephrosis
- prostatitis
- renal calculi (kidney stones)
- renal failure (acute and chronic).

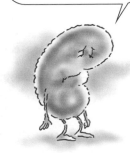

Trouble with my tubules can be traumatic—75% of all renal failure is caused by the destruction of my tubules.

Acute tubular necrosis

Acute tubular necrosis causes 75% of all cases of acute renal failure. Also called *acute tubulointerstitial nephritis*, this disorder destroys the tubular segment of the nephron, causing uremia (the excess accumulation of by-products of protein metabolism in the blood) and renal failure.

How it happens

Acute tubular necrosis may follow two types of kidney injury:

 ischemic injury, the most common cause

nephrotoxic injury, usually in such debilitated patients as the critically ill or those who have undergone extensive surgery.

The clock is ticking! The longer the disruption to blood flow, the worse the kidney damage.

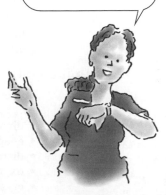

Disruption!

In ischemic injury, blood flow to the kidneys is disrupted. The longer the blood flow is interrupted, the worse the kidney damage. Blood flow to the kidneys may be disrupted by:
- circulatory collapse
- severe hypotension
- trauma

- hemorrhage
- dehydration
- cardiogenic or septic shock
- surgery
- anesthetics
- transfusion reactions.

Warning! Toxic materials

Nephrotoxic injury can result from:
- ingesting or inhaling toxic chemicals, such as carbon tetrachloride, heavy metals, and methoxyflurane anesthetics
- a hypersensitivity reaction of the kidneys to such substances as antibiotics and radiographic contrast agents.

Let's get specific

Some specific causes of acute tubular necrosis and their effects include:
- diseased tubular epithelium that allows glomerular filtrate (that should be excreted) to leak through the membranes and be reabsorbed into the blood
- obstructed urine flow from the collection of damaged cells, casts, RBCs, and other cellular debris within the tubular walls
- ischemic injury to glomerular epithelial cells, causing cellular collapse and poor glomerular capillary permeability
- ischemic injury to the vascular endothelium, eventually causing cellular swelling, and tubular obstruction.

A lesson on lesions

Deep or shallow lesions may occur in acute tubular necrosis. With ischemic injury, necrosis creates deep lesions, destroying the tubular epithelium and basement membrane (the delicate layer underlying the epithelium). Ischemic injury causes patches of necrosis in the tubules. Ischemia can also cause lesions in the connective tissue of the kidney.

With nephrotoxic injury, necrosis occurs only in the epithelium of the tubules, leaving the basement membrane of the nephrons intact. This type of damage may be reversible. (See *A close look at acute tubular necrosis.*)

Taking its toll

Toxicity takes a toll. Nephrotoxic agents can injure tubular cells by:
- direct cellular toxic effects
- coagulation and destruction (lysis) of RBCs
- disruption of normal function causing decreased perfusion
- oxygen deprivation (hypoxia)
- crystal formation of solutes.

Now I get it!

A close look at acute tubular necrosis

In acute tubular necrosis caused by ischemia, patches of necrosis occur, usually in the straight portion of the proximal tubules as shown below. In areas without lesions, tubules are usually dilated.

In acute tubular necrosis caused by nephrotoxicity, the tubules have a more uniform appearance as shown in the second illustration.

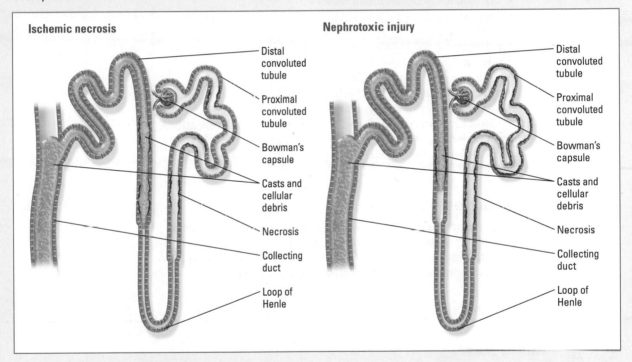

Ischemic necrosis

Nephrotoxic injury

Distal convoluted tubule

Proximal convoluted tubule

Bowman's capsule

Casts and cellular debris

Necrosis

Collecting duct

Loop of Henle

Getting complicated

There are several common complications of acute tubular necrosis:

• Infections (typically septicemia) complicate up to 70% of cases and are the leading cause of death.

• GI hemorrhage, fluid and electrolyte imbalance, and cardiovascular dysfunction may occur during the acute phase or the recovery phase.

• Neurologic complications are common in elderly patients and occur occasionally in younger patients.

• Excess blood calcium (hypercalcemia) may occur during the recovery phase.

What to look for

Early-stage acute tubular necrosis may be hard to spot because the patient's primary disease may obscure the signs and symptoms. The first recognizable sign may be decreased urine output, usually less than 400 ml/24 hours.

Other signs and symptoms depend on the severity of systemic involvement and may include:

- bleeding abnormalities
- vomiting of blood
- dry skin and mucous membranes
- lethargy
- confusion
- agitation
- edema
- fluid and electrolyte imbalances
- muscle weakness with hyperkalemia
- tachycardia and an irregular rhythm.

Mortality can be as high as 70%, depending on complications from underlying diseases. Nonoliguric forms of acute tubular necrosis have a better prognosis. (See *Treating acute tubular necrosis*.)

What tests tell you

Acute tubular necrosis is hard to diagnose except in advanced stages. These tests are commonly performed:

- Urinalysis shows dilute urine, low osmolality, high sodium levels, and urine sediment containing RBCs and casts.

Battling illness

Treating acute tubular necrosis

Acute tubular necrosis requires vigorous supportive measures during the acute phase until normal kidney function is restored.

- Initially, diuretics are given and fluids are infused to flush tubules of cellular casts and debris and replace lost fluids.
- Projected and calculated fluid losses require daily replacement.
- Transfusion of packed red blood cells is administered for anemia.
- Nonnephrotoxic antibiotics are given for infection.

- Hyperkalemia requires an emergency I.V. infusion of 50% glucose and regular insulin.
- Sodium bicarbonate may be needed to combat metabolic acidosis.
- Sodium polystyrene sulfonate is given by mouth or by enema to reduce potassium levels.
- Hemodialysis or peritoneal dialysis is used to prevent severe fluid and electrolyte imbalance and uremia.

- Blood studies reveal high blood urea nitrogen (BUN) and serum creatinine levels, low serum protein levels, anemia, platelet adherence defects, metabolic acidosis, and hyperkalemia.
- Electrocardiogram (ECG) may show arrhythmias from electrolyte imbalances and, with hyperkalemia, a widening QRS complex, disappearing P waves, and tall, peaked T waves.

Benign prostatic hyperplasia

Although most men older than age 50 have some prostate enlargement, in benign prostatic hyperplasia (BPH), the prostate gland enlarges enough to compress the urethra and cause urinary obstruction.

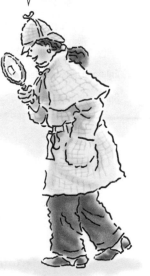

There's new evidence possibly linking a man's hormonal activity with benign prostatic hyperplasia.

How it happens

Recent evidence suggests a link between benign prostatic hyperplasia and hormonal activity. As men age, production of hormones that stimulate male characteristics (androgens) decreases and estrogen production increases. This causes an androgen-estrogen imbalance and high levels of dihydrotestosterone, the main prostatic intracellular androgen.

Other possible causes of prostate enlargement include:
- a tumor
- arteriosclerosis
- inflammation
- metabolic or nutritional disturbances.

Hormonal havoc

In BPH, here's what happens:
- Increased estrogen levels prompt androgen receptors in the prostate gland to increase.
- This causes an overgrowth of normal cells (hyperplasia) that begins around the urethra.
- Growth eventually causes areas of poor blood flow and tissue damage (necrosis) in adjacent prostatic tissue. The center and side lobes of the prostate usually grow but not the posterior lobe.
- As the prostate enlarges, it may extend into the bladder and decrease urine flow by compressing or distorting the urethra. (See *Prostatic enlargement*, page 290.)

Beyond benign

Urinary obstruction is a main complication that can lead to other complications. Enlargement that blocks the urethra and pushes up the bladder can stop urine flow and cause urinary tract infection (UTI) or calculi. Bladder muscles may thicken and a pouch (diverticulum) may form in the bladder that retains urine when the rest of the bladder empties.

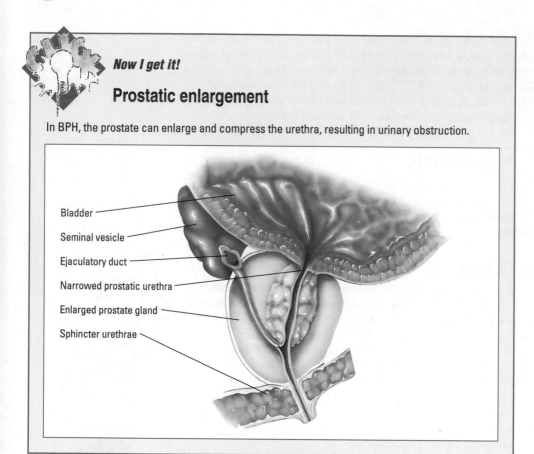

Now I get it!

Prostatic enlargement

In BPH, the prostate can enlarge and compress the urethra, resulting in urinary obstruction.

- Bladder
- Seminal vesicle
- Ejaculatory duct
- Narrowed prostatic urethra
- Enlarged prostate gland
- Sphincter urethrae

Other complications include:
- formation of a fibrous cord of connective tissue in the bladder wall (bladder wall trabeculation)
- detrusor muscle enlargement
- narrowing of the urethra
- incontinence
- acute or chronic renal failure
- distention of the innermost area of the kidney—the renal pelvis and calices—with urine (hydronephrosis).

What to look for

A patient's signs and symptoms depend on the extent of the prostate's enlargement and the lobes affected. Usually, the patient complains of a group of symptoms, known as *prostatism*. These include:
- decreased urine stream size and force
- interrupted urine stream

Battling illness

Treating benign prostatic hyperplasia

Conservative treatments for relieving symptoms of an enlarged prostate include:
- short-term fluid restriction to prevent bladder distention
- antimicrobials if infection occurs
- regular sexual intercourse to relieve prostatic congestion
- terazosin to improve urine flow rates
- finasteride to reduce prostate size.

Surgery
Surgery is the only effective therapy for acute urine retention, kidney distention (hydronephrosis), severe hematuria, recur-

rent urinary tract infections, or other intolerable symptoms. A transurethral resection—in which tissue is removed with a wire loop and an electric current—may be performed if the prostate weighs less than 2 oz (56.7 g).

Other transurethral procedures include vaporization of the prostate or a prostate incision with a scalpel or laser. Open surgical removal of the prostate is usually reserved for prostate cancers.

- urinary hesitancy causing straining and a feeling of incomplete voiding.

As the obstruction increases, the patient may report:
- frequent urination with nocturia
- dribbling
- urine retention
- incontinence
- blood in the urine.

An incompletely emptied and distended bladder is visible as a midline bulge, and an enlarged prostate is palpable with rectal digital examination.

Depending on the size of the prostate, the patient's age and health, and the extent of obstruction, this disorder may be treated surgically or symptomatically. (See *Treating benign prostatic hyperplasia*.)

What tests tell you

These tests are used to diagnose benign prostatic hyperplasia:
- Excretory urography may indicate urinary tract obstruction, hydronephrosis, calculi or tumors, and filling and emptying defects in the bladder.
- Elevated BUN and serum creatinine levels suggest impaired renal function.
- Urinalysis and urine culture show hematuria, pyuria, and UTI.
- Cystourethroscopy (performed when symptoms are severe to determine the best surgical procedure) can show prostate enlargement, bladder wall changes, calculi, and a raised bladder.
- Prostate-specific antigen test rules out prostatic cancer.

Glomerulonephritis

Glomerulonephritis is a bilateral inflammation of the glomeruli, commonly following a streptococcal infection.

In acute situations

Acute glomerulonephritis is most common in boys ages 3 to 7, but it can occur at any age. Up to 95% of children and 70% of adults recover fully; the rest, especially elderly patients, may progress to chronic renal failure within months.

This is all happening too quickly

Rapidly progressive glomerulonephritis most commonly occurs between ages 50 and 60. It may be idiopathic or associated with a proliferative glomerular disease such as poststreptococcal glomerulonephritis.

Goodpasture's syndrome, a type of rapidly progressive glomerulonephritis, is rare but occurs most commonly in men ages 20 to 30.

Chronic cases

Chronic glomerulonephritis is a slowly progressive disease characterized by inflammation, sclerosis, scarring, and eventual renal failure. It usually remains undetected until the progressive phase, which is irreversible.

How it happens

In nearly all types of glomerulonephritis, the epithelial layer of the glomerular membrane is disturbed.

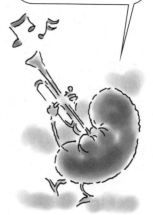

If this glomerulonephritis isn't detected, I'll soon be singing the blues!

Unwelcome lodger

Acute poststreptococcal glomerulonephritis results from an immune response that occurs in the glomerulus. The antigen, group A beta-hemolytic streptococci, stimulates antibody formation. As an antigen-antibody complex forms, it becomes lodged in the glomerular capillaries, causing an inflammatory response.

Glomerular injury occurs as a result of the inflammatory process when complexes initiate the release of immunologic substances that break down cells and increase membrane permeability. The severity of glomerular damage and renal insufficiency is related to the size, number, location, duration of exposure, and type of antigen-antibody complexes. (See *Immune complex deposits on the glomerulus.*)

What's so "good" about Goodpasture's?

In Goodpasture's syndrome, antibodies are produced against the pulmonary capillaries and glomerular basement membrane.

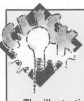

Now I get it!

Immune complex deposits on the glomerulus

The illustrations below show where the immune complex deposits appear in the glomerulus in glomerulonephritis.

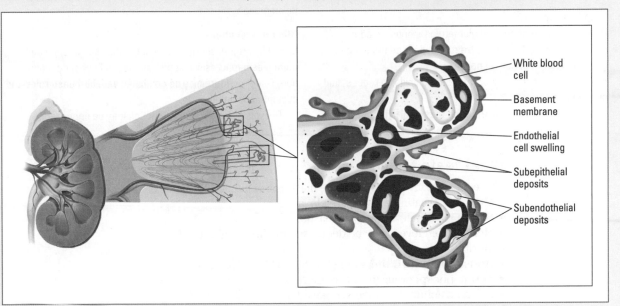

White blood cell

Basement membrane

Endothelial cell swelling

Subepithelial deposits

Subendothelial deposits

Glomerular filtration rate becomes reduced, and renal failure occurs within weeks or months.

What to look for

Possible signs and symptoms of glomerulonephritis include:
- decreased urination or oliguria
- smoky or coffee-colored urine
- shortness of breath
- orthopnea
- periorbital edema
- mild to severe hypertension
- bibasilar crackles on lung auscultation
- nausea
- malaise
- weight loss
- arthralgia. (See *Treating chronic glomerulonephritis*, page 294.)

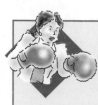

Battling illness

Treating chronic glomerulonephritis

Treatment focuses on the underlying disease.

Drug therapy
Drugs used to treat chronic glomerulonephritis include:
• antibiotics (7 to 10 days) to treat infections contributing to on-going antigen-antibody response
• diuretics, such as metalazone or furosemide, to reduce fluid overload
• vasodilators such as hydralazine to control hypertension

• corticosteroids to decrease antibody synthesis and suppress inflammation.

Other interventions
In rapidly progressive glomerulonephritis, the patient may require plasmaphoresis to suppress rebound antibody production. This procedure may be combined with corticosteroids and cyclophosphamide.
    Dialysis or kidney transplantation may be necessary.

What tests tell you

These blood study results aid in the diagnosis of glomerulonephritis:
• BUN and creatinine levels are elevated.
• Serum protein levels are decreased.
• Hemoglobin levels may be decreased in chronic glomerulo-nephritis.
• Antistreptolysin-O titers are elevated in 80% of patients.
• Serum phosphorous levels are increased.
• Serum calcium levels are decreased.
    These tests also help in the diagnosis of glomerulonephritis:
• Urinalysis reveals RBCs, white blood cells, mixed cell casts, and protein indicating renal failure.
• Kidney-ureter-bladder (KUB) radiography reveals bilateral kidney enlargement (acute glomerulonephritis).
• Renal biopsy confirms the diagnosis.

Hydronephrosis

An abnormal dilation of the renal pelvis and the calyces of one or both kidneys, hydronephrosis is caused by an obstruction of urine flow in the genitourinary tract.

How it happens

Almost any type of disease that results from obstruction of the urinary tract can result in hydronephrosis. The most common causes are:
• benign prostatic hyperplasia
• urethral strictures
• stenosis of the ureter or bladder outlet.

Less common causes include:
- congenital abnormalities
- abdominal tumors
- blood clots
- neurogenic bladder
- tumors of the ureter and bladder.

Instruction on obstruction

If the obstruction is in the urethra or bladder, hydronephrosis usually affects both kidneys; if the obstruction is in a ureter, it usually affects one kidney. Obstructions distal to the bladder cause the bladder to dilate and act as a buffer zone, delaying hydronephrosis. Total obstruction of urine flow with dilation of the collecting system ultimately causes complete atrophy of the cortex (the outer portion of the kidney) and cessation of glomerular filtration. (See *Renal damage in hydronephrosis*.)

Now I get it!

Renal damage in hydronephrosis

In hydronephrosis, the ureters dilate and kink, the renal pelvis dilates, and the parenchyma and papilla atrophy.

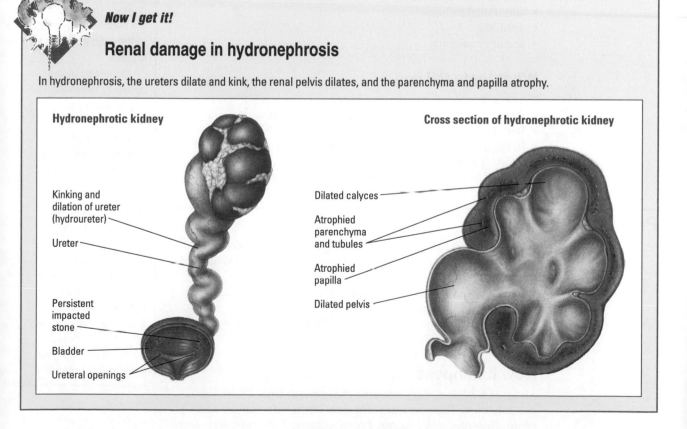

Hydronephrotic kidney

Kinking and dilation of ureter (hydroureter)

Ureter

Persistent impacted stone

Bladder

Ureteral openings

Cross section of hydronephrotic kidney

Dilated calyces

Atrophied parenchyma and tubules

Atrophied papilla

Dilated pelvis

From bad to worse

Untreated hydronephrosis can result in infection, or pyelonephritis, due to stasis that exacerbates renal damage and may create a life-threatening crisis. Paralytic ileus commonly accompanies acute obstructive disease of the urinary tract. (See *Treating hydronephrosis.*)

What to look for

Signs and symptoms depend on the cause of the obstruction. In mild cases, hydronephrosis produces either no symptoms or mild pain and slightly decreased urine flow. In more severe cases, it may produce severe, colicky renal pain or dull flank pain that may radiate to the groin and gross urinary abnormalities, such as hematuria, pyuria, dysuria, alternating polyuria and oliguria, and complete anuria.

Generally speaking

Other symptoms of hydronephrosis are more general and include:
- nausea and vomiting
- abdominal fullness
- dribbling
- urinary hesitancy.

What tests tell you

These tests are essential to the diagnosis of hydronephrosis:
- Excretory urography confirms hydronephrosis.
- Retrograde pyelography reveals hypdronephrosis.
- Renal ultrasonography reveals an obstruction and confirms hydronephrosis.
- Renal function studies demonstrate hydronephrosis.

Prostatitis

Prostatitis is an inflammation of the prostate gland. Types include:
- acute bacterial prostatitis, an ascending infection of the urinary tract
- chronic bacterial prostatitis, marked by recurrent UTI and persistent pathogenic bacteria
- prostatic inflammation without infection, the most common type of prostatitis.

How it happens

About 80% of bacterial prostatitis cases result from *Escherichia coli* infection. The remaining 20% result from infection by *Klebsiella, Enterobacter, Proteus, Pseudomonas, Serratia, Streptococ-*

Battling illness

Treating hydronephrosis

Treatment for hydronephrosis aims to preserve the patient's renal function and prevent infection.

Invasive interventions
Surgical removal of the obstruction is commonly necessary. Procedures, such as dilation for strictures of the urethra or prostatectomy for benign prostatic hyperplasia, are performed as soon as the patient is medically stable.

Inoperable obstructions may require decompression and drainage of the kidney, using a nephrostomy tube placed temporarily or permanently in the renal pelvis.

Other interventions
If renal function has already been affected, therapy may include a diet low in protein, sodium, and potassium. This is designed to stop the progression of renal failure before surgery.

Antibiotics are given if infection is present.

Now I get it!

Prostatic inflammation

The illustration below shows how an inflammed prostate can cause irritation in the urethra leading to urinary frequency and dysuria.

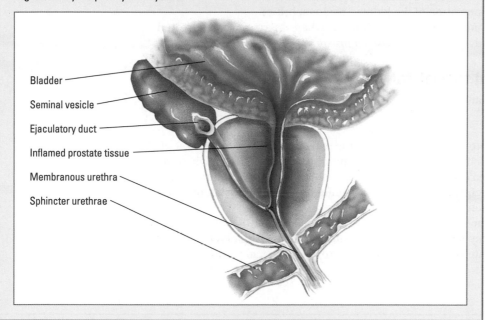

- Bladder
- Seminal vesicle
- Ejaculatory duct
- Inflamed prostate tissue
- Membranous urethra
- Sphincter urethrae

> Bacteria may spread to the prostate through the bloodstream.

cus, and *Staphylococcus* organisms, and diphtheroids, which are contaminants from normal flora of the urethra. (See *Prostatic inflammation*.)

On the road again

These organisms probably spread to the prostate gland by one of four methods:
- through the bloodstream
- from ascending urethral infection
- from invasion by rectal bacteria through the lymphatic vessels
- from reflux of infected urine from the bladder into prostatic ducts.

Invasion!

Chronic prostatitis is usually caused by bacterial invasion from the urethra. Less common means of acute or chronic infection are urethral procedures performed with instruments, such as cystoscopy and catheterization, and infrequent or excessive sexual intercourse.

Getting complicated

UTI is the most common complication of prostatitis. An untreated infection can progress to other problems, such as:
- prostatic abscess
- acute urine retention from prostatic edema
- inflammation of the kidney (pyelonephritis)
- inflammation of the epididymis, where spermatozoa are stored (epididymitis). (See *Treating prostatitis*.)

What to look for

Signs and symptoms vary according to the type of prostatitis.

Sneak attack

In acute bacterial prostatitis, the patient has the sudden onset of fever, chills, lower back pain, muscle pain (myalgia), pelvic or rectal area (perineal) fullness, joint pain (arthralgia), urinary urgency and frequency, cloudy urine, painful urination (dysuria), nocturia, and transient erectile dysfunction.

Some degree of urinary obstruction also may occur. The bladder may feel distended when palpated. When palpated rectally, the prostate is tender, abnormally hard, swollen, and warm.

Battling illness

Treating prostatitis

Treatment for prostatitis may include drug therapy, supportive measures, or surgery.

Drug therapy
Drugs used to treat prostatitis include:
- aminoglycosides in combination with penicillins or cephalosporins in severe acute cases
- co-trimoxazole to prevent chronic prostatitis
- co-trimoxazole, carbenicillin, nitrofurantoin, erythromycin, or tetracycline for *Escherichia coli* infections
- anticholinergics, analgesics, and minocycline, doxycycline, or erythromycin for nonbacterial prostatitis.

Supportive therapy
Supportive therapy includes bed rest, plenty of fluids, sitz baths, and stool softeners. Ejaculation or regular sexual intercourse using a condom to promote drainage of prostatic secretions is prescribed for chronic prostatitis.

Surgery
If drug therapy is unsuccessful, transurethral resection of the prostate may be done. This procedure may lead to retrograde ejaculation and sterility, so it usually isn't done on young men. Total prostatectomy is curative but may cause impotence and incontinence.

An extended stay

Chronic bacterial prostatitis may develop from acute prostatitis that doesn't clear up with antibiotics. Some patients are symptom-free, but usually the same signs and symptoms as in the acute form are present, although to a lesser degree.

Other signs and symptoms may include urethral discharge and painful ejaculation leading to sexual dysfunction. The prostate may feel soft, and a dry, crackling sound or sensation (crepitation) may be evident on palpation if prostatic calculi are present.

Things feel normal

The patient with nonbacterial prostatitis usually complains of dysuria, mild perineal or lower back pain, and nocturia. The patient may experience pain on ejaculation. The prostate gland usually feels normal on palpation.

What tests tell you

These tests confirm the diagnosis of prostatitis:
• X-ray of the pelvis may show prostatic calculi.
• Smears of prostatic secretions reveal inflammatory cells but usually no causative organism in nonbacterial prostatitis.
• Urodynamic evaluation may reveal detrusor muscle hyper-reflexia and pelvic floor myalgia from chronic spasms.

A firm diagnosis also depends on urine cultures, rectal examinations, and cultures for bacterial growth.

Renal calculi

Renal calculi, or *kidney stones*, may form anywhere in the urinary tract, but they usually develop in the renal pelvis or calices. Calculi form when substances that normally dissolve in the urine precipitate. They vary in size, shape, and number. (See *A close look at renal calculi*, page 300.)

About 1 in 1,000 Americans require hospitalization at some time for renal calculi. They're more common in men than women and rare in blacks and children.

How it happens

Renal calculi are particularly prevalent in specific geographic areas such as the southeastern United States. Although their exact cause is unknown, there are several predisposing factors:
• *Dehydration*—decreased water and urine excretion concentrates calculus-forming substances.
• *Infection*—infected, scarred tissue provides a site for calculus development. Calculi may become infected if bacteria are the nu-

Now I get it!

A close look at renal calculi

Renal calculi vary in size and type. Small calculi may remain in the renal pelvis or pass down the ureter as shown below left. A staghorn calculus, shown below right, is a cast of the innermost part of the kidney—the calyx and renal pelvis. A staghorn calculus may develop from a calculus that stays in the kidney.

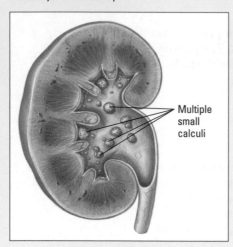

Multiple small calculi

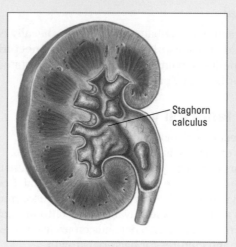

Staghorn calculus

cleus in calculi formation. Calculi that result from *Proteus* infections may lead to destruction of kidney tissue.

• *Changes in urine pH*—consistently acidic or alkaline urine provides a favorable medium for calculus formation.

• *Obstruction*—urinary stasis allows calculus constituents to collect and adhere, forming calculi. Obstruction also encourages infection, which compounds the obstruction.

• *Immobilization*—immobility from spinal cord injury or other disorders allows calcium to be released into the circulation and, eventually, to be filtered by the kidneys.

• *Diet*—increased intake of calcium or oxalate-rich foods encourages calculi formation.

• *Metabolic factors*—hyperparathyroidism, renal tubular acidosis, elevated uric acid (usually with gout), defective oxalate metabolism, a genetic defect in cystine metabolism, and excessive intake of vitamin D or dietary calcium may predispose a person to renal calculi.

This list of causes leaves no stone unturned!

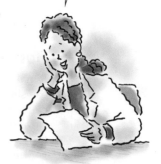

A delicate balance

Renal calculi usually arise because the delicate excretory balance breaks down.

Here's how it happens:

- Urine becomes concentrated with insoluble materials.
- Crystals form from these materials and then consolidate, forming calculi. These calculi contain an organic mucoprotein framework and crystalloids, such as calcium, oxalate, phosphate, urate, uric acid, struvite, cystine, and xanthine.
- Mucoprotein is reabsorbed by the tubules, establishing a site for calculi formation.
- Calculi remain in the renal pelvis and damage or destroy kidney tissue, or they enter the ureter.
- Large calculi in the kidneys may cause tissue damage (pressure necrosis).
- In certain locations, calculi obstruct urine, which collects in the renal pelvis (hydronephrosis). These calculi also tend to recur. Intractable pain and serious bleeding can result.
- Initially, hydrostatic pressure increases in the collection system near the obstruction, forcing nearby renal structures to dilate as well. The farther the obstruction is from the kidney, the less serious the dilation because the pressure is diffused over a larger surface area.
- With a complete obstruction, pressure in the renal pelvis and tubules increases, the GFR falls, and a disruption occurs in the junctional complexes between tubular cells. If left untreated, tubular atrophy and destruction of the medulla leave connective tissue in place of the glomeruli, causing irreversible damage.

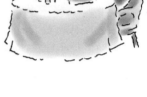

I'd like something... anything...to help prevent renal calculi, please!

What to look for

The key symptom of renal calculi is severe pain, which usually occurs when large calculi obstruct the opening of the ureter and increase the frequency and force of peristaltic contractions. Pain may travel from the lower back to the sides and then to the pubic region and external genitalia. Pain intensity fluctuates and may be excruciating at its peak.

The patient with calculi in the renal pelvis and calices may complain of more constant, dull pain. He also may report back pain from an obstruction within a kidney and severe abdominal pain from calculi traveling down a ureter. Severe pain is typically accompanied by nausea, vomiting and, possibly, fever and chills. (See *Treating renal calculi,* page 302.)

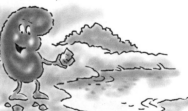

Oh, how I wish I could skip these stones! The pain they cause can be excruciating!

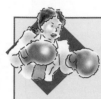

Battling illness

Treating renal calculi

Ninety percent of renal calculi are smaller than 5 mm in diameter and may pass naturally with vigorous hydration (more than 3 L/day). Other treatments may include drug therapy for infection or other effects of illness and measures to prevent recurrence of calculi. If calculi are too large for natural passage, they may be removed by surgery or other means.

Drug therapy

Drugs used to treat renal calculi include:
• antimicrobial agents for infection (varying with the cultured organism)
• analgesics, such as hydromorphone (Dilaudid) and morphine (Duramorph) for pain
• diuretics to prevent urinary stasis and further calculi formation
• thiazides to decrease calcium excretion into the urine
• methenamine (Hibrex) to suppress calculi formation when infection is present.

Preventive measures

Measures to prevent recurrence of renal calculi include:
• a low-calcium ion oxalate diet
• oxalate-binding cholestyramine for absorptive hypercalciuria
• parathyroidectomy for hyperparathyroidism
• allopurinol (Aloprim) for uric acid calculi
• daily oral doses of ascorbic acid to acidify the urine.

Removing calculi

Calculi lodged in the ureter may be removed by inserting a cystoscope through the urethra and then manipulating the calculi with catheters or retrieval instruments. A flank or lower abdominal approach may be needed to extract calculi from other areas, such as the kidney calyx or renal pelvis. Percutaneous ultrasonic lithotripsy and extracorporeal shock wave lithotripsy shatter the calculi into fragments for removal by suction or natural passage.

It's more than just a pain

Other signs and symptoms include:
• hematuria (when stones abrade a ureter)
• abdominal distention
• oliguria (from an obstruction in urine flow)
• dysuria
• frequency
• nausea and vomiting.

Most small calculi can be flushed out of a person's system by drinking lots of fluids.

What tests tell you

Diagnosis is based on clinical features and these tests:
• KUB radiography reveals most renal calculi.
• Excretory urography helps confirm the diagnosis and shows the size and location of calculi.
• Kidney ultrasonography is easy to perform, noninvasive, and nontoxic and detects obstructions not seen on the KUB radiography.

- Urinalysis may indicate pus in the urine (pyuria), a sign of UTI.
- 24-hour urine collection reveals calcium oxalate, phosphorus, and uric acid levels. Three separate collections, along with blood samples, are needed for accurate testing.
- Calculus analysis shows mineral content.
    These tests may identify the cause of calculus formation:
- Blood calcium and phosphorus levels detect hyperparathyroidism and show an increased calcium level in proportion to normal serum protein levels.
- Blood protein levels determine the level of free calcium unbound to protein.
- Differential diagnosis rules out appendicitis, cholecystitis, peptic ulcer, and pancreatitis as sources of pain.

Renal failure, acute

Acute renal failure is the sudden interruption of renal function. It can be caused by obstruction, poor circulation, or kidney disease. It's potentially reversible; however, if left untreated, permanent damage can lead to chronic renal failure.

How it happens

Acute renal failure may be classified as prerenal, intrarenal, or postrenal. Each type has separate causes. (See *Causes of acute renal failure*, page 304.)
- Prerenal failure results from conditions that diminish blood flow to the kidneys (hypoperfusion). Examples include hypovolemia, hypotension, vasoconstriction, or inadequate cardiac output. One condition, prerenal azotemia (excess nitrogenous waste products in the blood), accounts for 40% to 80% of all cases of acute renal failure. Azotemia occurs as a response to renal hypoperfusion. Usually, it can be rapidly reversed by restoring renal blood flow and glomerular filtration.
- Intrarenal failure, also called *intrinsic* or *parenchymal renal failure*, results from damage to the filtering structures of the kidneys, usually from acute tubular necrosis, a disorder that causes cell death, or from nephrotoxic substances such as certain antibiotics.
- Postrenal failure results from bilateral obstruction of urine outflow, as in prostatic hyperplasia or bladder outlet obstruction.

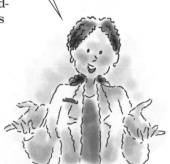

Postrenal failure is caused by any condition that blocks urine flow from both kidneys.

Causes of acute renal failure

Acute renal failure is classified as prerenal, intrarenal, or postrenal. All conditions that lead to prerenal failure impair blood flow to the kidneys (renal hypoperfusion), resulting in decreased glomerular filtration rate and increased tubular reabsorption of sodium and water. Intrarenal failure results from damage to the kidneys themselves; postrenal failure, from obstructed urine flow. This table shows the causes of each type of acute renal failure.

Prerenal failure
Cardiovascular disorders
- Arrhythmias
- Cardiac tamponade
- Cardiogenic shock
- Heart failure
- Myocardial infarction

Hypovolemia
- Burns
- Dehydration
- Diuretic overuse
- Hemorrhage
- Hypovolemic shock
- Trauma

Peripheral vasodilation
- Antihypertensive drugs
- Sepsis

Renovascular obstruction
- Arterial embolism
- Arterial or venous thrombosis
- Tumor

Severe vasoconstriction
- Disseminated intravascular coagulation
- Eclampsia
- Malignant hypertension
- Vasculitis

Intrarenal failure
Acute tubular necrosis
- Ischemic damage to renal parenchyma from unrecognized or poorly treated prerenal failure
- Nephrotoxins, including anesthetics such as methoxyflurane, antibiotics such as gentamicin, heavy metals such as lead, radiographic contrast media, and organic solvents
- Obstetric complications, such as eclampsia, postpartum renal failure, septic abortion, and uterine hemorrhage
- Pigment release, such as crush injury, myopathy, sepsis, and transfusion reaction

Other parenchymal disorders
- Acute glomerulonephritis
- Acute interstitial nephritis
- Acute pyelonephritis
- Bilateral renal vein thrombosis
- Malignant nephrosclerosis
- Papillary necrosis
- Periarteritis nodosa (inflammatory disease of the arteries)
- Renal myeloma
- Sickle cell disease
- Systemic lupus erythematosus
- Vasculitis

Postrenal failure
Bladder obstruction
- Anticholinergic drugs
- Autonomic nerve dysfunction
- Infection
- Tumor

Ureteral obstruction
- Blood clots
- Calculi
- Edema or inflammation
- Necrotic renal papillae
- Retroperitoneal fibrosis or hemorrhage
- Surgery (accidental ligation)
- Tumor
- Uric acid crystals

Urethral obstruction
- Prostatic hyperplasia or tumor
- Strictures

Going through phases

With treatment, each type of acute renal failure passes through three distinct phases:

 oliguric (decreased urine output)

 diuretic (increased urine output)

 recovery (glomerular filtration rate normalizes).

On the decrease...

The oliguric phase lasts from 2 weeks to several months. Oliguria is a decreased urine output (less than 400 ml/24 hours). Prerenal oliguria results from decreased blood flow to the kidney. Before damage occurs, the kidney responds to decreased blood flow by conserving sodium and water. After damage occurs, the kidney's ability to conserve sodium is impaired. Untreated prerenal oliguria may lead to acute tubular necrosis.

During this phase, BUN and creatinine levels rise, and the ratio of BUN to creatinine falls from 20:1 (normal) to 10:1. Hypervolemia occurs, causing edema, weight gain, and elevated blood pressure.

On the increase...

The diuretic phase may last from 1 to 3 weeks and is marked by urine output that can range from normal (1 to 2 L/day) to as high as 4 to 5 L/day. High urine volume has two causes:
• the kidney's inability to conserve sodium and water
• osmotic diuresis produced by high BUN levels.

During this phase, BUN and creatinine slowly rise, and hypovolemia and weight loss result. This phase lasts several days to 1 week. These conditions can lead to deficits of potassium, sodium, and water that can be deadly if left untreated. If the cause of the diuresis is corrected, azotemia gradually disappears and the patient improves greatly—leading to the recovery stage.

The recovery phase is reached when BUN and creatinine levels have returned to normal and urine output is between 1 and 2 L/day.

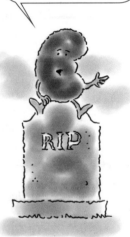

Acute renal failure is usually reversible with medical treatment but can be fatal without it.

Getting complicated

Primary damage to the renal tubules or blood vessels results in kidney failure (intrarenal failure). The causes of intrarenal failure are classified as nephrotoxic, inflammatory, or ischemic.

When the damage is caused by nephrotoxicity or inflammation, the delicate layer under the epithelium (basement membrane) becomes irreparably damaged, commonly proceeding to chronic renal failure. Severe or prolonged lack of blood flow (ischemia) may lead to renal damage (ischemic parenchymal injury) and excess nitrogen in the blood (intrinsic renal azotemia).

What to look for

The signs and symptoms of prerenal failure depend on the cause. If the underlying problem is a change in blood pressure and volume, the patient may have:
• oliguria
• tachycardia
• hypotension
• dry mucous membranes

- flat neck veins
- lethargy progressing to coma
- decreased cardiac output and cool, clammy skin in a patient with heart failure.

As renal failure progresses, the patient may show signs and symptoms of uremia, including:
- confusion
- GI complaints
- fluid in the lungs
- infection.

About 5% of all hospitalized patients develop acute renal failure. The condition is usually reversible with treatment, but if it isn't treated, it may progress to end-stage renal disease, excess urea in the blood (prerenal azotemia or uremia), and death. (See *Treating acute renal failure*.)

What tests tell you

These tests are used to diagnose acute renal failure:
- Blood studies reveal elevated BUN, serum creatinine, and potassium levels and decreased blood pH, bicarbonate, hematocrit (HCT), and hemoglobin levels.
- Urine specimens show casts, cellular debris, decreased specific gravity and, in glomerular diseases, proteinuria and urine osmolality close to serum osmolality. Urine sodium level is less than 20 mEq/L if oliguria results from decreased perfusion and more than 40 mEq/L if it results from an intrarenal problem.
- Creatinine clearance test measures the GFR and is used to estimate the number of remaining functioning nephrons.

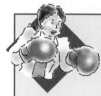

Battling illness

Treating acute renal failure

Supportive measures for acute renal failure include:
- a high-calorie diet, low in protein, sodium, and potassium
- fluid and electrolyte balance
- monitoring for signs and symptoms of uremia
- fluid restriction
- diuretic therapy during the oliguric phase
- prevention of infection
- renal-dose dopamine to improve renal perfusion.

Halting hyperkalemia
Meticulous electrolyte monitoring is needed to detect excess potassium in the blood (hyperkalemia). If symptoms occur, hypertonic glucose, insulin, and sodium bicarbonate are given I.V., and sodium polystyrene sulfonate is given by mouth or enema.

If these measures fail to control uremia, the patient may need hemodialysis, continuous renal replacement therapy, or peritoneal dialysis.

• ECG shows tall, peaked T waves, a widening QRS complex, and disappearing P waves if increased serum potassium (hyperkalemia) level is present.
• Other studies that help determine the cause of renal failure include kidney ultrasonography, plain films of the abdomen, KUB radiography, excretory urography, renal scan, retrograde pyelography, computed tomography scan, and nephrotomography.

Renal failure, chronic

Chronic renal failure, a usually progressive and irreversible deterioration, is the end result of gradual tissue destruction and loss of kidney function.

Blitz!

Occasionally, however, chronic renal failure results from a rapidly progressing disease of sudden onset that destroys the nephrons and causes irreversible kidney damage.

How it happens

Chronic renal failure typically progresses through four stages. (See *Stages of chronic renal failure.*)
    It may result from:
• chronic glomerular disease, such as glomerulonephritis, which affects the capillaries in the glomeruli
• chronic infections, such as chronic pyelonephritis and tuberculosis
• congenital anomalies such as polycystic kidney disease
• vascular diseases, such as hypertension and nephrosclerosis, which causes hardening of the kidneys
• obstructions such as renal calculi
• collagen diseases such as lupus erythematosus
• nephrotoxic agents such as long-term aminoglycoside therapy
• endocrine diseases such as diabetic neuropathy.

Fight to the finish

Nephron damage is progressive. Damaged nephrons can no longer function. Healthy nephrons compensate for destroyed nephrons by enlarging and increasing their clearance capacity. The kidneys can maintain relatively normal function until about 75% of the nephrons are nonfunctional.
    Eventually, the healthy glomeruli are so overburdened they become sclerotic and stiff, leading to their destruction as well. If this condition continues unchecked, toxins accumulate and produce potentially fatal changes in all major organ systems.

Stages of chronic renal failure

Chronic renal failure may progress through four stages:
• *Reduced renal reserve:* Glomerular filtration rate (GFR) is 35% to 50% of the normal rate.
• *Renal insufficiency:* GFR is 20% to 35% of the normal rate.
• *Renal failure:* GFR is 20% to 25% of the normal rate.
• *End-stage renal disease:* GFR is less than 20% of the normal rate.

Healthy nephrons work hard to keep me going, but, eventually, they're overwhelmed.

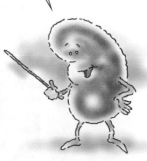

Getting complicated

Even if the patient can tolerate life-sustaining maintenance dialysis or a kidney transplant, he may still have anemia, nervous system effects (peripheral neuropathy), cardiopulmonary and GI complications, sexual dysfunction, and skeletal defects.

What to look for

Few symptoms develop until more than 75% of glomerular filtration is lost. Then the remaining normal tissue deteriorates progressively. Symptoms worsen as kidney function decreases. Profound changes affect all body systems. Major findings include:
- hypervolemia (abnormal increase in plasma volume)
- peripheral edema
- hyperphosphatemia
- hyperkalemia
- hypocalcemia
- azotemia
- metabolic acidosis
- anemia
- peripheral neuropathy.

Body count

Other signs and symptoms, by body system, include:
- *renal*—dry mouth, fatigue, nausea, hypotension, loss of skin turgor, listlessness that may progress to somnolence and confusion, decreased or dilute urine, irregular pulses, and edema
- *cardiovascular*—hypertension, irregular pulse, life-threatening arrhythmias, and heart failure
- *respiratory*—infection, crackles, and pleuritic pain
- *GI*—gum sores and bleeding, hiccups, metallic taste, anorexia, nausea, vomiting, ammonia smell to the breath, and abdominal pain on palpation
- *skin*—pallid, yellowish-bronze color; dry, scaly skin; thin, brittle nails; dry, brittle hair that may change color and fall out easily; severe itching; and white, flaky urea deposits (uremic frost) in critically ill patients
- *neurologic*—altered level of consciousness, muscle cramps and twitching, and pain, burning, and itching in legs and feet (restless leg syndrome)
- *endocrine*—growth retardation in children, infertility, decreased libido, amenorrhea, and impotence
- *hematologic*—GI bleeding and hemorrhage from body orifices, and easy bruising
- *musculoskeletal*—fractures, bone and muscle pain, abnormal gait, and impaired bone growth and bowed legs in children.

The progression of chronic renal failure can sometimes be slowed, but it's ultimately irreversible, culminating in end-stage renal disease. Although it's fatal without treatment, dialysis or a kidney transplant can sustain life. (See *Treating chronic renal failure.*)

What tests tell you

These tests are used to diagnose chronic renal failure:
• Blood studies show decreased arterial pH and bicarbonate levels, low HCT and low hemoglobin levels, and elevated BUN, serum creatinine, sodium, and potassium levels.
• Arterial blood gas analysis reveals metabolic acidosis.

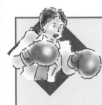

Battling illness

Treating chronic renal failure

Treatment for chronic renal failure may consist of one or more of these treatments, depending on the stage of failure.

Conservative measures
Conservative treatment includes:
• a low-protein diet to reduce end products of protein metabolism that the kidneys can't excrete
• a high-protein diet for patients on continuous peritoneal dialysis
• a high-calorie diet to prevent ketoacidosis (the accumulation of ketones, such as acetone, in the blood) and tissue atrophy
• sodium and potassium restrictions
• phosphorus restriction
• fluid restrictions to maintain fluid balance
• fat restrictions for patients with hyperlipidemia.

Drug therapy
Drugs used to treat chronic renal failure include:
• loop diuretics such as furosemide (if some renal function remains) to maintain fluid balance
• antihypertensives to control blood pressure and edema
• antiemetics to relieve nausea and vomiting
• histamine-2 receptor antagonists such as famotidine to decrease gastric irritation
• stool softeners to prevent constipation
• iron and folate supplements or red blood cell (RBC) infusion for anemia

• synthetic erythropoietin to stimulate the bone marrow to produce RBCs
• antipruritics, such as trimeprazine or diphenhydramine, to relieve itching
• aluminum hydroxide gel to lower serum phosphate levels
• supplementary vitamins, particularly B and D, and essential amino acids.

Dialysis
When the kidneys fail, kidney transplantation or dialysis may be the patient's only chance for survival. Dialysis options include:
• hemodialysis, which filters blood through a dialysis machine
• peritoneal dialysis, in which a catheter is placed in the peritoneal cavity for instillation of dialysate.

Emergency measures
Potassium levels in the blood must be monitored to detect hyperkalemia. Emergency treatment includes dialysis therapy, oral or rectal administration of cation exchange resins, such as sodium polystyrene sulfonate, and I.V. administration of calcium gluconate, sodium bicarbonate, 50% hypertonic glucose, and regular insulin.

Cardiac tamponade resulting from pericardial effusion may require emergency pericardiocentesis or surgery. Intensive dialysis and thoracentesis can relieve pulmonary edema and pleural effusion.

- Urine specific gravity becomes fixed at 1.010; urinalysis may show proteinuria, glycosuria, RBCs, leukocytes, casts, or crystals, depending on the cause.
- X-ray studies, including KUB radiography, excretory urography, nephrotomography, renal scan, and renal arteriography, show reduced kidney size.
- Renal biopsy is used to identify underlying disease.
- EEG shows changes that indicate brain disease (metabolic encephalopathy).

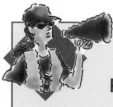

That's a wrap!

Renal system review

Understanding the renal system
The renal system collects the body's waste products and expels them as urine. The renal system includes:
- kidneys
- ureters
- urinary bladder
- urethra.

Kidneys
- Located on each side of the vertebral column in the upper abdomen outside the peritoneal cavity
- Work with the urinary system to collect the body's waste products and expel them as urine
- Filter about 45 gallons of fluid each day

Ureters
- Muscular tubes that contract rhythmically to transport urine from each kidney to the bladder

Urinary bladder
- A sac with muscular walls that collects and holds urine that's expelled from the ureters every few seconds

Urethra
- A narrow passageway from the bladder to the outside of the body through which urine is excreted

How the kidneys perform
- Maintain fluid and acid-base balance and regulate electrolyte concentration

- Detoxify the blood and eliminate wastes
- Regulate blood pressure
- Aid RBC production
- Regulate vitamin D and calcium formation

Controlling fluid balance
- Antidiuretic hormone: produced by the pituitary gland; controls the concentration of body fluids by altering the permeability of the kidneys
- Aldosterone: produced by the adrenal cortex; regulates water reabsorption by the distal tubules by increasing sodium reabsorption

Regulating acid-base balance
The kidneys:
- secrete hydrogen ions
- reabsorb sodium and bicarbonate ions
- acidify phosphate salts
- produce ammonia.

Collecting and eliminating waste
The kidneys:
- filter blood flowing through the glomeruli
- reabsorb filtered fluid through the tubules
- release the filtered substance from the tubules.

Regulating blood pressure
The kidneys:
- produce and secrete renin in response to a decline (actual or perceived) in extracellular fluid volume.

Renal system review (continued)

Producing RBCs
The kidneys:
• secrete erythropoietin (a hormone that prompts increased RBC production) when the oxygen supply in tissue blood drops.

Regulating vitamin D and calcium formation
• The kidneys help convert vitamin D to its active form.
• Active vitamin D helps regulate calcium and phosphorus.

Renal disorders
• *Acute tubular necrosis*—destruction of the tubular segment of the nephron, causing renal failure and uremia
• *Benign prostatic hyperplasia*—enlarged prostate gland that compresses the urethra and causes urinary obstruction

• *Glomerulonephritis*—bilateral inflammation of the glomeruli, commonly following a streptococcal infection
• *Hydronephrosis*—abnormal dilation of the renal pelvis and the calyces of one or both kidneys
• *Prostatitis*—inflammation of the prostate gland
• *Renal calculi*—substances that normally dissolve in the urine precipitate to form "kidney stones"
• *Renal failure, acute*—sudden interruption of renal function caused by obstruction, poor circulation, or kidney disease
• *Renal failure, chronic*—irreversible deterioration of tissue and eventual loss of kidney function

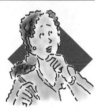

Quick quiz

1. Which of the following is the most accurate measurement of glomerular filtration?
    A. Blood pressure
    B. Intake and output
    C. Creatinine clearance
    D. BUN

Answer: C. This is because creatinine is only filtered by the glomeruli and not reabsorbed by the tubules.

2. Prerenal failure results from:
    A. bilateral obstruction of urine outflow.
    B. conditions that diminish blood flow to the kidneys.
    C. damage to the kidneys themselves.
    D. damage to the filtering systems of the kidneys.

Answer: B. One such condition, prerenal azotemia, accounts for between 40% and 80% of all cases of acute renal failure.

3. Which of the following is the main complication of benign prostatic hyperplasia?
    A. Urinary obstruction
    B. Renal calculi
    C. Prostatitis
    D. UTI

Answer: A. Depending on the size of the enlarged prostate and resulting complications, the obstruction may be treated surgically or symptomatically.

4.   The kidneys secrete erythropoietin when:
   A.   renin is secreted in response to a decrease in extra-cellular fluid volume.
   B.   calcium levels are insufficient.
   C.   vitamin D becomes inactive.
   D.   the oxygen supply in the blood circulating through the tissue drops.

Answer: D. Erythropoietin is secreted by the kidneys when there's a drop in the oxygen supply in tissue blood.

5.   Which factor can contribute to the formation of renal calculi?
   A.   Hypocalcemia
   B.   Changes in urine pH
   C.   Hypothyroidism
   D.   Hypophosphatemia

Answer: B. Urine that's consistently acidic or alkaline provides a favorable medium for stone formation.

Scoring

☆☆☆   If you answered all five items correctly, wow! Your ability to concentrate, absorb, and secrete data about the kidneys is amazing!

☆☆   If you answered four items correctly, fantastic! Your knowledge of things renal isn't venal.

☆   If you answered fewer than four items correctly, don't freak out. We recommend reading the chapter once more. After all, that's what reabsorption is all about.

9

Hematologic system

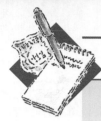

Just the facts

In this chapter, you'll learn:

♦ about blood and its components

♦ the function of blood

♦ pathophysiology, signs and symptoms, diagnostic tests, and treatments for common blood disorders.

Understanding blood

Blood is one of the body's major fluid tissues. Pumped by the heart, it continuously circulates through the blood vessels, carrying vital elements to every part of the body. Blood is made of:
• a liquid component—plasma
• cellular components—erythrocytes, leukocytes, and thrombocytes suspended in plasma.

A component list

Each of blood's components perform specific vital functions:
• Plasma carries antibodies and nutrients to tissues and carries wastes away.
• Erythrocytes, also called *red blood cells* (RBCs), carry oxygen to the tissues and remove carbon dioxide from them.
• Leukocytes, or *white blood cells* (WBCs), participate in the inflammatory and immune response.
• Thrombocytes, or platelets, along with the coagulation factors in plasma, are essential to normal blood clotting.
    A problem with any of these components may have serious and even deadly consequences.

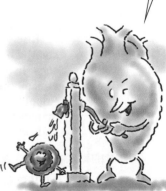

Thanks to the heart's pumping action, I can really "go with the flow."

Plasma

Plasma is a clear, straw-colored fluid that consists mainly of the proteins, albumin, globulin, and fibrinogen held in aqueous suspension. Plasma's fluid characteristics, including its osmotic pressure, viscosity, and suspension qualities, depend on its protein content.

Other components in plasma include glucose, lipids, amino acids, electrolytes, pigments, hormones, oxygen, and carbon dioxide. These components regulate acid-base balance and immune responses as well as carry nutrients to tissues and help to mediate coagulation.

Don't forget to digest this bit of info

Important products of metabolism that circulate in plasma include urea, uric acid, creatinine, and lactic acid.

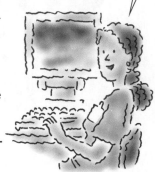

Plasma consists mostly of protein in water but also contains nutrients, gases, hormones, products of metabolism, and other substances.

Red blood cells

RBCs in adults are usually produced in the bone marrow. In the fetus, the liver and spleen also participate in RBC production. The RBC production process is called *erythropoiesis.*

All aboard

RBCs transport oxygen to body tissues and carbon dioxide away from them. Hemoglobin, an oxygen-carrying substance, gives RBCs this ability.

RBC production is regulated by the tissues' demand for oxygen and the blood cells' ability to deliver it. A lack of oxygen in the tissues (hypoxia) stimulates the formation and release of erythropoietin, a hormone that activates the bone marrow to produce RBCs. About 80% to 90% of erythropoietin is made in the kidneys; the remainder comes from the liver. Erythropoiesis may be enhanced by androgens. The life span for the typical RBC is 120 days.

The making of an erythrocyte

Erythrocyte formation begins with a precursor, called a *stem cell.* The stem cell eventually develops into an RBC. Development requires vitamin B_{12}, folic acid, and minerals, such as copper, cobalt, and—especially—iron.

Iron-clad facts

Iron is a component of hemoglobin and vital to the blood's oxygen-carrying capacity. Iron is found in food and, when consumed, is absorbed in the duodenum and upper jejunum. After iron is absorbed, it may be transported to the bone marrow for hemoglobin synthesis. Iron may also be transported to needy tissues such as muscle for myoglobin synthesis.

Unused iron is temporarily stored as ferritin and hemosiderin in specialized cells called *reticuloendothelial cells* (most commonly in the liver) until it's released for use in the bone marrow to form new RBCs.

Just think, I'm the body's primary defense against infection.

White blood cells

WBCs protect the body against harmful bacteria and infection. They're classified in one of two ways, as:

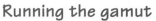 granular leukocytes (granulocytes), such as neutrophils, eosinophils, and basophils

nongranular leukocytes, such as monocytes and lymphocytes.

Most WBCs are produced in bone marrow. Lymphocytes complete their maturation in the lymph nodes.

Running the gamut

WBCs have a wide range of life spans; some granulocytes circulate for less than 6 hours, some monocytes may survive for weeks or months, and some lymphocytes last for years. Normally, the number of WBCs ranges from 5,000 to 10,000/µl.

It takes all types

Types of granulocytes include the following:
• Neutrophils, the predominant form of granulocyte, make up about 60% of WBCs. They surround and digest invading organisms and other foreign matter by phagocytosis.
• Eosinophils, minor granulocytes, defend against parasites, participate in allergic reactions, and fight lung and skin infections.
• Basophils, also minor granulocytes, release histamine into the blood and participate in delayed allergic reactions. They also contain heparin, an anticoagulant.

Call me T cell, and this is my fellow lymphocyte, B cell. We're just a couple of WBCs working hard to bolster your immunity.

Types of nongranular leukocytes include the following:
• Monocytes, along with neutrophils, devour invading organisms by phagocytosis. They also migrate to tissues where they develop into cells called *macrophages* that participate in immunity.
• Lymphocytes occur mostly in two forms: B cells and T cells. B cells produce antibodies while T cells regulate cell-mediated immunity.

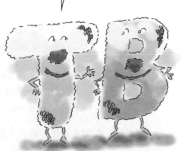

Platelets

Platelets are small (2 to 4 microns in diameter), colorless, disk-shaped cytoplasmic cells split from cells in bone marrow. They have a life span of 7 to 10 days.

Platelets perform three vital functions to help minimize blood loss:

They help constrict damaged blood vessels.

They form hemostatic plugs in injured blood vessels by becoming swollen, spiky, sticky, and secretory.

They provide substances that accelerate blood clotting, such as factors III and XIII and platelet factor 3.

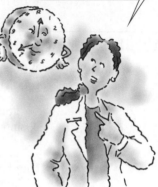

Clotting begins within minutes when a blood vessel is injured or severed.

It's a team effort

In a complex process called *hemostasis*, platelets, plasma, and coagulation factors interact to control bleeding. When tissue injury occurs, blood vessels at the injury site constrict and platelets mesh or clump to help prevent hemorrhage. (See *Understanding clotting.*)

Blood dyscrasias

Blood elements are prone to various types of dysfunction. An abnormal or pathologic condition of the blood is called a *dyscrasia*.

Erythrocytes, leukocytes, and platelets are manufactured in the bone marrow. Bone marrow cells and their precursors are especially vulnerable to physiologic changes that can affect cell production. Why? Because bone marrow cells reproduce rapidly and have a short life span. In addition, storage of circulating cells in the bone marrow is minimal.

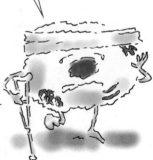

As a bone marrow cell, I can have it rough—my rapid reproduction coupled with a short life leaves me vulnerable to dysfunction.

Bringing some order to blood disorders

Blood disorders may be primary or secondary and quantitative or qualitative. They may involve some or all blood components.

A primary bleeding disorder occurs because of a problem within the blood itself. A secondary bleeding disorder results from a cause other than a defect in the blood.

Qualitative blood disorders stem from intrinsic cell abnormalities or plasma component dysfunction. Quantitative blood disorders result from increased or decreased cell production or cell destruction.

These can all end in bad blood

Blood disorders may be caused by:
• trauma

Now I get it!

Understanding clotting

When a blood vessel is severed or injured, clotting begins within minutes to stop loss of blood. Coagulation factors are essential to normal blood clotting. Absent, decreased, or excess coagulation factors may lead to a clotting abnormality. Coagulation factors are commonly designated by Roman numerals.

Arriving at clotting through two pathways

Clotting may be initiated through two different pathways, the intrinsic pathway or the extrinsic pathway. The intrinsic pathway is activated when plasma comes in contact with damaged vessel surfaces. The extrinsic pathway is activated when tissue thromboplastin, a substance released by damaged endothelial cells, comes in contact with one of the clotting factors.

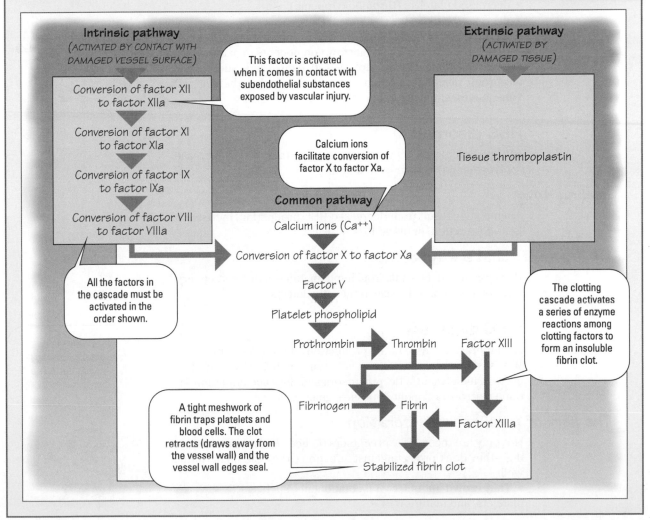

- chronic disease such as cirrhosis
- surgery
- malnutrition
- drugs
- toxins
- radiation
- genetic and congenital defects
- sepsis.

It's a no-win situation

Depressed bone marrow production or increased destruction of mature blood cells can result in:
- decreased RBCs (anemia)
- decreased platelets (thrombocytopenia)
- decreased leukocytes (leukopenia)
- all three components being decreased (pancytopenia).

The production of bone marrow components may increase. This results in myeloproliferative disorders, such as chronic myeloid leukemia, myelofibrosis, polycythemia vera, and essential thrombocytosis.

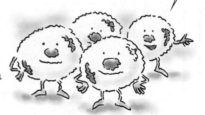

What to do! What to do! Decreasing our production can cause one set of problems and increasing production can cause other problems!

RBC disorders

RBC disorders may occur with a decrease (anemia) or increase (polycythemia) in their production.

Feeling down

Anemia may result from decreased RBC production, increased RBC destruction, or blood loss.

Up, up and...that's way too up

Polycythemia may result from hypoxia, tumors that secrete erythropoietin, kidney disease, or genetic defects.

WBC disorders

A temporary increase in the production and release of mature WBCs is a normal response to infection and inflammation. However, an increase in WBC precursors and their accumulation in bone marrow or lymphoid tissue signals leukemia.

The peril of precursor proliferation

Not only are these WBC precursors (called *blasts*) nonfunctioning—they don't protect against infection—they can be harmful as well:
- They crowd out other vital components, such as RBCs, platelets, and mature WBCs.

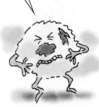

Blast those blasted blasts!!! And that's the censored version!

• They spill into the bloodstream, sometimes infiltrating organs and impairing their function.

Running at a deficit

The most common types of WBC deficiencies are neutropenia (decrease in the number of neutrophils in the blood) and lymphocytopenia (reduction in the number of lymphocytes in the blood). The latter is less common.

WBC deficiencies may result from:
• inadequate cell production
• drug reactions
• ionizing radiation
• infiltrated bone marrow (cancer)
• congenital defects
• aplastic anemias
• folic acid deficiency
• hypersplenism.

Platelet disorders

Disorders may occur with platelets when they're:

 too few (thrombocytopenia)

 too many (thrombocytosis)

 dysfunctional (thrombocytopathy).

> Decrease, excess, dysfunction ...it all leads to disorder.

Too few...

Thrombocytopenia may result from a congenital deficiency, or it may be acquired. Causes include:
• exposure to drugs such as heparin
• cancerous infiltration of bone marrow
• abnormal sequestration (blood accumulation and pooling) in the spleen
• infection
• exposure to ionizing radiation.

Too many...

Thrombocytosis occurs as a result of certain diseases such as cancer.

Too much trouble...

Thrombocytopathy usually results from disease, such as uremia or liver failure, or adverse effects of medications, such as salicylates and nonsteroidal anti-inflammatory drugs (NSAIDs). It can also be caused by some herbs, such as alfalfa, chamomile, clove, evening primrose oil, garlic, ginger, ginseng, and red clover.

Blood disorders

The disorders discussed in this section include:
- acid-base imbalances
- disseminated intravascular coagulation (DIC)
- idiopathic thrombocytopenic purpura (ITP)
- iron deficiency anemia
- thrombocytopenia.

> It's all about balance…acid-base balance is maintained by buffer systems and by the lungs and kidneys, which neutralize and eliminate acids as rapidly as the acids are formed.

Acid-base imbalances

Normally, the body's pH control mechanism is so effective that blood pH stays within a narrow range—7.35 to 7.45. Acid-base balance is maintained by buffer systems and by the lungs and kidneys, which neutralize and eliminate acids as rapidly as the acids are formed.

Buffer balancing act

The lungs influence acid-base balance by excreting carbon dioxide. The kidneys exert their effect by regulating bicarbonate. Dysfunction or interruption of a buffer system can cause an acid-base imbalance.

How it happens

Disturbances in acid-base balance can cause respiratory acidosis, respiratory alkalosis, metabolic acidosis, or metabolic alkalosis. (See *Understanding acid-base disorders*.)

Respiratory acidosis

When a patient hypoventilates, carbon dioxide builds up in the bloodstream. Retained carbon dioxide combines with water to form carbonic acid, which dissociates to release free hydrogen and bicarbonate ions. Increased partial pressure of arterial carbon dioxide ($Paco_2$) and free hydrogen ions stimulate the medulla to increase respiratory drive and expel carbon dioxide.

Hefty hemoglobin

As pH falls, 2,3-diphosphoglycerate accumulates in RBCs, where it alters hemoglobin to release oxygen. The hemoglobin picks up hydrogen ions and carbon dioxide and removes them from the serum.

Now I get it!

Understanding acid-base disorders

This chart provides an overview of selected acid-base disorders.

Disorder	ABG findings	Possible causes
Respiratory acidosis (excess carbon dioxide [CO_2] retention)	• pH < 7.35 • HCO_3^- > 26 mEq/L (if compensating) • $PaCO_2$ > 45 mm Hg	• Central nervous system depression from drugs, injury, or disease • Asphyxia • Hypoventilation from pulmonary, cardiac, musculoskeletal, or neuromuscular disease
Respiratory alkalosis (excess CO_2 excretion)	• pH > 7.45 • HCO_3^- < 22 mEq/L (if compensating) • $PaCO_2$ < 35 mm Hg	• Hyperventilation from anxiety, pain, or improper ventilator settings • Respiratory stimulation due to drugs, disease, hypoxia, or fever • Gram-negative bacteremia
Metabolic acidosis (bicarbonate [HCO_3^-] loss, acid retention)	• pH < 7.35 • HCO_3^- < 22 mEq/L • $PaCO_2$ < 35 mm Hg (if compensating)	• Bicarbonate depletion from diarrhea • Excess production of organic acids from hepatic disease, endocrine disorders, shock, or drug intoxication • Inadequate excretion of acids from renal disease
Metabolic alkalosis (HCO_3^- retention, acid loss)	• pH > 7.45 • HCO_3^- > 26 mEq/L • $PaCO_2$ > 45 mm Hg (if compensating)	• Loss of hydrochloric acid from prolonged vomiting or gastric suctioning • Loss of potassium from increased renal excretion (as in diuretic therapy) or steroids • Excessive alkali ingestion

As respiratory mechanisms fail, rising $PaCO_2$ stimulates the kidneys to retain bicarbonate and sodium ions and excrete hydrogen ions.

As the hydrogen ion concentration overwhelms compensatory mechanisms, hydrogen ions move into the cells and potassium ions move out. Without enough oxygen, anaerobic metabolism produces lactic acid.

Respiratory alkalosis

As pulmonary ventilation increases, excessive carbon dioxide is exhaled. Resulting hypocapnia leads to reduction of carbonic acid, excretion of hydrogen and bicarbonate ions, and rising serum pH.

Against rising pH, the hydrogen-potassium buffer system pulls hydrogen ions out of cells and into blood in exchange for potassium ions. Hydrogen ions entering blood combine with bicarbonate ions to form carbonic acid, and pH falls.

Hypocapnia causes an increase in heart rate, cerebral vasoconstriction, and decreased cerebral blood flow. After 6 hours, kidneys secrete more bicarbonate and less hydrogen.

Continued low $Paco_2$ and vasoconstriction increase cerebral and peripheral hypoxia. Severe alkalosis inhibits calcium ionization, increasing nerve and muscle excitability.

Metabolic acidosis

As hydrogen ions begin accumulating in the body, chemical buffers (bicarbonate and proteins) in cells and extracellular fluid bind them. Excess hydrogen ions decrease blood pH and stimulate chemoreceptors in the medulla to increase respiration. Consequent fall in $Paco_2$ frees hydrogen ions to bind with bicarbonate ions. Respiratory compensation occurs but isn't sufficient to correct acidosis.

Lots of movin' goin' on

Healthy kidneys compensate, excreting excess hydrogen ions, buffered by phosphate or ammonia. For each hydrogen ion excreted, renal tubules reabsorb and return to the blood one sodium ion and one bicarbonate ion.

Excess hydrogen ions in the extracellular fluid passively diffuse into cells. To maintain balance of charge across the cells' membrane, cells release potassium ions. Excess hydrogen ions change the normal balance of potassium, sodium, and calcium ions, impairing neural excitability.

Metabolic alkalosis

Chemical buffers in the extracellular fluid and intracellular fluid bind with bicarbonate in the body. Excess unbound bicarbonate raises blood pH, depressing chemoreceptors in the medulla, inhibiting respiration and raising $Paco_2$. Carbon dioxide combines with water to form carbonic acid. Low oxygen levels limit respiratory compensation.

When blood bicarbonate rises to 28 mEq/L, the amount filtered by the renal glomeruli exceeds the reabsorptive capacity of the renal tubules. Excess bicarbonate is excreted in the urine, and hydrogen ions are retained. To maintain electrochemical balance, sodium ions and water are excreted with bicarbonate ions.

When hydrogen ion levels in the extracellular fluid are low, hydrogen ions diffuse passively out of cells and extracellular potassium ions move into cells. As intracellular hydrogen levels fall, calcium ionization decreases, and nerve cells become permeable to sodium ions. Sodium ions moving into cells trigger neural impulses in the peripheral and central nervous systems.

What to look for

Each disturbance in acid-base balance has its own distinct signs and symptoms. (See *Treating disorders of acid-base balance*, page 324.)

Respiratory acidosis
Possible signs and symptoms of respiratory acidosis include:
- restlessness
- confusion
- apprehension
- somnolence
- asterixis (fine or flapping tremor)
- coma
- headaches
- dyspnea and tachypnea
- papilledema
- depressed reflexes
- hypoxemia
- tachycardia
- hypertension
- atrial and ventricular arrhythmias
- hypotension with vasodilation.

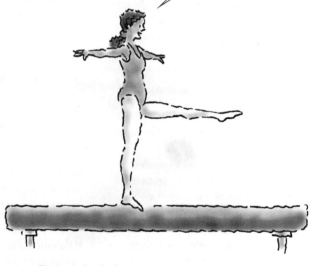

Each acid-base imbalance has its own distinct signs and symptoms and its own treatment plan. But I can't even think about imbalance now!

Respiratory alkalosis
Possible signs and symptoms of respiratory alkalosis include:
- deep, rapid respirations
- light-headedness or dizziness
- agitation
- circumoral and peripheral paresthesia
- carpopedal spasms, twitching, and muscle weakness.

Metabolic acidosis
Possible signs and symptoms of metabolic acidosis include:
- headache and lethargy progressing to drowsiness
- Kussmaul's respirations
- hypotension
- stupor and, if condition is severe and untreated, coma and death
- anorexia

Battling illness

Treating disorders of acid-base balance

The goal of treating all acid-base imbalances is reversing the underlying cause. In addition, each imbalance has its own individualized treatment plan.

Respiratory acidosis

Treatment of respiratory acidosis focuses on improving ventilation and lowering the partial pressure of arterial carbon dioxide. If hypoventilation can't be corrected, the patient should have an artificial airway inserted and be placed on mechanical ventilation. Bronchoscopy may be needed to remove retained secretions.

Treatment for respiratory acidosis with a pulmonary cause also includes:
• a bronchodilator to open constricted airways
• supplemental oxygen as needed
• drug therapy to treat hyperkalemia
• an antibiotic to treat infection
• chest physiotherapy to remove secretions from the lungs
• removal of a foreign body from the patient's airway if needed.

If respiratory acidosis stems from nonpulmonary conditions, such as neuromuscular disorders or a drug overdose, the underlying cause must be corrected.

Respiratory alkalosis

Treatment varies, depending on the cause.
• Treating the underlying condition may include removing the causative agent, such as a salicylate or other drugs, or taking steps to reduce fever and eliminate the source of sepsis.
• If acute hypoxemia is the cause, oxygen therapy is initiated. If anxiety is the cause, the patient may receive a sedative or an anxiolytic.
• Hyperventilation can be counteracted by having the patient breathe into a paper bag, which forces the patient to breathe exhaled carbon dioxide (CO_2), thereby raising the CO_2 level.
• If a patient's respiratory alkalosis is *iatrogenic* (caused by the effects of treatment), mechanical ventilator settings may be adjusted by decreasing the tidal volume or the number of breaths delivered per minute.

Metabolic acidosis

Treatment aims to correct the acidosis as quickly as possible by addressing both the symptoms and the underlying cause.
• Respiratory compensation is usually the first line of therapy, including mechanical ventilation if needed.
• For patients with diabetes, expect to administer rapid-acting insulin to reverse diabetic ketoacidosis and drive potassium back into the cell.
• For any patient with metabolic acidosis, monitor serum potassium levels. Even though high serum levels exist initially, serum potassium levels will drop when the acidosis is corrected, possibly resulting in hypokalemia. Any other electrolyte imbalances are evaluated and checked.
• Sodium bicarbonate is administered I.V. to neutralize blood acidity in patients with a pH lower than 7.1 and bicarbonate loss. Fluids are replaced parenterally as needed.
• Dialysis may be initiated in patients with renal failure or a toxic reaction to a drug. Such patients may receive an antibiotic to treat sources of infection or an antidiarrheal to treat diarrhea bicarbonate loss.

Metabolic alkalosis

Treatment for metabolic alkalosis may involve these interventions:
• Rarely, ammonium chloride is administered I.V. over 4 hours in severe cases.
• Thiazide diuretics and nasogastric suctioning are discontinued.
• An antiemetic may be administered to treat underlying nausea and vomiting.
• Acetazolamide may be administered to increase renal excretion of bicarbonate.

• nausea and vomiting
• diarrhea
• dehydration
• warm, flushed skin
• fruity-smelling breath.

Metabolic alkalosis

Possible signs and symptoms of metabolic alkalosis include:
- irritability
- carphology (picking at bedclothes)
- twitching
- confusion
- nausea and vomiting
- diarrhea
- cardiac arrhythmias
- slow, shallow respirations
- diminished peripheral blood flow
- carpopedal spasm in the hand
- Trousseau's sign (spasm of the wrist elicited by applying a blood pressure cuff to the upper arm and inflating it to a pressure 20 mm Hg above the patient's systemic blood pressure).

What tests tell you

Arterial blood gas results are the most commonly used laboratory tests to help diagnose acid-base imbalances.

Respiratory acidosis

These test results help diagnose respiratory acidosis:
- Chest X-ray may reveal the cause, such as heart failure, pneumonia, pneumothorax, or chronic obstructive pulmonary disease.
- Serum potassium level is greater than 5 mEq/L.
- Serum chloride level is low.
- Urine pH is acidic.

Respiratory alkalosis

These test results indicate respiratory alkalosis:
- Electrocardiogram (ECG) may reveal cardiac arrhythmias.
- Serum chloride level is low.
- Urine pH is basic.

Metabolic acidosis

These test results help confirm the diagnosis of metabolic acidosis:
- Urine pH is less than 4.5 in the absence of renal disease.
- Serum potassium level is greater than 5.5 mEq/L.
- Blood glucose level is greater than 150 mg/dl.
- Serum ketone bodies are present if the patient has diabetes.
- Plasma lactic acid is elevated, if lactic acidosis is present.
- Anion gap is greater than 14 mEq/L in high–anion gap metabolic acidosis, lactic acidosis, ketoacidosis, aspirin overdose, alcohol poisoning, renal failure, or other conditions characterized by accumulation of organic acids, sulfates, or phosphates. (The anion

gap is calculated by adding the chloride level and the bicarbonate level and then subtracting that total from the sodium level. The value normally ranges from 8 to 14 mEq/L and represents the level of unmeasured anions [negatively charged ions] in extracellular fluid.)
• Anion gap is 12 mEq/L or less in normal–anion gap metabolic acidosis from bicarbonate loss, GI or renal loss, increased acid load (from total parenteral nutrition fluids), rapid I.V. saline administration, or other conditions characterized by bicarbonate loss.

Metabolic alkalosis
The following findings suggest metabolic alkalosis:
• Serum potassium level is less than 3.5 mEq/L.
• Serum calcium level is less than 8.9 mg/dl.
• Serum chloride level is less than 98 mEq/L.
• Urine pH is 7; then, alkaline urine after renal compensatory mechanism begins to excrete bicarbonate.
• ECG may reveal depressed T wave, merging with a P wave, and atrial or sinus tachycardia.

Disseminated intravascular coagulation

In DIC, also called *consumption coagulopathy* or *defibrination syndrome*, clotting and hemorrhage occur at the same time in the vascular system.

A look at the DIC disaster area

DIC causes small blood vessel blockage, organ tissue damage (necrosis), depletion of circulating clotting factors and platelets, and activation of a clot-dissolving process called fibrinolysis. This, in turn, can lead to severe hemorrhage.

How it happens

There are five major precipitating causes of DIC:
• infection—gram-negative or gram-positive septicemia; viral, fungal, rickettsial, or protozoal infection
• obstetric complications—abruptio placentae, amniotic fluid embolism, retained dead fetus, eclampsia, septic abortion, postpartum hemorrhage
• neoplastic disease—acute leukemia, metastatic carcinoma, lymphomas
• disorders that produce necrosis—extensive burns and trauma, brain tissue destruction, transplant rejection, liver necrosis, anorexia

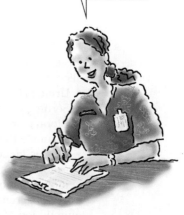

Here's a list of things that can lead to DIC.

• other disorders and conditions associated with massive insult to the body—heatstroke, shock, poisonous snakebite, cirrhosis, fat embolism, incompatible blood transfusion, drug reactions, cardiac arrest, surgery necessitating cardiopulmonary bypass, giant hemangioma, severe venous thrombosis, purpura fulminans, adrenal disease, acute respiratory distress syndrome, diabetic ketoacidosis, pulmonary embolism, multiple trauma, and sickle cell anemia.

DIC—a BIG mystery in many ways

No one is certain why these conditions and disorders lead to DIC. Furthermore, whether they lead to it through a common mechanism is also uncertain. In many patients, DIC may be triggered by the entrance of foreign protein into the circulation or by vascular endothelial injury.

DIC usually develops in association with three pathologic processes:

 damage to the endothelium

 release of tissue thromboplastin

 activation of factor X.

The play-by-play

DIC arises from the series of events described below:
• One of DIC's many causes triggers the coagulation system.
• Excess fibrin is formed (triggered by the action of thrombin, an enzyme) and becomes trapped in the microvasculature along with platelets, causing clots.
• Blood flow to the tissues decreases, causing acidemia, blood stasis, and tissue hypoxia; organ failure may result.
• Both fibrinolysis and antithrombotic mechanisms lead to anticoagulation.
• Platelets and coagulation factors are consumed and massive hemorrhage may ensue. (See *Understanding DIC*, page 328.)

What to look for

The most significant clinical feature of DIC is abnormal bleeding without a history of serious hemorrhagic disorder. Other signs and symptoms include:
• cutaneous oozing
• petechiae (microhemorrhages on the skin)
• bleeding from surgical or I.V. sites
• bleeding from the GI tract
• cyanosis of the extremities.

Now I get it!

Understanding DIC

The simplified illustration below shows the pathophysiology of disseminated intravascular coagulation (DIC). Circulating thrombin activates both coagulation and fibrinolysis, leading to paradoxical bleeding and clotting.

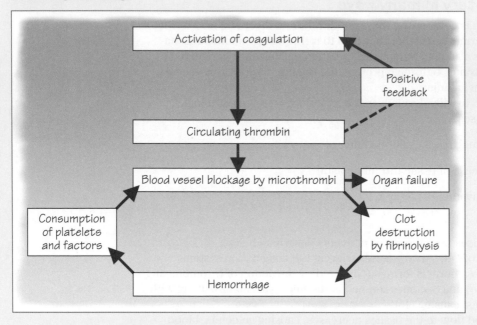

DIC is usually acute, although it may be chronic in cancer patients. The prognosis depends on the timeliness of detection, severity and site of the hemorrhage, and treatment of the underlying disease or condition. (See *Treating DIC*.)

What tests tell you

Abnormal bleeding with no other blood disorder suggests DIC. These test results support the diagnosis:
• Platelet count is decreased, usually to less than 100,000/µl, because platelets are consumed during thrombosis.
• Fibrinogen levels are decreased to less than 150 mg/dl because fibrinogen is consumed in clot formation. Levels may be normal if elevated by hepatitis or pregnancy.
• Prothrombin time (PT) is prolonged to more than 15 seconds.

Battling illness

Treating DIC

Successful management of disseminated intravascular coagulation (DIC) requires prompt treatment of the underlying disorder.

Support
Treatment may be highly specific or supportive. Supportive care is appropriate if the underlying disorder is self-limiting or if the patient isn't actively bleeding.

In case of bleeding
Active bleeding may require administration of fresh-frozen plasma, platelets, cryoprecipitate, or packed red blood cells to support hemostasis.

Drug therapy
Heparin therapy is controversial; it may be used early in the disease to prevent microclotting or as a last resort in a patient who's actively bleeding. If thrombosis occurs, heparin therapy is usually mandatory. In most cases, it's administered along with transfusion therapy. Amniocaproic acid may be given to inhibit fibrinolysis.

- Partial thromboplastin time (PTT) is prolonged to more than 60 to 80 seconds.
- Fibrin degradation products are increased, usually to greater than 45 mcg/ml. Increases are produced by excess fibrin clots broken down by plasmin.
- D-dimer test is positive at less than 1:8 dilution.
- Other blood test results include positive fibrin monomers, diminished levels of factors V and VIII, fragmentation of RBCs, and hemoglobin levels decreased to less than 10 g/dl.
- Renal status test results demonstrate reduced urine output (less than 30 ml/hour), elevated blood urea nitrogen levels (greater than 25 mg/dl), and elevated serum creatinine levels (greater than 1.3 mg/dl).

Confirmation can prove complicated

Final confirmation of the diagnosis may be difficult because similar test results also occur in other disorders such as primary fibrinolysis. However, fibrin degradation products and D-dimer tests are considered specific and diagnostic of DIC. Additional tests may determine the underlying cause.

Idiopathic thrombocytopenic purpura

Thrombocytopenia that results from immunologic platelet destruction is known as *ITP*. It occurs in two forms:

Acute ITP, also called *postviral thrombocytopenia*, usually affects children between ages 2 and 6.

Chronic ITP, also called *Werlhof's disease*, *purpura hemorrhagica*, *essential thrombocytopenia*, or *autoimmune thrombocytopenia*, affects adults younger than age 50, especially women between ages 20 and 40.

Acute ITP affects children ages 2 to 6 and usually follows a viral infection.

How it happens

ITP is an autoimmune disorder. Antibodies that reduce the life span of platelets appear in nearly all patients.

One follows infection, the other doesn't

Acute ITP usually follows a viral infection, such as rubella or chickenpox, and can result from immunization with a live vaccine.

Chronic ITP seldom follows infection and is commonly linked with immunologic disorders, such as systemic lupus erythematosus and human immunodeficiency virus infection. Chronic ITP affects women more commonly than men.

A plague on platelets

ITP occurs when circulating immunoglobulin G (IgG) molecules react with host platelets, which are then destroyed by phagocytosis in the spleen and, to a lesser degree, in the liver. Normally, the life span of platelets in circulation is 7 to 10 days. In ITP, platelets survive 1 to 3 days or less.

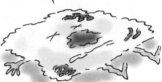

What hit me? It looked like my own immune system!

Getting complicated

Hemorrhage can severely complicate ITP. Potentially fatal purpuric lesions (caused by hemorrhage into tissues) may occur in vital organs, such as the brain and kidneys. ITP is usually a precursor of lymphoma.

What to look for

Signs and symptoms that indicate decreased platelets include:
- nosebleed
- oral bleeding
- purpura
- petechiae
- excessive menstruation.

Sudden bleeding here; creeping over there

In the acute form, sudden bleeding usually follows a recent viral illness, although it may not occur until 21 days after the virus strikes. In the chronic form, the onset of bleeding is insidious.

The prognosis for acute ITP is excellent; nearly four of five patients recover completely without specific treatment. The prognosis for chronic ITP is good; transient remissions lasting weeks or even years are common, especially in women. (See *Treating ITP*.)

What tests tell you

These tests help diagnose ITP:
- Platelet count less than 20,000/µl and prolonged bleeding time suggest ITP. Platelet size and appearance may be abnormal, and anemia may be present if bleeding has occurred.
- Bone marrow studies show an abundance of megakaryocytes (platelet precursors) and a circulating platelet survival time of only several hours to a few days.
- Humoral tests that measure platelet-associated IgG may help establish the diagnosis. However, they're nonspecific, so their usefulness is limited. One-half of patients with thrombocytopenia show an increased IgG level.

Memory jogger

To help you remember how **ITP** progresses, break down each of its initials this way:

Immune system makes antibodies against platelets.

Trapped platelets appear in the spleen and liver.

Phagocytosis causes thrombocytopenia.

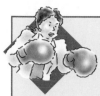

Battling illness

Treating ITP

Acute idiopathic thrombocytopenic purpura (ITP) may be allowed to run its course without intervention. Alternatively, it may be treated with glucocorticoids or immune globulin. Treatment with plasmapheresis or platelet pheresis with transfusion has met with limited success.

For chronic ITP, corticosteroids may be used to suppress phagocytic activity, promote capillary integrity, and enhance platelet production.

Splenectomy

Patients who don't respond spontaneously to treatment within 1 to 4 months or who require high doses of corticosteroids to maintain platelet counts require splenectomy. This procedure is up to 85% successful in adults when splenomegaly accompanies the initial thrombocytopenia.

Looking at alternatives

Alternative treatments include immunosuppressants, such as cyclophosphamide or vincristine, and high-dose I.V. immune globulin, which is effective in 85% of adults.

Immunosuppressant use requires weighing the risks against the benefits. Immune globulin has a rapid effect, raising platelet counts within 1 to 5 days, but this effect lasts only about 1 to 2 weeks. Immune globulin is usually administered to prepare severely thrombocytic patients for emergency surgery.

Iron deficiency anemia

Iron deficiency anemia is a disorder of oxygen transport in which the production of hemoglobin is inadequate. A common disease worldwide, iron deficiency anemia affects 10% to 30% of the adult population in the United States. Iron deficiency anemia occurs most commonly in premenopausal women, infants (particularly premature or low birth weight infants), children, and adolescents (especially girls).

How it happens

Iron deficiency anemia can result from:
• inadequate dietary intake of iron
• conditions resulting in iron malabsorption, such as chronic diarrhea and gastrectomy, and malabsorption syndromes such as celiac disease
• pregnancy, which diverts maternal iron to the fetus for RBC production
• blood loss secondary to drug-induced GI bleeding (from anticoagulants, aspirin, NSAIDs, or steroids)
• hemoglobulinurias (presence of hemoglobin in urine)
• mechanical RBC trauma caused by procedures such as cardiopulmonary bypass or devices such as ventricular assist devices or prosthetic heart valves.

In short supply

Iron deficiency anemia occurs when the supply of iron is too low for optimal RBC formation. This results in smaller (microcytic) cells that contain less color when they're stained for visualization under a microscope.

When the body's stores of iron, including plasma iron, become used up, the concentration of transferrin, which binds with and transports iron, decreases. Insufficient iron stores lead to smaller than normal RBCs that have a lower than normal hemoglobin concentration. In turn, the blood carries less oxygen.

What to look for

Iron deficiency anemia usually develops slowly, and therefore many patients are asymptomatic at first. By the time they develop symptoms, anemia is usually severe. These signs and symptoms include:

- generalized weakness and fatigue
- light-headedness and inability to concentrate
- palpitations
- dyspnea on exertion
- pica (craving for nonnutritive substances), especially for clay, cornstarch, and ice
- pallor, especially of the conjunctiva
- tachycardia
- dry, brittle, ridged nails with concave contours
- tender, pale, atrophic tongue (glossitis)
- cracking at the edges of the lips (angular stomatitis). (See *Treating iron deficiency anemia*.)

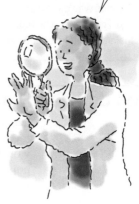

Iron deficiency anemia can cause dry, brittle nails.

Battling illness

Treating iron deficiency anemia

The first priority of treating iron deficiency anemia is determining the cause. After that's determined, replacement therapy can begin.

Drug options

If the cause was inadequate dietary intake, the treatment of choice is an oral preparation of iron or a combination of iron and ascorbic acid (which enhances iron absorption). In some cases, the iron may have to be administered parenterally; for example, if the patient is noncompliant to the oral preparation or in the case of malabsorption conditions.

Because total dose I.V. infusion of supplemental iron is painless and requires fewer injections, it's usually preferred over I.M. (which must be given by Z-track injection) administration.

What tests tell you

As iron deficiency anemia develops, it causes a predictable sequence of abnormalities in laboratory tests:
• In early stages, the total iron binding capacity may be elevated, and serum iron levels are decreased.
• Complete blood count shows a low hemoglobin level (males, less than 12 g/dl; females less than 10 g/dl) and low hematocrit (males, less than 47%; females, less than 42%). RBC counts may be normal in early stages, except in infants and children.
• Red cell indices reveal microcytic (smaller in size than normal) and hypochromic (contain less color than normal) cells.
• Bone marrow biopsy demonstrates depleted or absent iron stores and reduced production of precursors to RBCs. (See *Peripheral blood smear in iron deficiency anemia*.)

A hard nut to crack

The diagnosis of iron deficiency anemia is sometimes difficult due to coexisting conditions, such as infections, blood transfusions, and iron supplementation.

Now I get it!

Peripheral blood smear in iron deficiency anemia

This peripheral blood smear shows the cigar-shaped and microcytic hypochromic red blood cells of iron deficiency anemia.

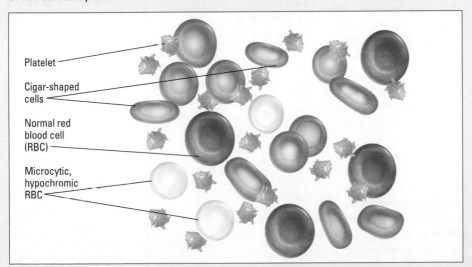

Platelet

Cigar-shaped cells

Normal red blood cell (RBC)

Microcytic, hypochromic RBC

Thrombocytopenia

Thrombocytopenia is characterized by a deficient number of circulating platelets. It's the most common cause of hemorrhagic disorders.

How it happens

Thrombocytopenia may be congenital or acquired, but the acquired form is more common. In either case, it usually results from:

- decreased or defective platelet production in the bone marrow
- increased destruction outside the marrow caused by an underlying disorder
- sequestration (increase in the amount of blood in a limited vascular area)
- blood loss. (See *Factors that decrease platelet count.*)

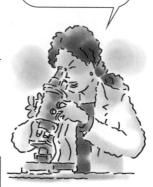

Platelets play a vital role in coagulation... that's why thrombocytopenia threatens the body's ability to control bleeding.

Factors that decrease platelet count

Decreased platelet count may result from diminished or defective platelet production, increased peripheral destruction of platelets, sequestration (separation of a portion of the circulating blood in a specific body part), or blood loss. More specific causes are listed below.

Diminished or defective production

Congenital
- Wiskott-Aldrich syndrome
- Maternal ingestion of thiazides
- Neonatal rubella

Acquired
- Aplastic anemia
- Marrow infiltration (acute and chronic leukemia, tumor)
- Nutritional deficiency (B_{12}, folic acid)
- Myelosuppressive agents
- Drugs that directly influence platelet production (thiazides, alcohol, hormones)
- Radiation
- Viral infections (measles, dengue)

Increased peripheral destruction

Congenital
- Nonimmune (prematurity, erythroblastosis fetalis, infection)
- Immune (drug-induced, especially with quinine and quinidine; posttransfusion purpura; acute and chronic idiopathic thrombocytopenic purpura; sepsis; alcohol)

Acquired
- Invasive lines or devices
- Ventricular assist devices, intra-aortic balloon pump, cardiopulmonary bypass
- Artificial hearts and prosthetic valves
- Heparin administration

Sequestration
- Hypersplenism
- Hypothermia

Loss
- Hemorrhage
- Bleeding

Let's meet the mechanisms responsible

In thrombocytopenia, lack of platelets can cause inadequate hemostasis. Four mechanisms are responsible:

- decreased platelet production
- decreased platelet survival
- pooling of blood in the spleen
- intravascular dilution of circulating platelets.

Fe, fi, fo, fum...

Platelets are produced by giant cells in bone marrow called *megakaryocytes*. Platelet production falls when the number of megakaryocytes is reduced or when platelet production becomes dysfunctional.

What to look for

Thrombocytopenia typically produces a sudden onset of petechiae in the skin and bleeding into any mucous membrane. Nearly all patients are otherwise symptom-free, although some may complain of malaise, fatigue, and general weakness.

In adults, large blood-filled blisters usually appear in the mouth. In severe disease, hemorrhage may lead to tachycardia, shortness of breath, loss of consciousness, and death.

Prognosis is excellent in drug-induced thrombocytopenia if the offending drug is withdrawn. Recovery may be immediate. In other cases, the prognosis depends on the patient's response to treatment of the underlying cause. (See *Treating thrombocytopenia*.)

What tests tell you

These tests help establish a diagnosis of thrombocytopenia:
- Platelet count is decreased, usually to less than 100,000/µl in adults.
- Bleeding time is prolonged.
- PT and PTT are normal.
- Platelet antibody studies can help determine why the platelet count is low and can also be used to select treatment.
- Platelet survival studies help differentiate between ineffective platelet production and platelet destruction as causes of thrombocytopenia.
- Bone marrow studies determine the number, size, and cytoplasmic maturity of megakaryocytes in severe disease. This helps identify ineffective platelet production as the cause and rules out malignant disease at the same time.

Battling illness

Treating thrombocytopenia

When treating thrombocytopenia, withdrawing the offending drug or treating the underlying cause, if possible, is essential. Other treatments include:
- administration of corticosteroids to increase platelet production
- administration of folate to stimulate bone marrow production of platelets
- I.V. administration of gamma globulin for severe or refractory thrombocytopenia (still experimental)
- platelet transfusion to stop episodic abnormal bleeding caused by a low platelet count (only minimally effective if platelet destruc-tion results from an immune disorder; may be reserved for life-threatening bleeding)
- splenectomy to correct disease caused by platelet destruction because the spleen acts as the primary site of platelet removal and antibody production.

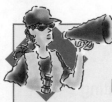

That's a wrap!

Hematologic system review

Plasma
- Consists of proteins, albumin, globulin, and fibrinogen
- Regulates acid-base balance and immune responses
- Mediates coagulation

RBCs
- Transport oxygen and carbon dioxide to and from body tissues
- Contain hemoglobin
- Decrease results in anemia
- Increase results in polycythemia

WBCs
- Protect against infection and inflammation
- Produced in bone marrow
- Increase and accumulation in bone marrow or lymphoid tissue indicates leukemia

Platelets
- Interact with plasma and coagulation factors to control bleeding
- Provide factors III and XIII and platelet factor 3 that accelerate blood clotting
- Decrease (thrombocytopenia), excess (thrombocytosis), or dysfunction (thrombocytopathy) cause platelet disorders

Understanding blood dyscrasias
Dyscrasias are abnormal conditions of the blood that are caused by the rapid reproduction and short life span of blood elements, such as:
- bone marrow cells
- erythrocytes
- leukocytes
- platelets.

Understanding blood disorders
- Primary—occur as a result of a problem within the blood itself
- Secondary—result from a cause other than a defect in the blood
- Quantitative—result from increased or decreased cell production or cell destruction
- Qualitative—stem from intrinsic cell abnormalities or plasma component dysfunction

Blood disorders
- *Acid-base imbalances*—disturbances in acid-base balance can cause respiratory acidosis, respiratory alkalosis, metabolic acidosis, or metabolic alkalosis
- *DIC*—clotting and hemorrhage occur in the vascular system at the same time; blood flow diminished to tissues and anticoagulation results, possibly hemorrhage
- *ITP*—antibodies develop against platelets; platelets are destroyed and may result in hemorrhage
- *Iron deficiency anemia*—occurs due to decreased iron supply and leads to blood cells becoming smaller, paler; results in less oxygen carried by blood
- *Thrombocytopenia*—results in a deficient number of platelets; occurs due to decreased platelet production, blood loss, sequestration, or destruction

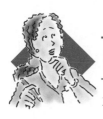

Quick quiz

1. A vital function of platelets is to:
- A. form hemostatic plugs in injured blood vessels.
- B. regulate acid-base balance and immune responses.
- C. protect the body against harmful bacteria and infection.
- D. carry oxygen to the tissues and remove carbon dioxide from them.

Answer: A. Platelets also minimize blood loss by causing damaged blood vessels to contract and provide materials that accelerate blood coagulation.

2. Which of the following is the normal life span of an RBC?
- A. 90 days
- B. 30 days
- C. 240 days
- D. 120 days

Answer: D. A normal RBC is viable for approximately 120 days.

3. Thrombocytopenia is characterized by:
- A. not enough circulating platelets.
- B. too many circulating platelets.
- C. decreased RBC production.
- D. decreased iron supply.

Answer: A. Platelet deficiency may be due to decreased or defective production of platelets or increased destruction of platelets.

4. The initial response to tissue injury in the extrinsic pathway is the release of which substance?
- A. Prothrombin
- B. Thrombin
- C. Tissue thromboplastin
- D. Fibrinogen

Answer: C. Tissue thromboplastin is also called *factor III*.

5. DIC is marked by:
- A. clotting deficiency and immune dysfunction.
- B. clotting and hemorrhage.
- C. hemorrhagic and fibrinolytic coagulopathy.
- D. excess carbon dioxide retention.

Answer: B. In DIC, clotting and hemorrhage occur simultaneously in the vascular system.

Scoring

⭐⭐⭐   If you answered all five items correctly, you're golden! Indeed, your knowledge of red and white blood cells has us green with envy!

⭐⭐   If you answered four items correctly, congrats! You're a connoisseur of liquid and formed components.

⭐   If you answered fewer than four items correctly, don't stop circulating. Never give up. Need inspiration? Think of the stem cell precursor that eventually emerges to become a mighty RBC.

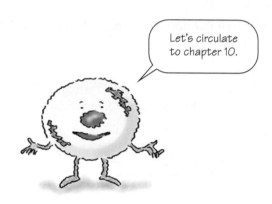

Let's circulate to chapter 10.

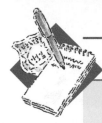

10

Immune system

Just the facts

In this chapter, you'll learn:

♦ the five structures of the immune system

♦ cell-mediated immunity, humoral immunity, and the complement system, and how they work

♦ the pathophysiology, signs and symptoms, diagnostic tests, and treatments for common immune system disorders.

Understanding the immune system

> We cells have a lot to do with the immune system.

The body protects itself from infectious organisms and other harmful invaders through an elaborate network of safeguards called the *host defense system*. This system has three lines of defense:

 physical and chemical barriers to infection

 the inflammatory response

 the immune response.

Physical barriers, such as the skin and mucous membranes, prevent most organisms from invading the body. Organisms that penetrate this first barrier simultaneously trigger the inflammatory and immune responses. Both responses involve stem cells in the bone marrow that form blood cells.

Structures of the immune system

These five structures in the body make up the immune system:

• bone marrow
• lymph nodes
• thymus

- spleen
- tonsils.

Bone marrow

B-cells are produced and develop in the bone marrow then migrate to the lymph nodes.

Lymph nodes

Lymph nodes are distributed along lymphatic vessels throughout the body. They filter lymphatic fluid, which drains from body tissues and later returns to the blood as plasma.

Double agents?

The lymph nodes also remove bacteria and toxins from the circulatory system. This means that, on occasion, infectious agents can be spread by the lymphatic system.

Thymus

The thymus, located in the mediastinal area (between the lungs), secretes a group of hormones that enable lymphocytes to develop into mature T cells.

"T" stands for "tough"

T cells attack foreign or abnormal cells and regulate cell-mediated immunity.

Spleen

The largest lymphatic organ, the spleen functions as a reservoir for blood. Cells in the splenic tissue, called *macrophages*, clear cellular debris and process hemoglobin.

Tonsils

The tonsils consist of lymphoid tissue and also produce lymphocytes.

Guarding against air raids

The location of the tonsils allows them to guard the body against airborne and ingested pathogens.

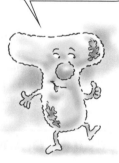

Basically, my job is to destroy target cells through the release of lymphokines.

Types of immunity

Certain cells have the ability to distinguish between foreign matter and what belongs to the body—a skill known as *immunocompetence.* When foreign substances invade the body, two types of immune responses are possible: cell-mediated immunity and humoral immunity.

Cell-mediated immunity

In cell-mediated immunity, T cells respond directly to antigens (foreign substances, such as bacteria or toxins, that induce antibody formation). This response involves destruction of target cells—such as virus-infected cells and cancer cells—through the secretion of lymphokines (lymph proteins). Examples of cell-mediated immunity are rejection of transplanted organs and delayed immune responses that fight disease.

Thirty-six percent of white blood cells (WBCs) are T cells. They are thought to originate from stem cells in the bone marrow; the thymus gland controls their maturity. In the process, a large number of antigen-specific cells are produced.

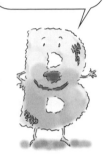

My job is to produce antibodies that, in turn, will attack an antigen.

A license to kill, help, or suppress

T cells can be killer, helper, or suppressor T cells.
• Killer cells bind to the surface of the invading cell, disrupt the membrane, and destroy it by altering its internal environment.
• Helper cells stimulate B cells to mature into plasma cells, which begin to synthesize and secrete immunoglobulin (proteins with known antibody activity).
• Suppressor cells reduce the humoral response.

Humoral immunity

B cells act in a different way than T cells to recognize and destroy antigens. B cells are responsible for humoral or immunoglobulin-mediated immunity. B cells originate in the bone marrow and mature into plasma cells that produce antibodies (immunoglobulin molecules that interact with a specific antigen). Antibodies destroy bacteria and viruses, thereby preventing them from entering host cells.

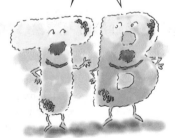

Keep in mind that I attack the antigen directly...

...while I produce antibodies that incapacitate the antigen.

Get to know your immunoglobulin

Five major classes of immunoglobulin exist:

Immunoglobulin G (IgG) makes up about 80% of plasma antibodies. It appears in all body fluids and is the major antibacterial and antiviral antibody.

Immunoglobulin M (IgM) is the first immunoglobulin produced during an immune response. It's too large to easily cross membrane barriers and is usually present only in the vascular system.

Immunoglobulin A (IgA) is found mainly in body secretions, such as saliva, sweat, tears, mucus, bile, and colostrum. It defends against pathogens on body surfaces, especially those that enter the respiratory and GI tracts.

Immunoglobulin D (IgD) is present in plasma and is easily broken down. It's the predominant antibody on the surface of B cells and is mainly an antigen receptor.

Immunoglobulin E (IgE) is the antibody involved in immediate hypersensitivity reactions, or allergic reactions that develop within minutes of exposure to an antigen. IgE stimulates the release of mast cell granules, which contain histamine and heparin.

Thanks for the complement

Part of humoral immunity, the complement system is a major mediator of the inflammatory response. It consists of proteins circulating as functionally inactive molecules.

The system causes inflammation by increasing:
- vascular permeability
- chemotaxis (movement of additional WBCs to an area of inflammation)
- phagocytosis (engulfing of foreign particles by cells called *phagocytes*)
- lysis of the foreign cell.

In most cases, an antigen-antibody reaction is necessary for the complement system to activate, a process called the *complement cascade*.

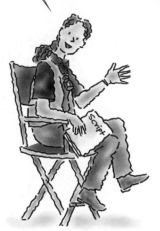

The *complement cascade* plays a crucial role in the inflammatory response.

Immune disorders

Common immune disorders include:
- allergic rhinitis
- anaphylaxis
- human immunodeficiency virus (HIV)
- lupus erythematosus
- rheumatoid arthritis.

What's the response?

Disorders of the immune response are of three main types:

 immunodeficiency disorders

 hypersensitivity disorders

 autoimmune disorders.

Absent or depressed

Immunodeficiency disorders result from an absent or depressed immune system. Some examples include HIV disease, DiGeorges syndrome, chronic fatigue syndrome, and immune dysfunction syndrome.

An allergen is the culprit

When an allergen (a substance the person is allergic to) enters the body, a hypersensitivity reaction occurs. It may be immediate or delayed. Hypersensitivity reactions are classified as:
- type I (IgE-mediated allergic reactions)
- type II (cytotoxic reactions)
- type III (immune complex reactions)
- type IV (cell-mediated reactions).

A body divided against itself

With autoimmune disorders, the body launches an immunologic response against itself. This leads to a sequence of tissue reactions and damage that may produce diffuse systemic signs and symptoms.

Examples of autoimmune disorders include rheumatoid arthritis, lupus erythematosus, dermatomyositis, and vasculitis.

Allergic rhinitis

Inhaled, airborne allergens may trigger an immune response in the upper airway. This causes two problems:
- rhinitis, or inflammation of the nasal mucous membrane
- conjunctivitis, or inflammation of the membrane lining the eyelids and covering the eyeball.

Hey, is this just hay fever?

When allergic rhinitis occurs seasonally, it's called *hay fever*, even though hay doesn't cause it and no fever occurs. When it occurs year-round, it's called *perennial allergic rhinitis*.

More than 20 million Americans suffer from this disorder, making it the most common allergic reaction. Although it can affect anyone at any age, it's most common in young children and adolescents.

How it happens

Allergic rhinitis is a type I, IgE-mediated hypersensitivity response to an environmental allergen in a genetically susceptible patient.

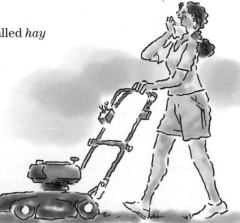

Ah-choo! Hay fever is usually caused by airborne pollens from trees, grass, and weeds, as well as by mold spores.

Hay fever occurs in the spring, summer, and fall, and is usually induced by airborne pollens from trees, grass, and weeds. In the summer and fall, mold spores also cause it.

Major perennial allergens and irritants include house dust and dust mites, feathers, molds, fungi, tobacco smoke, processed materials or industrial chemicals, and animal dander.

Swelling of the nasal and mucous membranes may trigger secondary sinus infections and middle ear infections, especially in perennial allergic rhinitis. Nasal polyps caused by edema and infection may increase nasal obstruction. Bronchitis and pneumonia are possible complications.

What to look for

In hay fever, the patient complains of sneezing attacks, rhinorrhea (profuse, watery nasal discharge), nasal obstruction or congestion, itching nose and eyes, and headache or sinus pain. An itchy throat and malaise also may occur.

Perennial allergic rhinitis causes chronic, extensive nasal obstruction or stuffiness, which can obstruct the eustachian tube, particularly in children. Conjunctivitis or other extranasal signs and symptoms can occur but are rare. (See *Types of rhinitis*.)

Would you look at that shiner!

Both conditions can cause allergic shiners (dark circles under the eyes) from venous congestion in the maxillary sinuses. The severity of signs and symptoms may vary from year to year. (See *Treating allergic rhinitis*.)

What tests tell you

IgE levels may be normal or elevated. Microscopic examination of sputum and nasal secretions shows a high number of eosinophils (granular leukocytes). The activity of eosinophils isn't completely

---

Types of rhinitis

Characteristics of the three common disorders of the nasal mucosa are listed below.

Chronic vasomotor rhinitis	Infectious rhinitis (common cold)	Rhinitis medicamentosa
• Eyes aren't affected.	• Nasal mucosa is beet red.	• Disorder is caused by excessive use of nasal sprays or drops.
• Nasal discharge contains mucus.	• Nasal secretions contain exudate.	• Nasal drainage and mucosal redness and swelling subside when the medication is discontinued.
• There's no seasonal variation.	• Fever and sore throat occur.	

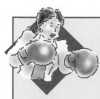

Treating allergic rhinitis

Treatment of allergic rhinitis involves controlling signs and symptoms and preventing infection. Treatment may include removing the environmental allergen. Drug therapy and immunotherapy may be used to treat perennial allergic rhinitis.

Annoying aftereffects
Antihistamines, such as chlorpheniramine, diphenhydramine, and promethazine, are effective in stopping a runny nose and watery eyes, but they usually produce sedation, dry mouth, nausea, dizziness, blurred vision, and nervousness. Nonsedating antihistamines, such as loratadine, desloratadine, fexofena-dine, and cetirizine, produce fewer annoying effects and have emerged as the treatment of choice.

Try these treatments, too
Topical intranasal corticosteroids may reduce local inflammation with minimal systemic adverse effects. Cromolyn sodium may help prevent allergic rhinitis, but it takes 4 weeks to produce a satisfactory effect and must be taken regularly during allergy season.

Long-term management may include immunotherapy or desensitization with injections of allergen extracts administered preseasonally, seasonally, or every year.

understood, but they're known to destroy parasitic organisms and play a role in allergic reactions.

Anaphylaxis

An acute type I allergic reaction, anaphylaxis causes sudden, rapidly progressive urticaria (hives) and respiratory distress. A severe reaction may lead to vascular collapse, systemic shock, and even death.

How it happens

Anaphylactic reactions result from systemic exposure to sensitizing drugs or other antigens, including:
- serums such as vaccines
- allergen extracts such as pollen
- enzymes such as L-asparaginase
- hormones
- penicillin and other antibiotics
- local anesthetics
- salicylates
- Latex (found in gloves, catheters, tubing, or balloons)
- polysaccharides such as iron dextran
- diagnostic chemicals such as radiographic contrast media
- foods, such as nuts and seafood
- sulfite-containing food additives
- insect venom, such as that from honeybees, wasps, and certain spiders

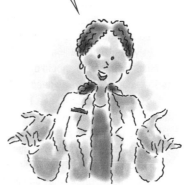

Anaphylaxis can result from contact with many common substances.

• a ruptured hydatid cyst (rare).

Penicillin is the most common anaphylaxis-causing antigen. It induces a reaction in 4 out of every 10,000 patients.

Reenacting the reaction

Here's how an anaphylactic reaction occurs:

• After initial exposure to an antigen, the immune system responds by producing IgE antibodies in the lymph nodes. Helper T cells enhance the process.

• Antibodies bind to membrane receptors located on mast cells in connective tissues and on basophils, which are a type of leukocyte.

• On reexposure, the antigen binds to adjacent IgE antibodies or cross-linked IgE receptors, activating inflammatory reactions such as the release of histamine.

Untreated anaphylaxis causes respiratory obstruction, systemic vascular collapse, and death—minutes to hours after the first symptoms occur. However, a delayed or persistent reaction may last up to 24 hours. (See *Treating anaphylaxis* and *Understanding anaphylaxis*.)

Battling illness

Treating anaphylaxis

Anaphylaxis is always an emergency. It requires an immediate injection of epinephrine 1:1,000 aqueous solution, 0.1 to 0.5 ml, subcutaneously (subQ) or I.M. If signs and symptoms persist, the injection should be repeated at 10- to 15-minute intervals as needed. Alternatively, 0.1 to 0.25 mg (1 to 2.5 ml of a 1:10,000 solution) may be given I.V. slowly over 5 to 10 minutes. The I.V. dose may be repeated every 5 to 15 minutes if needed or followed by an infusion at 1 to 4 mcg/minute. Diphenhydramine (Benadryl), 50 mg I.M. or I.V., may be given for allergic signs and symptoms. Aminophylline helps relieve bronchospasm.

Emphasis on epinephrine

In the early stages of anaphylaxis, when the patient remains conscious and normotensive, give epinephrine I.M. or subQ. Massage the injection site to speed the drug into the circulation. In severe reactions, when the patient is unconscious and hypotensive, give the drug I.V. as ordered. I.V. therapy is necessary to prevent vascular collapse after a severe reaction is treated.

Also, establish and maintain a patent airway. Watch for early signs of laryngeal edema, such as stridor, hoarseness, and dyspnea. If these occur, oxygen therapy along with endotracheal tube insertion or a tracheotomy is required.

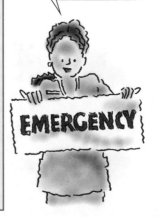

Act fast with anaphylaxis! An epinephrine injection is the first line of defense.

EMERGENCY

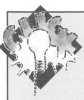

Now I get it!

Understanding anaphylaxis

The illustrations below teach the development of anaphylaxis

1. Response to antigen
Immunoglobulins (Ig) M and G recognize and bind the antigen.

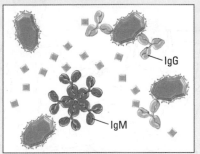

IgG

IgM

2. Release of chemical mediators
Activated IgE on basophils promotes the release of mediators: histamine, serotonin, and leukotrienes.

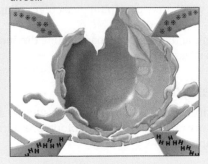

IgE

3. Intensified response
Mast cells release more histamine and ECF-A.

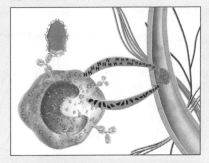

4. Respiratory distress
In the lungs, histamine causes endothelial cell destruction and fluid to leak into alveoli.

5. Deterioration
Meanwhile, mediators increase vascular permeability, causing fluid to leak from the vessels.

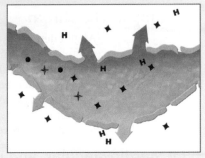

6. Failure of compensatory mechanisms
Endothelial cell damage causes basophils and mast cells to release heparin and mediator-neutralizing substances. However, anaphylaxis is now irreversible.

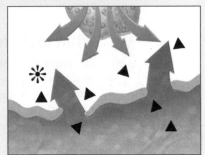

Key		
Complement cascade ▨	Serotonin ✦	ECF-A ◗
Histamine **H**	Leukotrienes ✳	Bradykinin ●
	Prostaglandins ✚	Heparin ▲

What to look for

Immediately after exposure, the patient may report a feeling of impending doom or fright, progressing to a fear of impending death, weakness, sweating, sneezing, dyspnea, nasal pruritus, and urticaria.

The skinny on skin effects

The skin may look cyanotic and pallid. Well-circumscribed, discrete, cutaneous wheals with red, raised wavy or indented borders and blanched centers usually appear and may merge to form giant hives.

A lump in the throat

Angioedema may cause the patient to complain of a lump in his throat; swelling of the tongue and larynx also occur. You may hear hoarseness, stridor, or wheezing. Chest tightness signals bronchial obstruction. These are all early signs of potentially fatal respiratory failure.

> In anaphylaxis, the degree of reaction is based on both the amount of allergen exposure and the number of prior exposures.

GI, cardiovascular, and neurologic effects

The patient may report severe stomach cramps, nausea, diarrhea, urinary urgency, and urinary incontinence.

Cardiovascular effects include hypotension, shock, and cardiac arrhythmias, which may precipitate vascular collapse if untreated.

Neurologic signs and symptoms may include dizziness, drowsiness, headache, restlessness, and seizures.

What tests tell you

The patient's history and signs and symptoms, such as increased heart and respiratory rate and decreased blood pressure, establish a diagnosis of anaphylaxis.

HIV disease

HIV is the infectious agent responsible for the immune system disorder HIV disease. The disease, characterized by progressive immune system impairment, destroys T cells and, therefore, the cell-mediated response. This immunodeficiency makes the patient more susceptible to infections and unusual cancers. (See *Facts about HIV infection and AIDS.*)

The Centers for Disease Control and Prevention (CDC) has established criteria for making a diagnosis of HIV disease. The course of HIV disease can vary, but it usually results in death from opportunistic infections. Most experts believe that virtually everyone infected with HIV will eventually develop acquired immunodeficiency syndrome (AIDS). (See *HIV infection classification*.)

How it happens

HIV is an RNA-based retrovirus that requires a human host to replicate. The average time between HIV infection and the development of AIDS is 8 to 10 years.

HIV destroys CD4+ cells—also known as *helper T cells*—that regulate the normal immune response. The CD4+ antigen serves as

---

HIV infection classification

The Centers for Disease Control and Prevention's revised classification system for human immu-nodeficiency virus (HIV)–infected adolescents and adults categorizes patients on the basis of three ranges of CD4+ T-lymphocyte counts along with three clinical conditions associated with HIV infection.

The classification system identifies where the patient lies in the progression of the disease and helps to guide treatment. Viral load indicates the amount of viral replication and helps predict the progress of the disease and the effectiveness of treatment.

Ranges of CD4+ T lymphocytes
- *Category 1:* CD4+ cell count greater than or equal to 500
- *Category 2:* CD4+ cell count 200 to 499
- *Category 3:* CD4+ cell count less than 200

Clinical categories
- *Category A* (conditions present in patients with documented HIV infection): asymptomatic HIV infection persistent, generalized lymph node enlargement or acute (primary) HIV infection with accompanying illness or history of acute HIV infection
- *Category B* (conditions present in patients with symptomatic HIV infection): bacillary angiomatosis, oropharyngeal or persistent vulvovaginal candidiasis, fever or diarrhea lasting

over 1 month, idiopathic thrombocytopenic purpura, pelvic inflammatory disease (especially with a tubo-ovarian abscess), and peripheral neuropathy
- *Category C* (conditions present in patients with acquired immunodeficiency syndrome): candidiasis of the bronchi, trachea, lungs, or esophagus; invasive cervical cancer; disseminated or extrapulmonary coccidioidomycosis; extrapulmonary cryptococcosis; chronic intestinal crypto-sporidiosis; cytomegalovirus (CMV) disease affecting organs other than the liver, spleen, or lymph nodes; CMV retinitis with vision loss; encephalopathy related to HIV; herpes simplex involving chronic ulcers or herpetic bronchitis, pneumonitis, or esophagitis; disseminated or extrapulmon-ary histoplasmosis; chronic, intestinal isosporiasis; Kaposi's sarcoma; Burkitt's lymphoma or its equivalent; immunoblastic lymphoma or its equivalent; primary brain lymphoma; disseminated or extrapulmonary *Mycobacterium avium* complex or *M. kansasii;* pulmonary or extrapulmonary *M. tuberculosis;* any other species of *Mycobacterium* (disseminated or extrapulmonary); *Pneumocystis carinii* pneumonia; recurrent pneumonia; progressive multifocal leukoencephalopathy; recurrent *Salmonella* septicemia; toxoplasmosis of the brain; wasting syndrome caused by HIV.

Facts about HIV infection and AIDS

Acquired immunodeficiency syndrome (AIDS) was first described by the Centers for Disease Control and Prevention (CDC) in 1981. By the end of 2005, approximately 437,000 people in the United States had been diagnosed with AIDS. It is estimated that more than 40,000 new infections occur each year.
- The AIDS epidemic is growing most rapidly among minority populations in the United States. It's the leading killer of Black males ages 25 to 44.
- According to the CDC, in the United States, AIDS affects nearly seven times more Blacks and three times more Hispanics than Whites.
- The prevalence of HIV infection isn't known, but the CDC estimates as many as 950,000 to 1.2 million U.S. residents may be infected, 30% of whom are unaware of their infection.

a receptor for HIV and allows it to invade the cell. Afterward, the virus replicates within the CD4+ cell, causing cell death.

On the surface

HIV can infect almost any cell that has the CD4+ antigen on its surface, including monocytes, macrophages, bone marrow progenitors, and glial, gut, and epithelial cells. The infection can cause dementia, wasting syndrome, and blood abnormalities.

Modes of transmission

HIV is transmitted three ways:

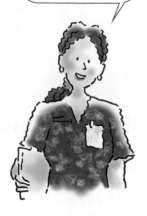

The CD4+ antigen on the cell surface allows HIV to infect the cell.

through contact with infected blood or blood products during transfusion or tissue transplantation (although routine testing of the blood supply since 1985 has cut the risk of contracting HIV this way) or by sharing a contaminated needle

through contact with infected body fluids, such as semen and vaginal fluids, during unprotected sex (anal intercourse is especially dangerous because it causes mucosal trauma)

across the placental barrier from an infected mother to a fetus, or from an infected mother to an infant either through cervical or blood contact at delivery or through breast milk.

Although blood, semen, vaginal secretions, and breast milk are the body fluids that most readily transmit HIV, it has also been found in saliva, urine, tears, and feces. However, there's no evidence of transmission through these fluids.

What to look for

After initial exposure, the infected person may have no signs or symptoms, or he may have a flulike illness (primary infection) and then remain asymptomatic for 10 or more years. As the syndrome progresses, he may have neurologic symptoms from HIV encephalopathy or symptoms of an opportunistic infection, such as *Pneumocystis carinii* pneumonia, cytomegalovirus, or cancer. Eventually, repeated opportunistic infections overwhelm the patient's weakened immune defenses, invading every body system. (See *Opportunistic diseases associated with AIDS.*)

(Text continues on page 356.)

Opportunistic diseases associated with AIDS

This chart describes some common diseases associated with acquired immunodeficiency syndrome (AIDS), their characteristic signs and symptoms, and their treatments.

Disease	Signs and symptoms	Treatment
BACTERIAL INFECTIONS		
Tuberculosis A disease caused by *Mycobacterium tuberculosis*, an aerobic, acid-fast bacillus spread through inhalation of droplet nuclei that are aerosolized by coughing, sneezing, or talking	Fever, weight loss, night sweats, and fatigue, followed by dyspnea, chills, hemoptysis, and chest pain	Isoniazid, rifampin, pyrazinamide, and ethambutol or streptomycin are given during the first 2 months of therapy, followed by rifampin and isoniazid for a minimum of 9 months and for at least 6 months after culture is negative for bacteria.
Mycobacterium avium *complex* A primary infection acquired by oral ingestion or inhalation; can infect the bone marrow, liver, spleen, GI tract, lymph nodes, lungs, skin, brain, adrenal glands, and kidneys; is chronic and may be localized and disseminated in its course of infection; incidence is decreasing because of changes in treatment of human immunodeficiency virus (HIV)	Multiple, nonspecific symptoms consistent with systemic illness: fever, fatigue, weight loss, anorexia, night sweats, abdominal pain, and chronic diarrhea; *physical examination findings:* emaciation, generalized lymphadenopathy, diffuse tenderness, jaundice, and hepato-splenomegaly; *laboratory findings:* anemia, leukopenia, and thrombocytopenia	Treatment includes clarithromycin or azithromycin and ethambutol. These drugs are given with one or more of the following: amikacin, ciprofloxacin, rifabutin, or rifampin.
Salmonellosis A disease acquired by ingestion of food or water contaminated by *Salmonella* but also linked to snake powders, pet turtles, and domestic turkeys; also can be spread by contaminated medications or diagnostic agents, direct fecal-oral transmission (especially during sexual activity), transfusion of contaminated blood products, and inadequately sterilized fiber-optic instruments used in upper GI endoscopic procedures	Nonspecific signs and symptoms, including fever, chills, sweats, weight loss, diarrhea, and anorexia	Although treatment of nontyphoid salmonellosis is usually unnecessary in immunocompetent individuals, it's required in persons with HIV. Antibiotic selection depends on drug sensitivities. However, treatment may include co-trimoxazole, amoxicillin, fluoroquinolones, ampicillin, or third-generation cephalosporins.

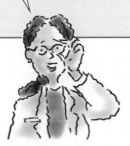

This chart can help you identify various infections that accompany AIDS.

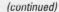

(continued)

Opportunistic diseases associated with AIDS (continued)

Disease	Signs and symptoms	Treatment
FUNGAL INFECTIONS		
Coccidioidomycosis An infectious disease caused by the fungus *Coccidioides immitis,* which grows in soil in arid regions in the southwestern United States, Mexico, Central America, and South America	Flulike illness (malaise, fever, back-ache, headache, cough, arthralgia), periarticular swelling in knees and ankles, meningitis, bony lesions, skin findings, and pulmonary or genitourinary involvement	Fluconazole, itraconazole, or ampho-tericin B is given.
Candidiasis A disease caused by the fungus *Candida albicans* that exists on teeth, gingivae, and skin and in the oropharynx, vagina, and large intestine; majority of infections are endogenous and related to interruption of normal defense mechanisms; possible human-to-human transmission, including congenital transmission in neo-nates, in whom thrush develops after vaginal delivery	*Thrush* (the most prevalent form in HIV-infected individuals): creamy, curdlike, white patches, surrounded by an erythematous base, found on any oral mucosal surface; *nail infection:* inflammation and tenderness of tissue surrounding the nails or the nail itself; *vaginitis:* intense pruritus of the vulva and curdlike vaginal discharge	Nystatin suspension and clotrimazole troches are administered for thrush; nystatin suspension or pastilles, clotrimazole troches, fluconazole, or itraconazole for esophagitis; topical clotrimazole, miconazole, or ketoconazole for cutaneous candidiasis; topical imidazole or oral fluconazole, ketoconazole, or both for candidiasis of nails; and topical clotrimazole, miconazole, or oral fluconazole for vaginitis.
Cryptococcosis An infectious disease caused by the fungus *Cryptococcus neoformans;* can be found in nature; can be aerosolized and inhaled; settles in the lungs, where it can remain dormant or spread to other parts of the body, particularly the central nervous system (CNS); responsible for three forms of infection: pulmonary, CNS, and disseminated; most pulmonary cases found serendipitously	*Pulmonary cryptococcosis:* fever, cough, dyspnea, and pleuritic chest pain; *CNS cryptococcosis:* fever, malaise, headaches, stiff neck, nausea and vomiting, and altered mentation; *disseminated cryptococcosis:* lymphadenopathy, multifocal cutaneous lesions; *other symptoms:* macules, papules, skin lesions, oral lesions, placental infection, myocarditis, prostatic infection, optic neuropathy, rectal abscess, and lymph node infection	Primary therapy for initial infection is amphotericin B, administered I.V. for 6 to 8 weeks; sometimes amphotericin B and flucytosine are used in combination. Fluconazole and itraconazole are also used. After initial treatment, the patient is typically maintained on lifelong fluconazole therapy.
Histoplasmosis A disease caused by the fungus *Histoplasma capsulatum* that exists in nature, is readily airborne, and can reach the bronchioles and alveoli when inhaled	*Most common:* fever, weight loss, hepatomegaly, splenomegaly, and pancytopenia; *less common:* diarrhea, cerebritis, chorioretinitis, meningitis, oral and cutaneous lesions, and GI mucosal lesions causing bleeding	Drug of choice is amphotericin B for acute treatment of illness and then for lifelong suppressive therapy. Itraconazole is also used.

Opportunistic diseases associated with AIDS *(continued)*

Disease	Signs and symptoms	Treatment
PROTOZOAN INFECTIONS		
Pneumocystis carinii *pneumonia* Pneumonia caused by *P. carinii;* also has properties of fungal infection, exists in human lungs, and is transmitted by airborne exposure; the most common life-threatening opportunistic infection in individuals with AIDS	Fever, fatigue, and weight loss for several weeks to months before respiratory symptoms develop; *respiratory symptoms:* dyspnea, usually noted initially on exertion and later at rest, and cough, usually starting out dry and nonproductive and later becoming productive	Co-trimoxazole may be given orally or I.V., although about 20% of AIDS patients are hypersensitive to sulfa drugs. I.V. pentamidine isethionate may be given but can cause many adverse effects, including permanent diabetes mellitus. Dapsone with trimethoprim, clindamycin, primaquine, atovaquone, or corticosteroids is also used. Prophylaxis for disease prevention and following treatment includes co-trimoxazole, atovaquone, or dapsone.
Cryptosporidiosis An intestinal infection by the protozoan *Cryptosporidium;* transmitted by person-to-person contact, water, food contaminants, and airborne exposure; most common site: small intestine	Abdominal cramping, flatulence, weight loss, anorexia, malaise, fever, nausea, vomiting, myalgia, and profuse, watery diarrhea	No effective therapy is known. Most medical therapy is palliative and directed toward symptom control, focusing on fluid replacement, occasionally total parenteral nutrition, correction of electrolyte imbalances, and analgesic, antidiarrheal, and antiperistaltic agents. Paromomycin, spiramycin, and octreotides are used.
Toxoplasmosis A disease caused by *Toxoplasma gondii;* major means of transmission through ingestion of undercooked meats and vegetables containing oocysts; causes focal or diffuse meningoencephalitis with cellular necrosis and progresses unchecked to the lungs, heart, and skeletal muscle	Localized neurologic deficits, fever, headache, altered mental status, and seizures	Sulfadiazine or clindamycin with pyrimethamine may be given; however, about 20% of AIDS patients are hypersensitive to sulfa drugs. Folinic acid may be given to prevent marrow toxicity from pyrimethamine. Patients must receive maintenance combination drug therapy in lower doses to prevent relapse.
Coccidiosis A disease caused by coccidian protozoan parasite *Isospora hominis* or *I. belli;* after ingestion, infects the small intes-tine and results in malabsorption and diarrhea	Watery, nonbloody diarrhea; crampy abdominal pain; nausea; anorexia; weight loss; weakness; occasional vomiting; and a low-grade fever	Fluconazole, itraconazole, or amphotericin B is used.

(continued)

Opportunistic diseases associated with AIDS (continued)

Disease	Signs and symptoms	Treatment
VIRAL INFECTIONS		
Herpes simplex virus Chronic infection caused by a herpes virus; often a reactivation of an earlier herpes infection	Red, blisterlike lesions occurring in oral, anal, and genital areas; also found on the esophageal and tracheobronchial mucosa; pain, bleeding, and discharge	Acyclovir, famciclovir, or valacyclovir is given I.V. or P.O. Lower maintenance doses may be given to prevent recurrence of symptoms.
Cytomegalovirus (CMV) A viral infection of the herpesvirus that may result in serious, widespread infection; most common sites: lungs, adrenal glands, eyes, CNS, GI tract, male GU tract, and blood	Unexplained fever, malaise, GI ulcers, diarrhea, weight loss, swollen lymph nodes, hepatomegaly, splenomegaly, blurred vision, floaters, dyspnea (especially on exertion), dry nonproductive cough, and vision changes leading to blindness in patients with ocular infection	Ganciclovir or foscarnet is used to treat CMV. Ganciclovir has shown some anti-HIV properties. Foscarnet or intraocular ganciclovir implants may be used to treat CMV retinitis.
Progressive multifocal leukoencephalopathy (PML) Progressive demyelinating disorder caused by hyperactivation of a papovavirus that leads to gradual brain degeneration	Progressive dementia, memory loss, headache, confusion, weakness, and other possible neurologic complications such as seizures	No form of therapy for PML has been effective, but attempted therapies include prednisone, acyclovir, and adenine arabinoside administered both I.V. and intrathecally.
Herpes zoster A disease also known as *acute posterior ganglionitis, shingles, zona,* and *zoster;* acute infection caused by reactivation of the chickenpox virus	Small clusters of painful, reddened papules that follow the route of inflamed nerves; may be disseminated, involving two or more dermatomes	Herpes zoster is most often treated with oral acyclovir capsules until healed. Treatment may have to continue at lower doses indefinitely to prevent recurrence. I.V. acyclovir is effective in disseminated varicella zoster lesions in some patients. Medications, such as capsaicin, may relieve pain associated with the infection and postherpetic neuropathies. Famciclovir and valacyclovir can also be used.

No bones about it! These infections can affect all my body systems.

Opportunistic diseases associated with AIDS *(continued)*

Disease	Signs and symptoms	Treatment
NEOPLASMS		
Kaposi's sarcoma A generalized disease with characteristic lesions involving all skin surfaces, including the face (tip of the nose, eyelids), head, upper and lower limbs, soles of the feet, palms of the hands, conjunctivae, sclerae, pharynx, larynx, trachea, hard palate, stomach, liver, small and large intestines, and glans penis	Manifested cutaneously and subcutaneously; usually painless, nonpruritic tumor nodules that are pigmented and violaceous (red to blue), nonblanching and palpable; patchy lesions appearing early and possibly mistaken for bruises, purpura, or diffuse cutaneous hemorrhages	Treatment isn't indicated for all individuals. Indications include cosmetically offensive, painful, or obstructive lesions or rapidly progressing disease. Systemic chemotherapy using single or multiple drugs may be given to alleviate symptoms. Radiation therapy may be used to treat lesions. Intralesional therapy with vinblastine may be given for cosmetic purposes to treat small cutaneous lesions, and laser therapy and cryotherapy may be used to treat small isolated lesions. Interferon alfa-2a and interferon alfa-2b are also used.
Malignant lymphomas Immune system cancer in which lymph tissue cells begin growing abnormally and spread to other organs; incidence in persons with AIDS: about 4% to 10%; diagnosed in HIV-infected individuals as widespread disease involving extranodal sites, most commonly in the GI tract, CNS, bone marrow, and liver	Unexplained fever, night sweats, or weight loss greater than 10% of patient's total body weight; signs and symptoms commonly confined to one body system: CNS (confusion, lethargy, and memory loss) or GI tract (pain, obstruction, changes in bowel habits, bleeding, and fever)	Individualized therapy may include a modified combination of methotrexate, bleomycin, doxorubicin, cyclophosphamide, vincristine, and dexamethasone. Radiation therapy—not chemotherapy—is used to treat primary CNS lymphoma.
Cervical neoplasm HIV-positive women appear to be at increased risk for cervical neoplasm associated with human papilloma virus infections. This has emerged as a significant gynecologic complication of HIV infection as more women become infected with HIV and live longer with illness because of antiretroviral therapy	*Possible indicators of early invasive disease:* abnormal vaginal bleeding, persistent vaginal discharge, or postcoital pain and bleeding; *possible indicators of advanced disease:* pelvic pain, vaginal leakage of urine and feces from a fistula, anorexia, weight loss, and fatigue	Treatment is tailored to the disease stage. Preinvasive lesions may require total excisional biopsy, cryosurgery, laser destruction, conization (and frequent Papanicolaou test follow-up) and, rarely, hysterectomy. Invasive squamous cell carcinoma may require radical hysterectomy and radiation therapy.

Child watch

In children, the incubation period averages only 17 months. Signs and symptoms resemble those for adults, except that children are more likely to have a history of bacterial infections, such as otitis media and lymphoid interstitial pneumonia, as well as types of pneumonia not caused by *P. carinii*, sepsis, and chronic salivary gland enlargement.

An infected person can test negative for HIV antibodies for up to 14 months after exposure.

What tests tell you

The CDC recommends testing for HIV 1 month after a possible exposure—the approximate length of time before antibodies can be detected in the blood. However, an infected patient can test negative for up to 14 months, although the average positive test occurs 3 to 7 weeks post-exposure. Antibody tests in neonates may also be unreliable because transferred maternal antibodies persist for up to 18 months, causing a false-positive result.

Standard HIV testing consists of the enzyme-linked immunosorbent assay (ELISA) which, if positive, is confirmed by the Western Blot Assay test. A rapid antigen test, called the P24, is used to screen donated blood. All of the commonly used tests react to HIV antibodies or antigens. Most people develop detectable HIV antibodies within 6 to 12 weeks of infection. In very rare cases, antibody development can take up to 6 months. It is extremely unusual for someone to take longer than 6 months to develop antibodies.

Testing earlier than 3 months after exposure may result in an unclear test result because the infected person may not yet have developed antibodies to HIV. If a person tests negative 3 months after a known exposure, some authorities recommend a follow-up test at 6 months post exposure.

Another test, the DNA/RNA test, detects the genetic material of HIV and can identify the virus within 1 week of infection; however, this test is very expensive and rarely used.

Other blood tests support the diagnosis and are used to evaluate the severity of immunosuppression. They include CD4+ and CD8+ cell (killer T cell) subset counts, erythrocyte sedimentation rate (ESR), complete blood count (CBC), serum beta (sub 2) microglobulin, p24 antigen, neopterin levels, and anergy testing.

Many opportunistic infections in AIDS patients are reactivations of previous infections. Therefore, patients may also be tested for syphilis, hepatitis B, tuberculosis, toxoplasmosis, and histoplasmosis. (See *Treating HIV disease*.)

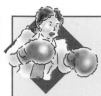

Battling illness

Treating HIV disease

There is no cure for human immunodeficiency virus (HIV) disease; however, several types of drugs are used to treat the disease and prolong life.

Antiretrovirals

Antiretroviral drugs are used to control the reproduction of the virus and to slow the progression of HIV-related disease. Highly Active Antiretroviral Therapy, commonly referred to as HAART, is the recommended treatment for HIV infection. HAART combines three or more antiretroviral medications in a daily regimen. The Food and Drug Administration has approved five classes of antiretroviral drugs.

  Nonnucleoside reverse transcriptase inhibitors—bind to and disable reverse transcriptase, a protein that HIV needs to make more copies of itself. Such drugs as delavirdine, efavirenz, and nevirapine are included in this class.

  Nucleoside reverse transcriptase inhibitors—are faulty versions of building blocks that HIV requires to make more copies of itself. When HIV uses one of these drugs instead of a normal building block, reproduction of the virus is halted. Abacavir, didanosine, emtricitabine, lamivudine, stavudine, tenofovir DF, zalcitabine, and zidovudine are included in this class.

  Protease inhibitors—disable protease, a protein that HIV needs to make more copies of itself. These drugs include amprenavir, atazanavir, fosamprenavir, indinavir, lopinavir, nelfinavir, ritonavir, and saquinavir.

  Fusion inhibitors—block HIV entry into cells. Enfuvirtide is the only currently approved fusion inhibitor.

  Integrase inhibitors—inhibit the insertion of HIV DNA into human DNA via the integrase enzyme. Isentress is the only approved integrase inhibitor.

Anti-infectives and antineoplastics

In addition to antiretroviral drugs, anti-infective drugs are prescribed to treat opportunistic infections. Antineoplastic drugs are used to treat associated cancers.

Lupus erythematosus

A chronic, inflammatory, autoimmune disorder affecting the connective tissues, lupus erythematosus takes two forms: discoid and systemic. The first type affects only the skin; the second type affects multiple organs and can be fatal.

Discoid lupus erythematosus causes superficial lesions—typically over the cheeks and bridge of the nose—that leave scars after healing. Systemic lupus erythematosus (SLE) is characterized by recurrent remissions and exacerbations.

About 16,000 new cases of SLE are diagnosed each year. Lupus erythematosus strikes women 8 times more often than men and occurs 15 times more often during the childbearing years. It occurs worldwide but is most prevalent among Native Americans, Blacks, Hispanics, and Asians.

Battling illness

Treating SLE

Drugs are the mainstay of treatment for systemic lupus erythematosus (SLE). In patients who have mild disease, nonsteroidal anti-inflammatory drugs such as ibuprofen usually control arthritis and arthralgia. Skin lesions require sun protection and topical corticosteroid creams, such as triamcinolone and hydrocortisone.

Fluorinated steroids may control acute or discoid lesions. Stubborn lesions may respond to intralesional or systemic corticosteroids or antimalarials, such as hydroxychloroquine, chloroquine, and dapsone. Because hydroxychloroquine and chloroquine can cause retinal damage, patients receiving them should have an ophthalmologic examination every 6 months.

More medication information

Corticosteroids are the treatment of choice for systemic symptoms, acute generalized exacerbations, and injury to vital organs from pleuritis, pericarditis, nephritis, vasculitis, and central nervous system involvement. With initial prednisone doses of 60 mg or more, the patient's condition usually improves noticeably within 48 hours. After symptoms are under control, the drug dosage is gradually reduced and then discontinued.

In patients whose kidneys or central nervous system is affected by SLE, immunosuppressive drugs, such as cyclophosphamide and mycophenolate, may be used. In addition, methotrexate is sometimes effective in controlling the disease.

Get to it early

Although there's no cure for lupus, the prognosis improves with early detection and treatment. Prognosis remains poor for patients who develop cardiovascular, renal, or neurologic complications or severe bacterial infections. (See *Treating SLE.*)

How it happens

The exact cause of lupus erythematosus remains a mystery, but autoimmunity is probably the primary cause, along with environmental, hormonal, genetic and, possibly, viral factors. (See *The lowdown on lupus.*)

In autoimmunity, the body produces antibodies against its own cells. The formed antigen-antibody complexes can suppress the body's normal immunity and damage tissues. A significant feature of patients with SLE is their ability to produce antibodies against many different tissue components, such as red blood cells, neutrophils, platelets, lymphocytes, or almost any organ or tissue in the body.

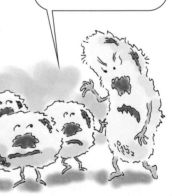

We didn't do anything wrong! Why are you attacking your own cells?!

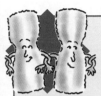

The genetic link

The lowdown on lupus

Apoptosis

Researchers are currently trying to identify genes that play a role in the development of lupus. They suspect that a genetic defect in a cellular process called *apoptosis* is present in people with lupus. Apoptosis allows the body to eliminate cells that have fulfilled their function and need to be replaced. If a problem with apoptosis occurs, harmful cells may linger, causing damage to the body's own tissue.

Complement

Researchers are also studying genes for *complement*, a series of proteins in the blood that play an important role in the immune system. Complement acts as a backup for antibodies, helping them destroy foreign substances that invade the body. A decrease in the amount of complement makes the body less able to fight or destroy foreign substances. If these substances aren't removed from the body, the immune system may become overactive and make autoantibodies.

SLE susceptibility

Most people with SLE have a genetic predisposition. Other predisposing factors include stress, streptococcal or viral infections, exposure to sunlight or ultraviolet light, immunization, pregnancy, and abnormal estrogen metabolism. Drugs may also trigger or aggravate the disease. (See *Drugs that spark SLE.*)

What to look for

The onset of SLE may be acute or insidious, but the disease has no characteristic clinical pattern. Patients may complain of fever, anorexia, weight loss, malaise, fatigue, abdominal pain, nausea, vomiting, diarrhea, constipation, rashes, and polyarthralgia (multiple joint pain).

Blood disorders, such as anemia, leukopenia, lymphopenia, thrombocytopenia, and an elevated ESR, occur because of circulating antibodies. Women may report irregular menstruation or amenorrhea, particularly during exacerbations.

About 90% of patients have joint involvement that resembles rheumatoid arthritis. About 40% have Raynaud's phenomenon—intermittent, severe pallor of the fingers, toes, ears, or nose.

Drugs that spark SLE

Many drugs can cause symptoms that resemble those of systemic lupus erythematosus (SLE). Other drugs may actually trigger SLE or activate it. These drugs include:
• procainamide
• hydralazine
• isoniazid
• methyldopa
• anticonvulsants
• penicillins, sulfa drugs, and hormonal contraceptives (less common).

Shedding light on lupus

The skin eruption characteristic of lupus erythematosus is a rash on areas exposed to light. The rash varies in severity from red areas to disc-shaped plaque. The classic "butterfly" rash occurs on about 50% of the patients with this disorder. Patchy alopecia is also common in SLE.

Cardiopulmonary effects

Cardiopulmonary signs and symptoms occur in about 50% of patients. They include chest pain, indicating pleuritis; dyspnea, suggesting parenchymal infiltrates and pneumonitis; tachycardia; central cyanosis; and hypotension. These signs and symptoms may signal pulmonary embolism.

Neurologic effects

Seizure disorders and confusion may indicate neurologic damage. Other central nervous system signs and symptoms include emotional lability, psychosis, headaches, irritability, stroke, and depression.

Urinary system effects

Be especially alert for infrequent urination, which may signal renal failure, and urinary frequency, painful urination, and bladder spasms, which are signs and symptoms of urinary tract infection (UTI). UTIs and renal failure are the leading causes of death for SLE patients.

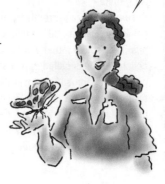

Approximately 50% of SLE patients develop the classic "butterfly" rash.

What tests tell you

These tests are used to diagnose lupus erythematosus:
• CBC with differential may show anemia and a reduced WBC count.
• Serum electrophoresis may show hypergammaglobulinemia.
• Other blood tests may show a decreased platelet count and an elevated ESR. Active disease is diagnosed by decreased serum complement levels, leukopenia, mild thrombocytopenia, and anemia.
• Chest X-rays may reveal pleurisy or lupus pneumonitis.
• Antinuclear antibodies are elevated.

Rheumatoid arthritis

A chronic, systemic, inflammatory disease, rheumatoid arthritis usually attacks peripheral joints and surrounding muscles, tendons, ligaments, and blood vessels. Spontaneous remissions and unpredictable exacerbations mark the course of this potentially crippling disease.

Rheumatoid arthritis affects 2.1 million Americans—1.5 million women and 600,000 men—and although it occurs in all age-groups, the peak onset is between ages 20 and 50.

Lifelong treatment

Rheumatoid arthritis usually requires lifelong treatment and some-times surgery. In most patients, the disease is intermittent, allow-ing for periods of normal activity. However, 10% of patients suffer total disability from severe joint deformity, associated symptoms, or both. The prognosis worsens with the development of nodules, vasculitis (inflammation of a blood or lymph vessel), and high titers of rheumatoid factor.

How it happens

The cause of rheumatoid arthritis isn't known, but infections, ge-netics, and endocrine factors may play a part. (See *RA marker*.)

When exposed to an antigen, a person susceptible to rheuma-toid arthritis may develop abnormal or altered IgG antibodies. The body doesn't recognize these antibodies as "self," so it forms an antibody known as *rheumatoid factor* against them. By aggregat-ing into complexes, rheumatoid factor causes inflammation.

Eventually, inflammation causes cartilage damage. Immune re-sponses continue, including complement system activation. Com-plement system activation attracts leukocytes and stimulates the release of inflammatory mediators, which then exacerbate joint destruction. (See *Treating rheumatoid arthritis*, page 362.)

Four-alarm inflammation

If unarrested, joint inflammation occurs in four stages:

First, synovitis develops from congestion and edema of the synovial membrane and joint capsule.

Formation of pannus (thickened layers of granulation tis-sue) marks the onset of the second stage. Pannus covers and in-vades cartilage and eventually destroys the joint capsule and bone.

The third stage is characterized by fibrous ankylosis (fi-brous invasion of the pannus and scar formation that occludes the joint space). Bone atrophy and misalignment cause visible deformities and restrict movement, causing muscle atrophy, im-balance, and, possibly, partial dislocations.

In the fourth stage, fibrous tissue calcifies, resulting in bony ankylosis (fixation of a joint) and total immobility. Pain associ-ated with movement may restrict active joint use and cause fi-brous or bony ankylosis, soft-tissue contractures, and joint defor-

The genetic link

RA marker

Researchers suspect that viruses may trigger rheumatoid arthritis (RA) in some people who have an inherited ten-dency for the disease. Many people with RA have a genetic marker called *HLA-DR4*. Re-searchers also suspect that other genes may be implicated in RA.

IgG appears in all body fluids and is the major antibacterial and antiviral antibody.

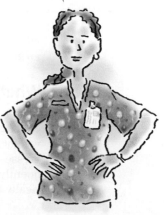

Battling illness

Treating rheumatoid arthritis

Treatment measures are used to reduce pain and inflammation and preserve the patient's functional capacity and quality of life.

Drug therapy

Nonsteroidal anti-inflammatory drugs (NSAIDs), which include the traditional NSAIDs (such as ibuprofen), COX-2 inhibitors (celecoxib [Celebrex] and valdecoxib [Bextra]), and salicylates (aspirin) are the mainstay of therapy because they decrease inflammation and relieve joint pain.

Other drugs that can be used are hydroxychloroquine, gold salts, penicillamine, and corticosteroids such as prednisone. Immunosuppressants—cyclophosphamide, methotrexate, and azathioprine—are used in the early stages of the disease.

A new class of drugs, tumor necrosis factor (TNF) alpha-blockers, is now available for the treatment of rheumatoid arthritis. Drugs such as infliximab (Remicade), adalimumab (Humira), and etanercept (Embrel) are proving to be effective in both adult and juvenile RA, as well as in other autoimmune disorders.

Protein-A immunoadsorption therapy

Patients with moderate to severe rheumatoid arthritis who haven't responded well to drug therapy may opt for protein-A immunoadsorption therapy. During this therapy, blood is drawn from a vein in the patient's arm and pumped into an apheresis machine, which separates plasma from the blood cells. Plasma then passes through a PROSORBA column (a plastic cylinder about the size of a coffee mug that contains a sandlike substance coated with protein A). Protein A in the cylinder binds with the antibodies produced in rheumatoid arthritis. After the plasma passes through the PROSORBA column, it's returned to the body through a vein in the patient's other arm.

This procedure typically lasts 2 hours. The recommended regimen is one treatment weekly for 12 weeks.

Physical and other therapies

Joint function can be preserved through range-of-motion exercises and a carefully individualized physical and occupational therapy program. Surgery is available for joints that are damaged or painful.

mities. (See *The effects of rheumatoid arthritis in certain joints.*)

What to look for

At first, the patient may complain of nonspecific symptoms, including fatigue, malaise, anorexia, persistent low-grade fever, weight loss, and vague articular symptoms. As inflammation progresses through the four stages, specific symptoms develop, frequently in the fingers. They usually occur bilaterally and symmetrically and may extend to the wrists, elbows, knees, and ankles.

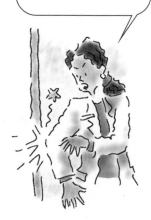

Pain from rheumatoid arthritis can occur in the elbow. I can make it happen without having the disorder!

Now I get it!

The effects of rheumatoid arthritis on certain joints

Many joints can be affected by RA, including the knee, hand and wrist, and hip.

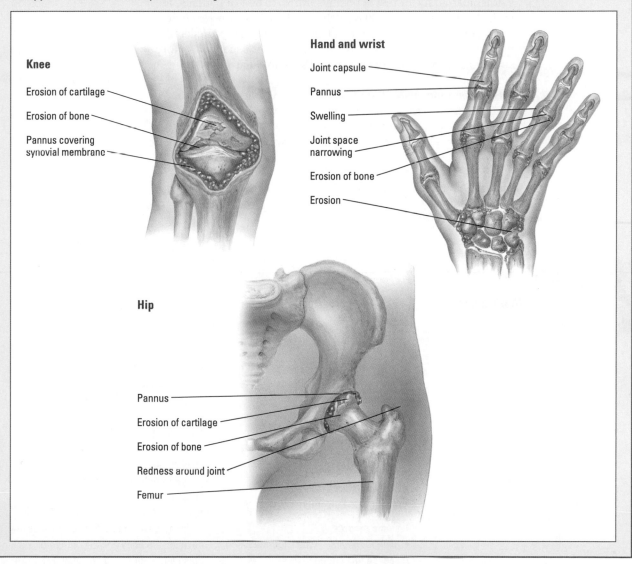

Knee

Erosion of cartilage

Erosion of bone

Pannus covering synovial membrane

Hand and wrist

Joint capsule

Pannus

Swelling

Joint space narrowing

Erosion of bone

Erosion

Hip

Pannus

Erosion of cartilage

Erosion of bone

Redness around joint

Femur

What tests tell you

Although no test can be used to definitively diagnose rheumatoid arthritis, these tests are useful:

• X-rays may show bone demineralization and soft-tissue swelling and help determine the extent of cartilage and bone destruction, erosion, subluxations, and deformities.

• Rheumatoid factor test is positive in 75% to 80% of patients, as indicated by a titer of 1:160 or higher. Although the presence of rheumatoid factor doesn't confirm the disease, it helps in determining the prognosis. A patient with a high titer usually has more severe and progressive disease with extra-articular signs and symptoms.

• Synovial fluid analysis shows increased volume and turbidity but decreased viscosity and complement levels. The WBC count often exceeds $10,000/mm^3$.

• Serum protein electrophoresis may show elevated serum globulin levels.

• ESR is elevated in 85% to 90% of patients. Because an elevated rate often parallels disease activity, this test helps monitor the patient's response to therapy.

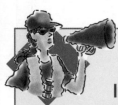

That's a wrap!

Immune system review

Understanding the immune system

The body protects itself from infectious organisms through the host defense system. Three lines of defense include:

• physical and chemical barriers to infection

• the inflammatory response

• the immune response.

Structures

• Bone marrow

• Lymph nodes

• Thymus

• Spleen

• Tonsils

Types of immunity

• Cell-mediated immunity—T cells respond to antigen

• Humoral immunity—B cells respond to antigen

Types of disorders

• Immunodeficiency disorders

• Hypersensitivity disorders

• Autoimmune disorders

Immune disorders

• *Allergic rhinitis*—type I, IgE-mediated response to allergen

• *Anaphylaxis*—type I allergic reaction from systemic exposure to antigen

• *Human immunodeficiency virus disease*—ribonucleic acid retrovirus replicates within the CD4+ cell, resulting in cell death

• *Lupus erythematosus*—antibodies are produced against body's own cells; normal immunity suppressed by formed antigen-antibody complex that results in tissue damage

• *Rheumatoid arthritis*—exposure to an antigen causes altered IgG antibodies to develop; the body doesn't recognize these antibodies, and an antibody known as *rheumatoid factor* forms against them

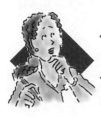

Quick quiz

1. The CDC recommends that HIV antibody testing take place:
    A.   immediately after a possible exposure.
    B.   1 month after a possible exposure.
    C.   3 months after a possible exposure.
    D.   35 months after a possible exposure.

Answer: C. Testing earlier than 3 months after exposure may give unclear test results because the infected person may not have developed antibodies to HIV.

2. Which immunoglobulin is responsible for the hypersensitivity reaction?
    A.   IgA
    B.   IgG
    C.   IgE
    D.   IgM

Answer: C. IgE is the immunoglobulin involved in the immediate hypersensitivity reactions of humoral immunity.

3. Which type of rhinitis is caused by excessive use of nasal sprays or drops?
    A.   Allergic rhinitis
    B.   Chronic vasomotor rhinitis
    C.   Infectious rhinitis
    D.   Rhinitis medicamentosa

Answer: D. Rhinitis medicamentosa can be resolved by discontinuing these medications.

4. Which of the following is the most common anaphylaxis-causing antigen?
    A.   Bee sting
    B.   Penicillin
    C.   Shellfish
    D.   Nuts

Answer: B. Penicillin is the most common anaphylaxis-causing antigen because of its systemic effects on the body.

5. Lupus erythematosus is characterized by:
    A.   ulnar rotation of the hand.
    B.   butterfly rash.
    C.   flulike syndrome.
    D.   dark circles under the eyes.

Answer: B. About half of all patients get the characteristic butterfly rash over their noses and cheeks.

6.   Common complaints associated with rheumatoid arthritis include:

    A.   painful joints, weak muscles, and peripheral neuropathy.

    B.   dizziness, dyspnea, and tachycardia.

    C.   anemia, Raynaud's phenomenon, and amenorrhea.

    D.   headache, emotional lability, and patchy alopecia.

Answer: A. These symptoms typically develop in the fingers and extend bilaterally to the wrists, elbows, knees, and ankles.

Scoring

☆☆☆   If you answered all six items correctly, bravo! Your performance is immune to criticism.

☆☆   If you answered four or five items correctly, congratulations! Clearly, the Quick quiz provided a stimulus that evoked an effective and appropriate response.

☆   If you answered fewer than four items correctly, that's okay. We still have plenty of body systems to cover, so now is no time to become hypersensitive.

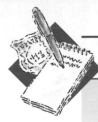

11

Infection

Just the facts

In this chapter, you'll learn:

♦ the body's defense mechanisms against infection

♦ the four types of infective microorganisms and how they invade the body

♦ the causes, pathophysiology, diagnostic tests, and treatments for several common infectious diseases.

Understanding infection

An infection is a host organism's response to a pathogen, or disease-causing substance. It results when tissue-destroying microorganisms enter and multiply in the body. Some infections take the form of minor illnesses, such as colds and ear infections. Others result in a life-threatening condition called *sepsis*, which causes widespread vasodilation and multiple-organ-dysfunction syndrome (MODS).

Infection-causing microbes

Four types of microorganisms can enter the body and cause infection:

 viruses

 bacteria

 fungi

 parasites.

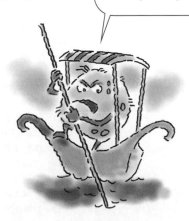

There are four different types of us microorganisms that can glide in and ruin your day!

Viruses

Viruses are microscopic genetic parasites that may contain genetic material, such as deoxyribonucleic acid (DNA) or ribonucleic acid (RNA). They have no metabolic capability and need a host cell to replicate.

Viral hide-and-seek

Viral infections occur when normal inflammatory and immune responses fail. The virus develops in the cell and "hides" there. After it's introduced into the host cell, the inner capsule releases genetic material, causing the infection. Some viruses surround the host cell and preserve it; others kill the host cell on contact.

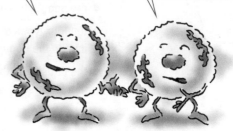

Viruses contain genetic material and need a host cell to replicate.

Bacteria are single-celled organisms that reproduce by cell division and may contain harmful proteins.

Bacteria

Bacteria are one-celled microorganisms that have no true nucleus and reproduce by cell division. Pathogenic bacteria contain cell-damaging proteins that cause infection. These proteins come in two forms:
• exotoxins—released during cell growth
• endotoxins—released when the bacterial cell wall decomposes. These endotoxins cause fever and aren't affected by antibiotics.

   Bacteria are classified several other ways, such as by their shape, growth requirements, motility, and whether they're aerobic (requiring oxygen) or anaerobic (don't require oxygen to survive).

Fungi

Fungi are nonphotosynthetic microorganisms that reproduce asexually (by division). They're large compared to other microorganisms and contain a true nucleus. Fungi are classified as:
• yeasts—round, single-celled, facultative anaerobes, which can live with or without oxygen
• molds—filament-like, multinucleated, aerobic microorganisms.

There's a fungus among us

Although fungi are part of the human body's normal flora, they can overproduce, especially when the normal flora is compromised. For example, vaginal yeast infections can occur with antibiotic treatment because normal flora are killed by the antibiotic, allowing yeast to reproduce. Infections caused by fungi are called *mycotic infections* because pathogenic fungi release mycotoxin. Most of these infections are mild unless they become systemic or the patient's immune system is compromised.

Parasites

Parasitic infections are uncommon except in hot, moist climates. *Parasites* are single-celled or multicelled organisms that depend on a host for food and a protective environment. Most common parasitic infections, such as tapeworm and tick infestations, occur in the intestines.

Barriers to infection

A healthy person can usually ward off infections with the body's own defense mechanisms. The body has many built-in infection barriers, such as the skin and secretions from the eyes, nasal passages, prostate gland, testicles, stomach, and vagina. Most of these secretions contain bacteria-killing particles called *lysozymes*. Other body structures, such as cilia in the pulmonary airways that sweep foreign material from the breathing passages, also offer infection protection.

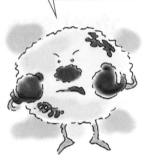

The body has built-in defense mechanisms against pathogens.

Trillions of harmless inhabitants

Normal flora are harmless microorganisms that reside on and in the body. They're found on the skin and in the nose, mouth, pharynx, distal intestine, colon, distal urethra, and vagina. The skin contains 10,000 microorganisms per square centimeter. Trillions of microorganisms are secreted from the GI tract daily.

Many of these microorganisms provide useful, protective functions. For example, the intestinal flora help synthesize vitamin K, which is an important part of the body's blood-clotting mechanism.

The infection process

Infection occurs when the body's defense mechanisms break down or when certain properties of microorganisms, such as virulence or toxin production, override the defense system.

Other factors that create a climate for infection include:
- poor nutrition
- stress
- humidity
- poor sanitation
- crowded living conditions
- pollution
- dust
- medications
- hospitalization (health care–associated infection).

Enter, attach, and spread

Infection results when a pathogen enters the body through direct contact, inhalation, ingestion, or an insect or animal bite. The pathogen then attaches itself to a cell and releases enzymes that destroy the cell's protective membrane. Next, it spreads through the bloodstream and lymphatic system, finally multiplying and causing infection in the target tissue or organ.

Striking while there's opportunity

Infections that strike people with altered, weak immune systems are called *opportunistic infections.* For example, patients with acquired immunodeficiency syndrome (AIDS) are plagued by opportunistic infections such as *Pneumocystis carinii* pneumonia.

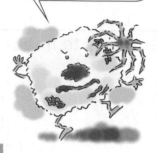

A pathogen may attach itself to a cell and release enzymes that destroy the cell's protective membrane.

Infectious disorders

The infections discussed in this section include:
- herpes simplex
- herpes zoster
- infectious mononucleosis
- Lyme disease
- rabies
- respiratory syncytial virus
- rubella
- salmonellosis
- toxoplasmosis.

Herpes simplex

A recurrent viral infection, herpes simplex occurs as two types:

Type 1 primarily affects the skin and mucous membranes and commonly produces cold sores, also known as *fever blisters.*

Type 2 primarily affects the genital area, causing painful clusters of small ulcerations.

Both types of herpes simplex virus can infect the eyes and other organs in the body. In addition, both types can result in localized or generalized infection.

Herpes simplex occurs worldwide and is equally common in men and women. It's most prevalent in lower socioeconomic groups, probably because of crowded living conditions.

The risk of recurrent attacks

Although herpes simplex may be latent for years, initial infection makes the patient a carrier susceptible to recurrent attacks. Outbreaks may be provoked by fever, menses, stress, heat, cold, lack of sleep, or sun exposure.

Potentially serious

Pregnant women should avoid exposure to herpes simplex because it can cause severe congenital anomalies in neonates. These abnormalities range from localized skin lesions to disseminated infection of major organs. Some examples of common complications in neonates are seizures, mental retardation, blindness, and deafness.

Herpes may also cause severe illness in immunocompromised patients; examples include pneumonias, hepatitis, and neurologic complications. Women with herpes simplex type 2 may have an increased risk of cervical cancer.

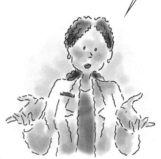

Herpes simplex type 1, spread by oral and respiratory secretions, causes cold sores (also known as *fever blisters*) in the skin and mucous membranes.

How it happens

Herpesvirus hominis, a widespread infectious agent, causes both types of herpes simplex. Type 1 is transmitted by oral and respiratory secretions, and type 2 is transmitted by sexual contact. However, cross-infection may result from orogenital sex. The average incubation for generalized infection is 2 to 12 days; for localized genital infection, 3 to 7 days.

The herpes simplex virus is a linear, double-stranded DNA molecule with an outer coating of lipid-type membrane. Here's what happens during exposure:
- The virus fuses to the host cell membrane.
- The virus releases proteins, turning off the host cell's protein production or synthesis.
- The virus replicates and synthesizes structural proteins.
- The virus pushes its nucleocapsid (protein coat and nucleic acid) into the cytoplasm of the host cell and releases the viral DNA.
- Complete virus particles capable of surviving and infecting a living cell (called *virion*) are transported to the cell's surface.

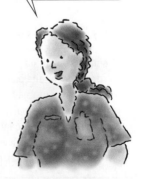

Type 2 herpes simplex mainly affects the genital area and is spread by sexual contact.

It's not over

Herpes simplex infection doesn't end in cell death. Instead, the virus enters a latent state during which it's maintained by the cell. Viral replication and redevelopment of herpetic lesions is called *reactivation*.

What to look for

Type 1 herpes simplex may cause generalized or localized infection as the virus invades the cells around the mouth. Generalized infection begins with fever and a sore, red, swollen throat. In addition to characteristic vesicles, the patient may develop submaxillary lymphadenopathy, increased salivation, halitosis, and anorexia. The patient usually reports severe mouth pain. After a brief prodromal period, primary lesions erupt.

Examination of the mouth may reveal edema and small vesicles (blisters) on a red base. These vesicles eventually rupture, leaving a painful ulcer and then yellow crusting. Common sites for vesicles are the tongue, gingiva, and cheeks, but they may occur anywhere in or around the mouth. The cervical glands may also be swollen. A generalized infection usually lasts 4 to 10 days. (See *What's a vesicle?*)

With primary genital, or type 2 herpes simplex, the patient usually complains first of tingling in the area involved, malaise, dysuria, dyspareunia (painful intercourse) and, in females, leukorrhea (white vaginal discharge containing mucus and pus cells).

Next, localized, fluid-filled vesicles appear and may last for weeks. In women, they occur on the cervix, labia, perianal skin, vulva, and vagina. In men, they develop on the glans penis, foreskin, and penile shaft. Lesions may also occur on the mouth or anus. After rupture, vesicles become shallow, painful ulcers with redness, edema, and oozing, yellow centers. Inguinal swelling may also be present.

Patients should be taught how to care for themselves during a herpes outbreak and how to avoid infecting others. (See *Treating herpes simplex.*)

What's a vesicle?

A *vesicle* is a raised, circumscribed, fluid-filled lesion, less than ¼" (0.6 cm) in diameter. It's the typical lesion of chickenpox and herpes simplex.

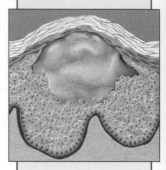

Battling illness

Treating herpes simplex

A generalized primary herpes infection usually requires drugs to reduce fever and pain. Anesthetic mouthwashes, such as viscous lidocaine, may help the patient with oral lesions eat and drink with less pain.

Acyclovir, the drug most commonly used to treat herpes, may reduce symptoms, viral shedding, and healing time. It's available in topical, oral, and I.V. forms. Valacyclovir, do-

cosanol, or famciclovir may also be given. Foscarnet may be used in patients who have shown resistance to acyclovir.

Don't pass it on
Patients with genital herpes should avoid sexual intercourse until lesions completely heal. They should also inform sexual partners of their condition.

What tests tell you

Confirmation of herpes simplex requires isolating the virus from local lesions and performing a tissue biopsy. In primary infection, an increase in antibodies and a moderate increase in white blood cell (WBC) count support the diagnosis.

Herpes zoster

Also called *shingles*, herpes zoster is an acute inflammation of dorsal root ganglia—nerve cell clusters found on the dorsal root of each spinal nerve.

The patient acquires the virus after having chickenpox as a child, so shingles can occur in all age groups. The prognosis is good and most patients recover completely unless the infection spreads to nerve roots that originate in the brain.

How it happens

The same virus that causes chickenpox, *herpesvirus varicella zoster*, causes this disorder. Because the disease affects nerves at their roots, localized, vesicular skin lesions are usually confined to an area of skin supplied by branches from a single nerve (called a *dermatome*). The patient may have severe pain in peripheral areas innervated by the inflamed nerve root. Chronic pain—called *postherpetic neuralgia*—is the most common persisting adverse effect.

Coming around

Reactivation of the varicella zoster virus is what causes shingles, but what triggers the reactivation is unknown.

The varicella zoster virus reactivates after lying dormant in the cerebral ganglia or the ganglia of posterior nerve roots. Some believe that the virus multiplies as it reactivates and that antibodies from the initial chickenpox infection usually neutralize it. However, without opposition from effective antibodies, the virus will continue to multiply in the ganglia, destroying neurons and spreading down the sensory nerves to the skin.

What to look for

The first symptom of herpes zoster is pain within the dermatome. Patients may also have fever and malaise.

What happens next

After 2 to 4 days, severe, intermittent, or continuous, deep pain may occur. Pruritus, paresthesia (unusual skin sensations, such as prickling), or hyperesthesia (heightened skin sensitivity) in the

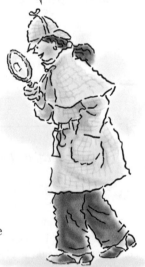

The exact cause of shingles is a mystery, but antibodies from a childhood chickenpox infection usually neutralize it.

trunk, arms, or legs may also occur as more nerves are affected. The patient may also develop chills and a low-grade fever.

And then...

After the pain starts, small, red, nodular skin lesions erupt on painful areas and spread unilaterally around the thorax or vertically over the arms or legs. They change rapidly into pus- or fluid-filled vesicles, which may become infected or even gangrenous. Bacterial infection of the skin is usually caused by *Staphylococcus aureus* or *Streptococcus pyogenes*, and may result from scratching. (See *A look at herpes zoster.*)

10 to 21 days later

About 10 to 21 days after the rash appears, the vesicles dry and form scabs.

Nerve specific

When branches of the trigeminal nerve are involved, lesions appear on the face, in the mouth, or in the eyes. When the sensory branch of the facial nerve is involved, lesions appear in the ear canal and on the tongue. (See *Treating herpes zoster.*)

A look at herpes zoster

The illustration below shows the umbilicated vesicles present on the skin in herpes zoster.

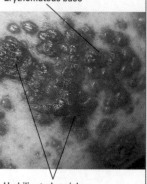

Erythematous base

Umbilicated vesicles

Battling illness

Treating herpes zoster

Primary treatment includes antipruritics, such as calamine lotion, to relieve itching and analgesics, such as aspirin, acetaminophen, codeine, or capsaicin to relieve pain. A systemic corticosteroid, such as cortisone or corticotropin, may also be used to relieve pain and reduce inflammation.

Tincture of benzoin applied to unbroken lesions helps prevent a secondary infection. If lesions rupture and become infected with bacteria, systemic antibiotics are given. Herpes zoster affecting the trigeminal nerve and cornea calls for idoxuridine ointment or another antiviral agent. Other medications used are tranquilizers, sedatives, and tricyclic antidepressants with phenothiazines.

Acyclovir may be prescribed for immunocompromised patients and those with infections of the ophthalmic branch of the trigeminal nerve. The drug stops the rash from spreading, reduces the duration of viral shedding and acute pain, and prevents visceral complications. Valacyclovir and famciclovir also are used for the treatment of most herpes infections.

If other pain relief measures fail, transcutaneous peripheral nerve stimulation, patient-controlled analgesia, or a small dose of radiotherapy may be effective.

What tests tell you

Vesicular fluid analysis is used to diagnose herpes zoster. This test differentiates herpes zoster from localized herpes simplex.

Infectious mononucleosis

An acute infectious disease, infectious mononucleosis has three hallmarks:

 fever

 sore throat

 swollen cervical lymph nodes.

It also may cause liver dysfunction, increased numbers of lymphocytes and monocytes, and the development and persistence of heterophil antibodies.

Infectious mononucleosis mainly affects young adults and children, although it's usually so mild in children that it's commonly overlooked. It's fairly prevalent in the United States, Canada, and Europe, and both sexes are affected equally.

Here's the good news

Major complications of infectious mononucleosis are uncommon. About 90% of children older than age 4 have acquired antibodies. Other types of mononucleosis are caused by cytomegalovirus and are benign and self-limiting.

How it happens

Infectious mononucleosis is caused by the Epstein-Barr virus, a member of the herpesvirus group. Most cases are spread by the oropharyngeal route; however, transmission by blood transfusion and during cardiac surgery is also possible. The disease is contagious before symptoms develop and remains contagious until the patient's fever subsides and oropharyngeal lesions disappear.

The disorder develops this way:

• The virus invades the B cells of the oropharyngeal lymphoid tissues and then replicates.

• As the B cells die, the virus is released into the blood, causing fever and other symptoms.

• During this period, antiviral antibodies appear and the virus disappears from the blood, lodging mainly in the parotid gland, one of the salivary glands.

• Reproduction of the virus occurs in the parotid gland, accounting for its presence in saliva. (See *Glands affected by Epstein-Barr virus*, page 376.)

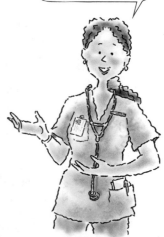

Infectious mononucleosis is known as the *kissing disease* because it's spread by the oropharyngeal route.

Glands affected by Epstein-Barr virus

The illustration shows the different glands that are affected by mononucleosis or the Epstein-Barr virus.

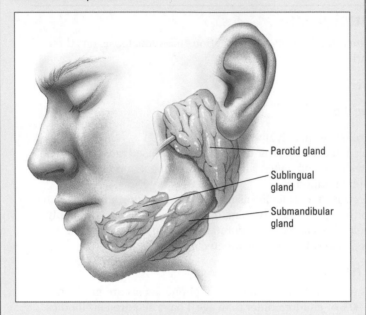

Parotid gland

Sublingual gland

Submandibular gland

What to look for

After an incubation period of about 10 days in children and 30 to 50 days in adults, the patient experiences headache, malaise, profound fatigue, anorexia, myalgia (muscle tenderness), and abdominal discomfort. Three to 5 days later, he develops an extremely sore throat and dysphagia (difficulty swallowing). Fever usually peaks in the late afternoon or evening, reaching 101° to 102° F (38.3° to 38.9° C).

Inspection of the pharynx reveals exudative tonsillitis and pharyngitis. Petechiae on the palate, swollen eyes, a raised and red rash that resembles rubella, and jaundice also may occur. Cervical lymph nodes swell and are mildly tender when palpated. Inguinal and axillary nodes as well as the spleen and liver also may be swollen.

The prognosis for patients with infectious mononucleosis is excellent. (See *Treating infectious mononucleosis.*)

Battling illness

Treating infectious mononucleosis

Because mononucleosis is hard to prevent and resists standard antimicrobial treatment, therapy is mainly supportive. It includes relief of symptoms, bed rest during the acute febrile period, and acetamino-phen or ibuprofen for fever, headache, and sore throat.

Don't give aspirin to children because of its association with Reye's syndrome, a serious illness that can lead to death.

In cases of severe inflammation and airway obstruction, steroids can relieve swelling and prevent the need for a tracheotomy. About 20% of patients also have a streptococcal infection and need antibiotic therapy for at least 10 days. Sports, physical activities, or exercise of any kind should be avoided for 3 to 4 weeks after the onset of symptoms to avoid splenic rupture.

What tests tell you

These diagnostic tests confirm infectious mononucleosis:
• WBC count is abnormally high (10,000 to 20,000/µl) during the second and third weeks of illness. From 50% to 70% of the total count consists of lymphocytes and monocytes, and 10% of the lymphocytes are atypical.
• Heterophil antibodies in serum drawn during the acute phase and at 3- to 4-week intervals increase to four times normal.
• Indirect immunofluorescence shows antibodies to Epstein-Barr virus and cellular antigens. This test is usually more definitive than that for heterophil antibodies.

Lyme disease

Lyme disease occurs chiefly in the United States and is named for the Connecticut town in which it was first recognized in 1975. It affects multiple body systems and usually appears in summer or early fall with a skin lesion called *erythema chronicum migrans* or a "bull's-eye." Weeks or months later, cardiac, neurologic, or joint abnormalities may develop, sometimes followed by arthritis. The incidence has increased in most states over the past 10 years.

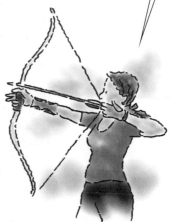

The bull's-eye–shaped rash is the beginning of the Lyme disease syndrome.

How it happens

Lyme disease is caused by the spirochete *Borrelia burgdorferi*, which is carried by deer ticks. Here's how the disease develops:
• The tick injects spirochete-laden saliva into the bloodstream or deposits fecal matter on the skin.
• After incubating for 3 to 32 days, the spirochetes migrate outward, causing a rash.
• Spirochetes disseminate to other skin sites or organs through the bloodstream or lymphatic system. They may survive for years in the joints, or they may die after triggering an inflammatory response in the host.

What to look for

Lyme disease occurs in three stages. Signs and symptoms may take years to fully develop.

Stage 1

In stage one, a red lesion forms at the site of the tick bite—usually the axilla, thigh, or groin—and may expand to more than 20″ (50.8 cm) in diameter. The lesion has a white center and a bright red outer rim, and it may itch, sting, or burn. It usually disappears within 1 month. (See *Looking at the bull's-eye of Lyme disease*.)

After a few days, more lesions may erupt in addition to a migratory, ringlike rash and conjunctivitis. In 3 to 4 weeks, the lesions fade to small red blotches, which persist for several more weeks.

The rash is commonly accompanied by fatigue, headache, chills, fever, sore throat, stiff neck, nausea, and muscle and joint pain. In children, body temperature may rise to 104° F (40° C) and be accompanied by chills. At this stage, 10% of patients report symptoms, such as palpitations and mild dyspnea. Severe headache and stiff neck, which suggest meningeal irritation, may also occur.

Stage 2

Weeks to months later, patients who aren't treated may enter the second stage of the disease. Meningitis, cranial nerve palsies, and peripheral neuropathy may occur. Fewer than 10% of patients have cardiac signs and symptoms. With neurologic involvement, neck stiffness usually occurs only with extreme flexion.

Stage 3

In the final stage, arthritis occurs 6 weeks to several years after the tick bite. Usually, only one or a few joints are affected, especially large ones, such as the knees. Recurrent attacks may lead to chronic arthritis with severe cartilage and bone erosion. One-half of patients who aren't treated progress to this stage. (See *Treating Lyme disease*.)

What tests tell you

These tests are used to diagnose Lyme disease:
• Blood tests, including antibody titers, enzyme-linked immuno-sorbent assay, and Western blot assay, may be used to identify *Borrelia burgdorferi*. Unfortunately, blood tests don't always confirm Lyme disease, especially in the early stages before the body produces antibodies or seropositivity for *B. burgdorferi*. Mild anemia and elevated erythrocyte sedimentation rate, WBC count, serum immunoglobulin M (IgM) level, and aspartate aminotransferase level support the diagnosis.
• Cerebrospinal fluid (CSF) analysis may be used to detect antibodies to *B. burgdorferi* if the disease has affected the central nervous system (CNS).

Looking at the bull's-eye of Lyme disease

The characteristic bull's-eye red rash appears at the site of the tick bite; however, many people don't notice the rash especially if it's in an area where it's hard to see.

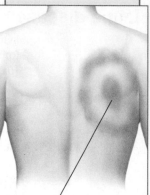

Characteristic erythema chronicum migrans lesion

Half of all patients with Lyme disease who aren't treated progress to stage 3 of the disease.

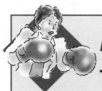

Battling illness

Treating Lyme disease

A 3- to 4-week course of oral amoxicillin or doxycycline is the treatment of choice for adults infected with Lyme disease. Cefuroxime or erythromycin can be used for patients who are allergic to penicillin or who can't take tetracyclines. These drugs can minimize complications if taken early in the disease. In later stages of the disease, particularly when neurologic symptoms are present, treatment with I.V. ceftriaxone or penicillin for 4 weeks or more may be necessary. Analgesics and antipyretics reduce inflammation and fever.

Memory jogger

To help you remember the progression of signs and symptoms, use the acronym **LIME:**

Lesions, lymph node swelling, like the flu (stage 1)

Innervation problems, such as meningitis and peripheral neuropathy (stage 2)

Movement problems such as arthritis (stage 3)

Everything else, such as myocarditis and arrhythmias (stage 3).

Rabies

An acute CNS infection, rabies is transmitted by an animal bite and is almost always fatal after symptoms occur. Fortunately, immunization soon after infection may prevent death.

How it happens

Rabies is caused by the rabies virus, a rhabdovirus. It's transmitted to a human from the bite of an infected animal through the skin or mucous membranes. Airborne droplets and infected tissue occasionally transmit the virus. Increased domestic animal control and vaccination in the United States has reduced cases of rabies in humans. Consequently, most human rabies can be traced to dog bites that occurred in other countries or bites from wild animals such as raccoons.

Here's how the disease progresses:
• The rabies virus begins replicating in the striated muscle cells at the bite site.
• The virus spreads along the nerve pathways to the spinal cord and brain, where it replicates again.
• The virus moves through the nerves into other tissues, including the salivary glands.

The incubation period for the rabies virus is hours to weeks.

Increased domestic animal control and vaccination in the United States has reduced cases of rabies in humans.

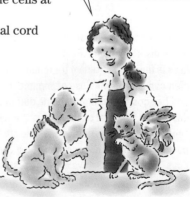

What to look for

Signs and symptoms of rabies begin appearing in 1 to 3 months in patients who don't receive immunization in time.

Prodromal symptoms

At first, the patient complains of local or radiating pain or burning and a sensation of cold, pruritus, and tingling at the bite site. He may also report malaise, headache, anorexia, nausea, sore throat, a persistent loose cough, nervousness, anxiety, irritability, hyperesthesia, sensitivity to light and loud noises, and excessive salivation, tearing, and perspiration. He may have a temperature of 100° to 102° F (37.8° to 38.9° C). (See *Treating rabies*.)

Excitation phase

About 2 to 10 days after prodromal signs and symptoms begin, an excitation phase occurs. This is marked by intermittent hyperactivity, anxiety, apprehension, pupillary dilation, shallow respirations, and altered level of consciousness. Cranial nerve dysfunction may cause ocular palsies, strabismus (deviation of the eye), asymmetrical pupillary dilation or constriction, absence of corneal reflexes, facial muscle weakness, and hoarseness. Temperature also rises to about 103° F (39.4° C).

Hydrophobia

About 50% of patients have hydrophobia, which causes forceful, painful pharyngeal muscle spasms that expel fluids from the mouth, resulting in dehydration and, possibly, apnea, cyanosis, and death. Swallowing problems cause frothy drooling, and soon the sight, sound, or thought of water triggers uncontrollable pharyngeal muscle spasms and excessive salivation. Nuchal rigidity (rigidity of the neck muscles) and seizures accompanied by cardiac arrhythmias or arrest may occur.

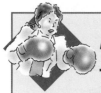

Battling illness

Treating rabies

There's no treatment for rabies after symptoms of the disease appear. Postexposure prophylaxis is the most effective treatment. This regimen consists of one dose of immune globulin and five doses of rabies vaccine during a 28-day period. The first dose of rabies vaccine should be given as soon as possible after exposure. Additional doses should be given on days 3, 7, 14, and 28 days after the first vaccine.

The wound should immediately be washed with soap and water. Further wound care should be based on the extent of the injury.

If the patient develops symptoms, isolate the patient and wear a gown, gloves, mask, and protective eyewear when handling saliva and articles contaminated with saliva. Take precautions to avoid being bitten or scratched by the patient during the excitation phase. Provide supportive care.

Between excitatory and hydrophobic episodes, the patient usually remains cooperative and lucid. After about 3 days, these phases subside, and progressive paralysis leads to coma and death.

What tests tell you

There are no diagnostic tests for rabies before its onset. Histologic examination of brain tissue from human rabies victims shows perivascular inflammation of the gray matter, degeneration of neurons, and characteristic minute bodies, called *Negri bodies*, in the nerve cells.

Respiratory syncytial virus infection

Respiratory syncytial virus (RSV) infection occurs almost exclusively in infants and young children. In this population, it's the leading cause of lower respiratory tract infections, pneumonia, tracheobronchitis, bronchiolitis, otitis media, and fatal respiratory diseases.

Antibody titers suggest that most children younger than age 4 have contracted some form of RSV infection, although it may be mild. In fact, bronchiolitis associated with this disease peaks at age 2 months, making it the only viral disease that has its maximum impact during the first few months of life.

How it happens

RSV infection results from an organism that belongs to a subgroup of a large group of viruses called the *myxoviruses*. Here are the key facts about RSV pathophysiology:
• The organism is transmitted from person to person by respiratory secretions.
• It has an incubation period of 4 to 5 days.
• Bronchiolitis or pneumonia occurs and, in severe cases, may damage the bronchiolar epithelium.
• Interalveolar thickening and filling of alveolar spaces with fluid may occur.

What to look for

Signs and symptoms vary in severity. They include nasal congestion, coughing, wheezing, malaise, sore throat, earache, dyspnea, and fever. Although uncommon, signs of CNS infection, such as weakness, irritability, and nuchal rigidity, may also be observed.

Along with severe respiratory distress caused by increased mucus production, you may note nasal flaring, retraction, cyanosis, and tachypnea. With a lower respiratory tract infection, you may

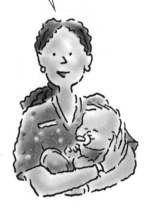

RSV infection is the only viral disease that has its maximum impact during the first few months of life.

auscultate wheezes, rhonchi, and crackles caused by interstitial lung edema and bronchial spasm.

Reinfection is common and produces milder symptoms than the primary infection. School-age children, adolescents, and young adults with mild reinfections are probably the source of infection for infants and young children. (See *Treating RSV infection*.)

What tests tell you

These tests are used to diagnose RSV infection:
• Cultures of nasal and pharyngeal secretions may reveal the virus; however, this infection is so labile that cultures aren't always reliable.
• Serum antibody titers may be elevated, but in infants younger than age 6 months, the presence of maternal antibodies may nullify test results.

Rubella

Commonly called *German measles*, rubella is an acute, mildly contagious viral disease that produces a distinctive 3-day rash and enlarged lymph nodes. Worldwide in distribution, rubella flourishes during the spring, particularly in cities, with epidemics occurring sporadically.

Rubella occurs most commonly in children ages 5 to 9, adolescents, and young adults. The disease is self-limiting, and the prognosis is excellent except for congenital rubella, which can cause serious birth defects.

How it happens

The rubella virus is transmitted through contact with the blood, urine, stool, or nasopharyngeal secretions of an infected person. It's communicable from about 10 days before the rash appears until 5 days after. It can also be transmitted transplacentally.

The virus replicates first in the respiratory tract and then spreads through the bloodstream. It has been detected in blood as early as 8 days before and up to 2 days after the rash appears. Shedding of virus from the oropharynx persists for up to 8 days after the onset of symptoms.

Battling illness

Treating RSV infection

Treatment measures for RSV support respiratory function, maintain fluid balance, and relieve symptoms. Riba-virin, a broad-spectrum antiviral agent, is used in infants with severe lower respiratory tract infection. The drug is given in aerosol form by way of a tent, oxygen hood, mask, or ventilator for 2 to 5 days, 12 to 18 hours per day. This therapy reduces the severity of symptoms and improves oxygen saturation.

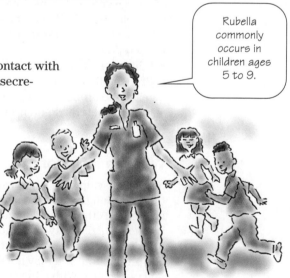

Rubella commonly occurs in children ages 5 to 9.

What to look for

The patient's history may reveal inadequate immunization, exposure to someone with a recent rubella infection, or recent travel to an endemic area without reimmunization.

Examination reveals a maculopapular, mildly itchy rash that usually begins on the face and then spreads rapidly, commonly covering the trunk and extremities within hours. Small, red macules on the soft palate *(Forschheimer spots)* may precede or accompany the rash. By the end of the second day, the rash begins to fade in the opposite order in which it appeared. It usually disappears on the third day, but may persist for 4 or 5 days. The rapid appearance and disappearance of the rubella rash distinguishes it from rubeola (measles).

A low-grade fever (99° to 101° F [37.2° to 38.3° C]) may occur, but it usually disappears after the first day of the rash. Rarely, a patient's temperature may reach 104° F (40° C).

Children usually don't have prodromal symptoms, but adolescents and adults may have a headache, malaise, anorexia, sore throat, and cough before the rash appears. Palpation reveals suboccipital, postauricular, and postcervical lymph node enlargement, a hallmark sign.

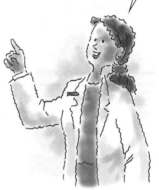

Palpable enlarged lymph nodes—or swollen glands—are a classic sign of rubella.

Congenital risk

In congenital rubella, the virus is transmitted through the placenta to the fetus by an infected mother. The fetus may have the virus in utero and for 6 to 31 months after birth.

Serious and potentially fatal complications include growth retardation, infiltration of the liver and spleen by hematopoietic tissue (tissue that forms blood cells), interstitial pneumonia, a decreased number of megakaryocytes (giant cells in the bone marrow that produce mature blood platelets), and structural malformations of the cardiovascular and central nervous systems. (See *Treating rubella*, page 384.)

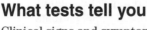

What tests tell you

Clinical signs and symptoms are usually sufficient to make a diagnosis, so laboratory tests are seldom performed. However, these tests may be used:

• Cell cultures of the throat, blood, urine, and CSF, along with convalescent serum that shows a fourfold rise in antibody titers, confirms the diagnosis.

• Blood tests confirm rubella-specific IgM antibody. In congenital rubella, rubella-specific IgM antibody appears in umbilical cord blood.

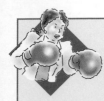

Battling illness

Treating rubella

Because the rubella rash is self-limiting and only mildly pruritic, it doesn't require topical or systemic medication. Treatment consists of antipyretics and analgesics for fever and joint pain. Bed rest isn't necessary, but the patient should be isolated until the rash disappears.

Immunization with the live rubella virus prevents the disease. The vaccine should be given along with measles and mumps vaccines at age 15 months. Repeat immunizations should be given to anyone immunized before 1960 and then every 10 years thereafter.

Take precautions

Only hospital workers not at risk for rubella should provide patient care, and they should use isolation precautions until 5 days after the rash disappears. Infants with congenital rubella need to be isolated for 3 months, until three throat cultures are negative. Be sure to report confirmed cases of rubella to local public health officials.

Immune globulin may be administered I.M. or I.V. to staff and visitors who haven't been immunized. Before giving the vaccine to anyone, precautionary steps should be taken.

Before immunizing anyone with the rubella vaccine:
• make sure that they aren't allergic to neomycin
• make sure that they aren't pregnant
• advise women of childbearing age to avoid pregnancy by using an effective birth control method for at least 3 months after receiving the vaccine.

Salmonellosis

Every year approximately 40,000 cases of salmonellosis are reported in the United States. Because many milder cases aren't diagnosed or reported, the actual number of cases may be greater.

Salmonellosis, occurring more commonly in the spring than winter, is typically found in children. However, young children, elderly people, and immunocompromised patients are the most likely to contract severe infections.

Salmonellosis occurs as enterocolitis, bacteremia (bacteria in the blood), localized infection, typhoid fever and, rarely, paratyphoid fever. Enterocolitis and bacteremia are especially common and virulent in infants, the elderly, and those already weakened by other infections, especially AIDS. It's estimated that 1,000 patients die each year of acute salmonellosis.

Got the fever

Typhoid fever, the most severe form of salmonellosis, usually lasts from 1 to 4 weeks. Most patients are younger than age 30, but most carriers are women older than age 50. Typhoid fever is on the rise in this country because of travel to endemic areas.

How it happens

Salmonellosis is caused by gram-negative bacilli of the genus *Salmonella*, a member of the Enterobacteriaceae family. The most common species of *Salmonella* include *S. typhi*, which causes typhoid fever; *S. enteritidis*, which causes enterocolitis; and *S. choleraesuis*, which causes bacteremia. Many *Salmonella* bacteria can survive for weeks in water, ice, sewage, and food.

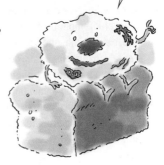

Salmonella bacteria can survive for weeks in water, ice, sewage, and food.

Watch what you eat

Nontyphoidal salmonellosis usually follows ingestion of contaminated dry milk, chocolate bars, pharmaceuticals of animal origin, or contaminated or inadequately processed foods, especially eggs, chicken, turkey, and duck. Proper cooking reduces the risk but doesn't eliminate it.

The disease may also spread through contact with infected people or animals and, in young children, through fecal-oral spread. Typhoid fever usually results from drinking water contaminated by the excretions of a carrier.

Typhoid fever progresses this way: After contaminated food is ingested, the bacteria pass the gastric barrier and invade the upper small bowel, causing a transient bacteremia that produces no symptoms. The bacteria are ingested by mononuclear phagocytes and must survive and multiply within them to cause illness.

What to look for

All infections resulting from bacteria other than *S. typhi* can cause acute diarrhea, septicemic syndrome, focal abscesses, meningitis, osteomyelitis, endocarditis, or mycotic aneurysm (an aneurysm infected by a fungus).

Persistent bacteremia kicks off the clinical phase of infection. The bacteria continue to multiply in the cells, and when the number passes a critical threshold, secondary bacteremia occurs, resulting in invasion of the gallbladder and intestine. Sustained bacteremia causes a persistent fever. Inflammatory responses to tissue invasion result in cholecystitis, intestinal hemorrhage, or perforation.

Nontyphoidal forms of salmonellosis usually produce mild to moderate illness, with low mortality. Mortality caused by typhoid fever is about 3% in people who are treated and 10% in those who aren't treated. An attack of typhoid fever confers lifelong immunity. (See *Treating salmonellosis*, page 386.)

What tests tell you

These tests are used to diagnose salmonellosis:
• Blood cultures isolate the organism in typhoid fever, paratyphoid fever, and bacteremia.
• Stool cultures isolate the organism in typhoid fever, paratyphoid fever, and enterocolitis.

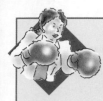

Use extreme caution when handling materials that could be contaminated with *Salmonella* microbes.

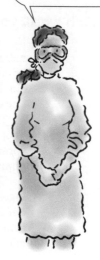

Battling illness

Treating salmonellosis

Drugs used to treat typhoid fever, paratyphoid fever, or bacteremia include ampicillin, amoxicillin, chloramphenicol, ciprofloxacin, ceftriaxone, cefotaxime, and co-trimoxazole for extremely toxemic patients. Localized abscesses may need surgical drainage.

Camphorated opium tincture, kaolin and pectin mixtures, diphenoxylate, codeine, or small doses of morphine can relieve diarrhea and control cramps for patients who remain active.

When caring for a patient with salmonellosis, wear gloves and a gown when disposing of feces-contaminated materials, and wash your hands thoroughly after contact with the patient. Continue enteric precautions until three consecutive stool cultures are negative after antibiotic treatment. *Report all salmonellosis cases to public health officials.*

• Cultures of urine, bone marrow, pus, and vomitus may show the presence of *Salmonella* organisms.

In endemic areas, symptoms of enterocolitis allow a working diagnosis before the cultures are positive. *S. typhi* in stools 1 or more years after treatment indicates that the patient is a carrier (about 3% of patients).

Toxoplasmosis

Seventy percent of people in the United States are infected with *Toxoplasma gondii*. Although it usually causes a localized infection, it may produce a generalized infection in neonates, patients with AIDS or lymphoma, patients who have undergone recent organ transplants, and those on immunosuppressive therapy.

Warn pregnant and hoping-to-be-pregnant women to have someone else change Fluffy's litter box.

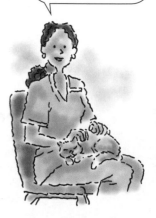

Congenital and deadly

Congenital toxoplasmosis, characterized by CNS lesions, may cause stillbirth or serious birth defects. It's transmitted transplacentally from a mother who acquires primary toxoplasmosis shortly before or during pregnancy. The infection is more severe when it's acquired early in pregnancy.

How it happens

Toxoplasmosis is caused by the intracellular parasite *Toxoplasma gondii*, which affects both birds and mammals. It's transmitted to humans by ingestion of tissue cysts in raw or undercooked meat or by fecal-oral contamination from infected cats. An infected cat may excrete as many as 100 million parasites per day, but a single cyst can cause infection.

Direct transmission can also occur during blood transfusions or organ transplants. The disease also occurs in people who don't eat meat and aren't exposed to cats, so an unknown means of transmission exists.

Here's how the infection develops:
• When tissue cysts are ingested, parasites are released, which quickly invade and multiply within the GI tract.

Let's head for the GI tract!

• The parasitic cells rupture the invaded host cell and then disseminate to the CNS, lymphatic tissue, skeletal muscle, myocardium, retina, and placenta.
• As the parasites replicate and invade adjoining cells, cell death and focal necrosis occur, surrounded by an acute inflammatory response—the hallmarks of this infection.
• After the cyst reaches maturity, the inflammatory process becomes undetectable, and the cysts remain latent within the brain until they rupture.

In the normal host, the immune response checks the infection, but this isn't what happens in immunocompromised or fetal hosts. In these patients, focal destruction results in necrotizing encephalitis, pneumonia, myocarditis, and organ failure.

What to look for

A patient with mild, localized toxoplasmosis may complain of malaise, myalgia, headache, fatigue, and sore throat. He'll also have a fever.

A patient with fulminating, generalized infection may complain of headache, vomiting, cough, and dyspnea. His temperature may run as high as 106° F (41.1° C). He may also have delirium and seizures (signs of encephalitis), a maculopapular rash (except on the palms, soles, and scalp), and cyanosis.

An infant with congenital toxoplasmosis may have hydrocephalus or microcephalus, seizures, jaundice, purpura, and rash. Other defects, which may not be apparent until months or years later, include strabismus, blindness, epilepsy, and mental retardation.

Once infected with toxoplasmosis, the patient may carry the organism for life. Reactivation of the acute infection can also occur. (See *Treating toxoplasmosis.*)

Battling illness

Treating toxoplasmosis

Most effective during the acute stage, treatment for toxoplasmosis consists of drug therapy with a sulfonamide and pyrimethamine for 4 to 6 weeks. The patient may also receive folic acid to counteract the drugs' adverse effects, such as anemia and bone marrow toxicity. Unfortunately, these drugs don't eliminate tissue cysts that are already developed. Therefore, patients with acquired immunodeficiency syndrome (AIDS) need toxoplasmosis treatment for life.

An AIDS patient who can't tolerate sulfonamides may receive clindamycin instead. This drug is also the primary treatment in ocular toxoplasmosis.

Report all cases of toxoplasmosis to the local public health department.

What tests tell you

Blood tests for the detection of a specific toxoplasma antibody is the primary diagnostic tool for detection of active infection.

Another test, which isolates the *T. gondii* in mice after their inoculation with human body fluids, reveals antibodies for the disease and confirms toxoplasmosis.

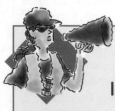

That's a wrap!

Infection review

Infection facts
• Infection is a host's response to a pathogen.
• Viruses, bacteria, fungi, and parasites cause infection.
• Infection results when a pathogen enters the body; the pathogen attaches to a cell and destroys the cell's protective membrane, spreads through blood and lymph, multiplies, and causes infection in target organ or tissue.

Understanding infection
• Results when a host organism responds to a pathogen or disease-causing substance
• Develops when tissue-destroying microorganisms enter and multiply in the body
• Takes the form of minor illnesses, such as colds and ear infections, or results in a life-threatening condition called *sepsis,* which causes widespread vasodilation and MODS
• Caused by four types of microorganisms:
  – viruses
  – bacteria
  – fungi
  – parasites.

Development
Infection occurs when the body's defense mechanisms break down or when microorganisms override the defense system. Other factors include:
• poor nutrition
• stress
• humidity
• poor sanitation
• crowded living conditions
• pollution
• dust
• medications.
  Infection results when a pathogen enters the body through direct contact, inhalation, ingestion, or an insect or animal bite.

Infectious disorders
• *Herpes simplex*—virus fuses to host cell membrane, turns off host's protein synthesis, and replicates; viral DNA is released
• *Herpes zoster*—reactivation of varicella-zoster virus; trigger of reactivation unknown
• *Infectious mononucleosis*—virus invades B cells of oropharyngeal lymph; B cells die, and virus is released in blood; fever and other symptoms occur

• *Lyme disease*—tick injects spirochete into blood or deposits feces on skin; after incubation, spirochetes migrate, cause a rash, and disseminate to other skin areas and organs
• *Rabies*—bite transmits virus through skin; the virus replicates and spreads to the spinal cord and brain, where it replicates again
• *RSV infection*—virus transmitted through respiratory secretions; bronchiolitis or pneumonia occurs (severe cases may lead to bronchiolar epithelial damage); alveolar spaces may fill with fluid
• *Rubella*—virus transmitted through body fluid contact; the virus replicates in respiratory tract and spreads to the bloodstream
• *Salmonellosis*—gram-negative bacilli are ingested through contaminated food or water, or through contact with an infected person or animal; the bacilli then invade the upper small bowel and cause bacteremia
• *Toxoplasmosis*—intracellular parasites are ingested; parasites are then released and invade and multiply in the GI tract; the parasitic cell ruptures host and disseminates throughout the body

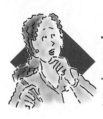

Quick quiz

1. The four types of microorganisms that cause infection are:
    A.   bacteria, flora, microbes, and viruses.
    B.   bacteria, viruses, fungi, and parasites.
    C.   fungoids, spirochetes, mycoplasms, and parasites.
    D.   bacteria, yeast, flora, and parasites.

    Answer: B. Bacteria, viruses, fungi, and parasites are pathogens that enter the body and cause infections.

2. An opportunistic infection occurs because:
    A.   the host has an altered, weak immune system.
    B.   the pathogen is especially persistent.
    C.   a large number of pathogens attack the host cells.
    D.   the host has a fever.

    Answer: A. Opportunistic infections occur in AIDS patients and others whose immune systems aren't functioning effectively.

3. The type of herpesvirus that causes cold sores is:
    A.   herpes simplex type 2.
    B.   herpes simplex type 1.
    C.   herpes zoster.
    D.   herpes varicella.

    Answer: B. The herpes simplex type 1 virus commonly causes cold sores, but it can also be spread to the genital area, eyes, and other organs.

4. The most severe form of salmonellosis is:
    A.   enterocolitis.
    B.   bacteremia.
    C.   paratyphoid fever.
    D.   typhoid fever.

    Answer: D. Typhoid fever has a 3% mortality rate in people who are treated and a 10% mortality rate in those who aren't treated.

Scoring

☆☆☆   If you answered all four items correctly, give yourself a hand! Your enthusiasm for bacteria, viruses, and parasites is infectious!

☆☆   If you answered three items correctly, give yourself a pat on the back! Your knowledge and understanding is thriving like parasites in the tropics!

☆   If you answered fewer than three items correctly, practice, practice, and pump up on parasite power.

12

Cancer

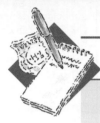

Just the facts

In this chapter, you'll learn:

♦ the causes of abnormal cell growth

♦ the warning signs of cancer

♦ classifications of cancer

♦ the process of cancer metastasis

♦ pathophysiology, tests, and treatments for common types of cancer.

Understanding cancer

Cancer ranks second to cardiovascular disease as the leading cause of death in the United States. One out of four deaths is due to cancer. Some epidemiologists predict that it will outrank cardiovascular disease by the year 2010. Every year, more than 1 million cancer cases are diagnosed in the United States, and 550,000 people die of cancer-related causes. One-third of these deaths are related to nutrition problems, physical inactivity, obesity, and other lifestyle factors and could have been prevented.

The importance of early detection

In most cases, early detection of cancer enables more effective treatment and a better prognosis for the patient. A careful assessment, beginning with history, is critical. In gathering assessment information, you need to ask the patient about risk factors, such as cigarette smoking, a family history of cancer, and exposure to potential hazards, such as asbestos.

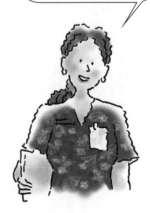

In most cases, early detection of cancer is key to achieving an optimal outcome.

Abnormal cell growth

Cancer is classified by the tissues or blood cells in which it originates. Most cancers derive from epithelial tissues and are called
carcinomas. Others arise from these tissues and cells:
- glandular tissues (adenocarcinomas)
- connective, muscle, and bone tissues (sarcomas)
- tissue of the brain and spinal cord (gliomas)
- pigment cells (melanomas)
- plasma cells (myelomas)
- lymphatic tissue (lymphomas)
- leukocytes (leukemia)
- erythrocytes (erythroleukemia).

Uncontrolled growth

Cancer cells first develop from a mutation in a single cell. This cell
grows without the control that characterizes normal cell growth.
At a certain stage of development, the cancer cell fails to mature
into the type of normal cell from which it originated. (See *Histologic characteristics of cancer cells*.) In addition to this uncontrolled localized growth, cancer cells can spread from the site of
origin, a process called *metastasis*. (See *How cancer metastasizes*.)

Memory jogger

When asking assessment questions, remember the American Cancer Society's mnemonic device, **CAUTION**.

Change in bowel or bladder habits

A sore that doesn't heal

Unusual bleeding or discharge

Thickening or lump

Indigestion or diffi-culty swallowing

Obvious changes in a wart or mole

Nagging cough or hoarseness

Histologic characteristics of cancer cells

Cancer is a destructive (malignant) growth of cells, which invades nearby tissues and may metastasize to other areas of the body. Dividing rapidly, cancer cells tend to be extremely aggressive.

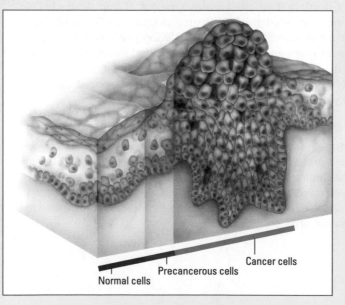

Normal cells   Precancerous cells   Cancer cells

Now I get it!

How cancer metastasizes

Cancer cells may invade nearby tissues or metastasize (spread) to other organs. They may move to other tissues by any or all of the three routes described below.

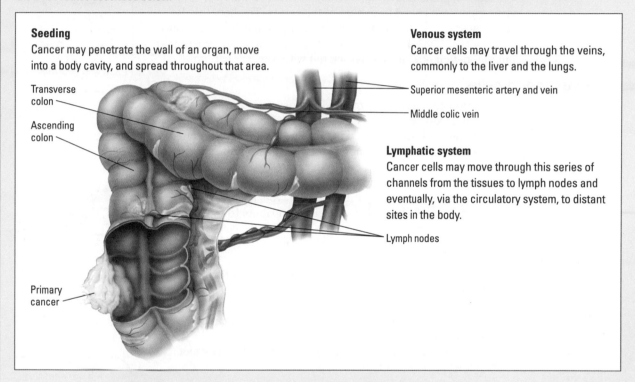

Seeding
Cancer may penetrate the wall of an organ, move into a body cavity, and spread throughout that area.

Transverse colon

Ascending colon

Primary cancer

Venous system
Cancer cells may travel through the veins, commonly to the liver and the lungs.

Superior mesenteric artery and vein

Middle colic vein

Lymphatic system
Cancer cells may move through this series of channels from the tissues to lymph nodes and eventually, via the circulatory system, to distant sites in the body.

Lymph nodes

Cancer cells metastasize three ways:

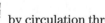 by circulation through the blood and lymphatic system

by accidental transplantation during surgery

by spreading to adjacent organs and tissues.

What causes cancer?

All cancers involve the malfunction of genes that control cell growth and division. A cell's transformation from normal to cancerous is called *carcinogenesis*. Carcinogenesis has no single cause but probably results from complex interactions between viruses, physical and chemical carcinogens, and genetic, dietary, immunologic, metabolic, and hormonal factors.

The virus factor

Animal studies show that viruses can transform cells. The Epstein-Barr virus that causes infectious mononucleosis is associated with Burkitt's lymphoma, Hodgkin's disease, and nasopharyngeal cancer. Human papillomavirus, cytomegalovirus, and herpes simplex virus type 2 are linked to cancer of the cervix. The hepatitis B virus causes hepatocellular carcinoma, the human T-cell lymphotropic virus (HTLV-1) causes adult T-cell leukemia, and the human immunodeficiency virus is associated with Kaposi's sarcoma.

Always use a sunscreen with an SPF of 15 or higher to help protect against the sun's ultraviolet rays.

Overexposed cells

The relationship between excessive exposure to the sun's ultraviolet rays and skin cancer is well established. Damage caused by ultraviolet light and subsequent sunburn are linked to skin cancers, such as squamous cell carcinoma, basal cell carcinoma, and melanoma.

Radiation exposure may induce tumor development. Other factors, such as the patient's tissue type, age, length of exposure, and hormonal status, also contribute to the carcinogenic effect.

Something in the air

Substances in the environment can cause cancer by damaging deoxyribonucleic acid in the cells. Examples of common carcinogens and related cancers are:
- tobacco (lung, pancreatic, kidney, bladder, mouth, and esophageal cancer)
- asbestos and airborne aromatic hydrocarbons (lung cancer)
- alkylating agents (leukemia).

You are what you eat! A high-protein and high-fat diet is associated with colorectal cancer.

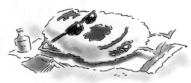

Immune factor

Evidence suggests that a severely compromised immune system can lead to the development of certain cancers. Transplant recipients receiving immunosuppressants and those with acquired immunodeficiency syndrome have an increased risk of certain cancers, such as Kaposi's sarcoma, non-Hodgkin's lymphoma, and skin cancer.

Danger at the diner

Colorectal cancer is associated with high-protein and high-fat diets. Food additives, such as nitrates, and food preparation methods, such as charbroiling, may also contribute to the development of cancer.

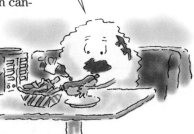

The genetic factor

About 5% to 10% of all cancers are clearly hereditary in that an inherited faulty gene predisposes the person to a very high risk of particular cancers. These cancers may be autosomal recessive, X-linked, or autosomal dominant disorders. (See chapter 13, Genetics.) Such cancers share these characteristics:
• early onset
• increased incidence of bilateral cancer in paired organs (breasts, adrenal glands, and kidneys)
• increased incidence of multiple primary cancers in nonpaired organs
• abnormal chromosome complement in tumor cells
• unique tumor site combinations
• two or more family members in the same generation with the same cancer.

Hormones: Helping or hurting?

The role hormones play in cancer is controversial. Excessive hormone use, especially of estrogen, may contribute to certain forms of cancer while reducing the risk of other forms.

The best defense

One theory suggests that the body develops cancer cells continuously but that the immune system recognizes them as foreign and destroys them. According to the theory, this defense mechanism, called *immunosurveillance*, promotes antibody production, cellular immunity, and immunologic memory. Therefore, an interruption in immunosurveillance could lead to the overproduction of cancer cells and, possibly, a tumor.

Through immunosurveillance, the rest of the immune system and I recognize cancer cells as foreign and destroy them.

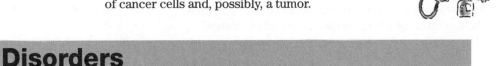

Disorders

Types of cancer discussed in this section include:
• basal cell carcinoma
• breast cancer
• cervical cancer
• colorectal cancer
• endometrial cancer
• Hodgkin's disease
• leukemia
• lung cancer
• malignant melanoma
• multiple myeloma

- prostate cancer
- testicular cancer.

Basal cell carcinoma

Basal cell carcinoma, also known as basal cell epithelioma, is a slow-growing, destructive skin tumor that usually occurs in people older than age 40. Basal cell carcinoma is most prevalent in blond, fair-skinned males, and it's the most common malignant tumor that affects whites. The two major types of basal cell carcinoma are noduloulcerative and superficial.

How it happens

Prolonged sun exposure is the most common cause of basal cell carcinoma—90% of tumors occur on sun-exposed areas of the body. Arsenic ingestion, radiation exposure, burns, immunosuppression and, rarely, vaccinations are other possible causes.

Although the pathogenesis is uncertain, some experts hypothesize that basal cell carcinoma originates when undifferentiated basal cells become carcinomatous instead of differentiating into sweat glands, sebum, and hair.

What to look for

The patient history may reveal that the patient became aware of an odd-looking skin lesion, which prompted him to seek medical examination. The history may also disclose prolonged exposure to the sun sometime in the patient's life or other risk factors for this disease. Inspection may reveal:
- small, smooth, pinkish, and translucent papules lesions
- telangiectatic vessels cross the surface of the lesion

I'm depressed
- as the lesions enlarge, their centers become depressed and their borders become firm and elevated

Chest and back
- multiple oval or irregularly shaped, lightly pigmented plaques
- sharply defined, slightly elevated, threadlike borders

Head and neck
- waxy, sclerotic, yellow to white plaques without distinct borders. (See *Looking at basal cell carcinoma*.)

Now I get it!

Looking at basal cell carcinoma

The illustration below shows the central crater and papule characteristic of basal cell carcinoma.

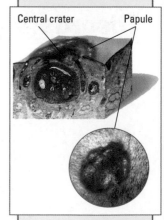

Central crater   Papule

Battling illness

Treating basal cell carcinoma

Depending on the size, location, and depth of the lesion, treatment may include curettage and electrodesiccation, chemotherapy, surgical excision, irradiation, or chemosurgery:
• Curettage and electrodesiccation offer good cosmetic results for small lesions.
• Topical fluorouracil is often used for superficial lesions. This medication produces marked local irritation or inflammation in the involved tissue but no systemic effects.
• Microscopically controlled surgical excision carefully removes recurrent lesions until a tu-

mor-free plane is achieved. After removal of large lesions, skin grafting may be required.
• Irradiation is used if the tumor location requires it. It's also preferred for elderly or debilitated patients who might not tolerate surgery.
• Chemosurgery may be necessary for persistent or recurrent lesions. It consists of periodic applications of a fixative paste (such as zinc chloride) and subsequent removal of fixed pathologic tissue. Treatment continues until tumor removal is complete.
• Cryotherapy, using liquid nitrogen, freezes the cells and kills them.

What tests tell you

All types of basal cell carcinomas are diagnosed by clinical appearance.
•   Incisional or excisional biopsy and histologic study may help to determine the tumor type and histologic subtype. (See *Treating basal cell carcinoma.*)

Breast cancer

Breast cancer is the most common cancer in women. Although the disease may develop any time after puberty, 70% of cases occur in women older than age 50. Breast cancer ranks second among cancer deaths in women, behind cancer of the lung and bronchus.

How it happens

The exact causes of breast cancer remain elusive. Scientists have discovered specific genes linked to approximately 5% of all cases of breast cancer (called *BRCA1* and *BRCA2*), which confirms that the disease can be inherited from a person's mother or father. Those who inherit either of these genes have an 80% chance of developing breast cancer. (See *Susceptibility to breast cancer*, page 398.)

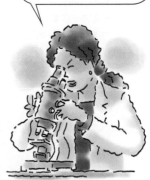

Numerous risk factors for breast cancer have been identified, but the exact cause remains unknown.

Other significant risk factors have been identified. These include:

- a family history of breast cancer
- radiation exposure
- being a premenopausal woman older than age 45
- obesity
- age
- recent use of hormonal contraceptives
- early onset of menses or late menopause
- nulligravida (never pregnant)
- first pregnancy after age 30
- high-fat diet
- colon, endometrial, or ovarian cancer
- postmenopausal progestin and estrogen therapy
- alcohol use (one or more alcoholic beverages per day)
- benign breast disease.

About one-half of all breast cancers develop in the upper outer quadrant. (See *Breast quadrants.*)

Understanding classification

Breast cancer is generally classified by the tissue of origin and the location of the lesion:

- Lobular cancer develops within the lobes.
- Ductal cancer, the most common form, develops within the ducts.
- Less than 1% of breast cancers originate in the nonepithelial connective tissue.
- Inflammatory cancer (rare) grows rapidly and causes the overlying skin to become edematous, inflamed, and indurated.

Susceptibility to breast cancer

Patients with BRCA1 and BRCA2 account for approximately 5% of all breast cancer cases. General screening of the population for these genes isn't recommended. However, screening women with a strong family history of breast cancer is recommended when genetic counseling is available.

Recent studies suggest that prophylactic removal of the breasts in BRCA1 and BRCA2 carriers greatly decreases the risk of breast cancer in these individuals. Recent studies also show that removing the ovaries and fallopian tubes in premenopausal BRCA1 and BRCA2 carriers reduces the risk of breast cancer.

Breast quadrants

This illustration shows the quadrants of the right breast and the Tail of Spence. The upper outer quadrant is the most common site of breast cancer.

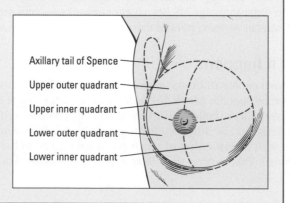

Axillary tail of Spence

Upper outer quadrant

Upper inner quadrant

Lower outer quadrant

Lower inner quadrant

- Paget's disease is the growth of cancerous cells within the breast ducts beneath the nipple.

Breast cancer is also classified as invasive or noninvasive. *Invasive tumor cells*, which make up 90% of all breast cancers, break through the duct walls and encroach on other breast tissues. *Noninvasive tumor cells* remain confined to the duct in which they originated. (See *Types of breast cancer*.)

What to look for

Typically, the patient discovers a thickening of the breast tissue or a painless lump or mass in her breast. A mass may be detected on a mammogram before a lesion becomes palpable. Inspection may reveal nipple retraction, scaly skin around the nipple, skin changes, erythema, and clear, milky, or bloody discharge. Edema in the arm indicates advanced nodal involvement.

Palpation may identify a hard lump, mass, or thickening of breast tissue. Palpation of the cervical supraclavicular and axillary nodes may reveal lumps or enlargement.

Although growth rates vary, a lump may take up to 8 years to become palpable at ⅜″ (1 cm). Breast cancers can spread via the lymphatic system and bloodstream, through the right side of the heart to the lungs and, eventually, to the other breast, chest wall, liver, bone, and brain. (See *Treating breast cancer*, page 400.)

What tests tell you

These tests are used to diagnose breast cancer:
- Breast self-examination (done regularly) followed by a clinical breast examination, is one method for detecting breast lumps early.
- Mammography—the primary test for breast cancer—can be used to detect tumors that are too small to palpate.
- Fine-needle aspiration and excisional biopsy provide cells for histologic examination to confirm diagnosis.
- Hormone receptor assay can be used to pinpoint whether the tumor is estrogen- or progesterone-dependent so that appropriate therapy can be chosen.
- Ultrasonography can be used to distinguish between a fluid-filled cyst and a solid mass.
- Chest X-rays can be used to pinpoint chest metastasis.

> Let's review proper breast self-examination techniques.

Now I get it!

Types of breast cancer

The illustrations below show ductal carcinoma in situ and infiltrating or invasive ductal carcinoma.

Ductal carcinoma in situ

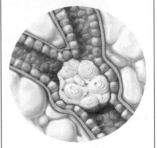

Infiltrating (invasive) ductal carcinoma

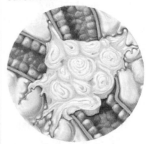

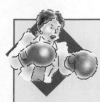

Treating breast cancer

Treatment for breast cancer may include a combination of surgery, radiation, chemotherapy, and hormonal therapy, depending on the disease stage and type, the woman's age and menopausal status, and the disfiguring effects of the surgery. Each treatment is explained here.

Lumpectomy

Through a small incision, the surgeon removes the tumor, surrounding tissue and, possibly, nearby lymph nodes. The patient usually undergoes radiation therapy afterward.

Lumpectomy is used for small, well-defined lesions. Studies show that lumpectomy and radiation are as effective as mastectomy in early-stage breast cancer.

Partial mastectomy

The surgeon removes the tumor along with a wedge of normal tissue, skin, fascia, and axillary lymph nodes. Radiation therapy or chemotherapy is usually used after surgery to destroy undetected disease in other breast areas.

Total mastectomy

A total mastectomy involves removal of the breast tissue. This procedure is used if the cancer is confined to breast tissue and no lymph node involvement is detected. Chemotherapy or radiation therapy may follow. If the patient doesn't have advanced disease, reconstructive surgery can be used to create a breast mound.

Modified radical mastectomy

The surgeon removes the entire breast, axillary lymph nodes, and the lining that covers the chest muscles. If the lymph nodes contain cancer cells, radiation therapy and chemotherapy follow. Modified radical mastectomy has largely replaced the radical mastectomy because it preserves the pectoral muscles.

Before or after tumor removal, radiation therapy may be used to destroy a small, early-stage tumor without distant metastasis. It can also be used to prevent or treat local recurrence. Preoperative radiation therapy to the breast also "sterilizes" the area, making the tumor more manageable surgically, especially in inflammatory breast cancer.

Chemotherapy

Cytotoxic drugs may be used either as adjuvant therapy or primary therapy. Decisions to start chemotherapy are based on several factors, such as the stage of the cancer and hormone receptor assay results.

Chemotherapy may be administered in a hospital, doctor's office, clinic, or patient's home. The drugs may be given orally, or by I.M., subQ, or I.V. injection

Chemotherapy commonly involves the use of a combination of drugs. A typical regimen makes use of cyclophosphamide, methotrexate, doxorubicin, and fluorouracil.

Hormone therapy

Hormone therapy lowers the levels of estrogen and other hormones suspected of nourishing breast cancer cells. Anti-estrogen therapy, with tamoxifen or raloxifene, is used in women at increased risk for developing breast cancer. Other commonly used drugs include the antiandrogen aminoglutethimide, the androgen fluoxymesterone, the estrogen diethylstilbestrol, and the progestin megestrol.

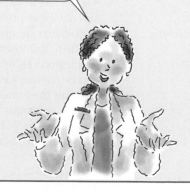

In choosing therapy for breast cancer treatment, the doctor considers the stage of the disease, the patient's age and menopausal status, and possible body image alteration.

- Scans of the bone, brain, liver, and other organs can be used to detect distant metastasis.
- Laboratory tests, such as alkaline phosphatase levels and liver function tests, can uncover distant metastasis.
- Ductoscopy reveals small intraductal lesions that aren't palpable or visible on mammography.
- Ductal lavage identifies cancerous cells in the milk ducts of the breast.

Cervical cancer

Cervical cancer is the third most common cancer of the female reproductive system. It's classified as either preinvasive or invasive.

Preinvasive cancer ranges from minimal cervical dysplasia, in which the lower third of the epithelium contains abnormal cells, to carcinoma in situ, in which the full thickness of epithelium contains abnormally proliferating cells. Preinvasive cancer is curable in 75% to 90% of patients with early detection and proper treatment. If untreated, it may progress to invasive cervical cancer, depending on the form.

In invasive disease, usually squamous cell carcinoma, cancer cells penetrate the basement membrane and can spread directly to contiguous pelvic structures or disseminate to distant sites by way of lymphatic routes. Invasive cancer typically occurs between ages 30 and 50; it rarely occurs younger than age 20. (See *Looking at cervical cancer*, page 402.)

How it happens

The human papillomavirus (HPV) is accepted as the cause of virtually all cervical dysplasias and cervical cancers. Certain strains of HPV (16, 18, 31) are associated with an increased risk of cervical cancer. A recently approved vaccine, HPV recombinant vaccine (Gardasil), is recommended for women and girls ages 9 to 26 years to protect against cervical cancer. Several predisposing factors have been related to the development of cervical cancer:
- intercourse at a young age (younger than age 16)
- multiple sexual partners
- herpes virus 2
- other bacterial or viral venereal infections.

What to look for

Preinvasive cancer produces no symptoms or other clinical changes. In early invasive cervical cancer, the patient history includes:
- abnormal vaginal bleeding, such as a persistent vaginal discharge that may be yellowish, blood-tinged, and foul-smelling

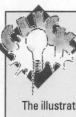

Looking at cervical cancer

The illustrations below show cervical carcinoma in situ and squamous cell carcinoma of the cervix.

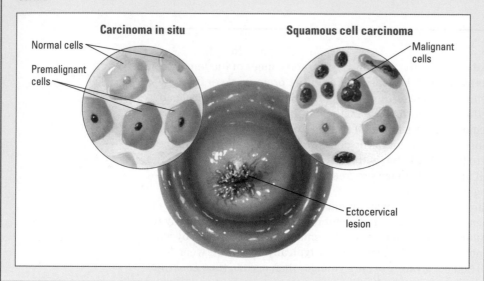

- postcoital pain and bleeding
- bleeding between menstrual periods
- unusually heavy menstrual periods.

The patient history may suggest one or more of the predisposing factors for this disease.

Advancement

If the cancer has advanced into the pelvic wall, the patient may report:
- gradually increasing flank pain, which can indicate sciatic nerve involvement.
- leakage of urine, which may point to metastasis into the bladder with formation of a fistula.
- leakage of stool, which may indicate metastasis to the rectum with fistula development.

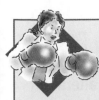

Battling illness

Treating cervical cancer

Accurate clinical staging will determine the type of treatment. Preinvasive lesions may be treated with total excisional biopsy, cryosurgery, laser destruction, conization (followed by frequent Pap test follow-ups) or, rarely, hysterectomy. Therapy for invasive squamous cell carcinoma may include radical hysterectomy and radiation therapy (internal, external, or both). Rarely, pelvic exenteration may be performed for recurrent cervical cancer.

Complications

Complications of surgery include:
• bladder dysfunction
• formation of lymphocytes or seromas after lymphadenectomy
• pulmonary embolism.

Complications of radiation therapy include:
• diarrhea
• abdominal cramping
• dysuria
• leukopenia.

Combined surgery and irradiation in the abdomen and pelvis may lead to small bowel obstruction, stricture and fibrosis of the intestine or rectosigmoid, and rectovaginal or vesicovaginal fistula.

What tests tell you

• Papanicolaou (Pap) test identifies abnormal cells.
• Colposcopy determines the source of the abnormal cells seen on the Pap test.
• Cone biopsy is performed if endocervical curettage is positive.
• The Vira/Pap test permits examination of the specimen's deoxyribonucleic acid (DNA) structure to detect HPV.
• Lymphangiography, cystography, and major organ and bone scans, can detect metastasis. (See *Treating cervical cancer*.)

Colorectal cancer

Colorectal cancer accounts for 10% to 15% of all new cancer cases in the United States. It occurs equally in both sexes and is the third most common cause of cancer death. It strikes most commonly in people older than age 50.

The importance of a thorough assessment

Because colorectal cancer progresses slowly and remains localized for a long time, early detection is key to recovery. Unless the tumor metastasizes, the 5-year survival rate is 80% for rectal cancer and 85% for colon cancer.

How it happens

The primary risk factor for colorectal cancer is age. Several disorders and preexisting conditions are also linked to colorectal cancer, including:

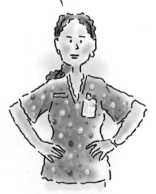

Because colorectal cancer progresses slowly, early detection is key.

- ulcerative colitis
- Crohn's disease
- Turcot's syndrome
- hereditary nonpolyposis colorectal carcinoma
- other pelvic cancers treated with abdominal radiation
- genetic abnormality.

Polyp wallop

Colorectal polyps are closely tied to colon cancer. The larger the polyp, the greater the risk.

The genetic angle

The cause of colorectal cancer may be related to genetic factors—deletions on chromosomes 17 and 18—that may promote mutation and transition of the mucosal cells to a malignant state. (See *Gene alteration and colon cancer.*)

High fat, low fiber

A high-fat, low-fiber diet is thought to contribute to colorectal cancer by slowing fecal movement through the bowel. This results in prolonged exposure of the bowel mucosa to digested materials and may encourage mucosal cells to mutate.

The couch potato factor

Other risk factors include:
- smoking
- alcohol consumption
- obesity
- physical inactivity.

Recent studies suggest that estrogen replacement therapy and nonsteroidal anti-inflammatory drugs, such as aspirin, may reduce the risk of colorectal cancer. (See *Types of colorectal cancer.*)

What to look for

In its early stages, colorectal cancer usually causes no symptoms. Rectal bleeding, blood in the stool, a change in bowel habits, and cramping pain in the lower abdomen may signal advanced disease. (See *Treating colorectal cancer*, page 406.)

What tests tell you

Several tests are used to diagnose colorectal cancer:
- Digital rectal examination (DRE) is used to detect 15% of colorectal cancers, specifically rectal and perianal lesions.
- Fecal occult blood test is used to detect blood in stool.

The genetic link

Gene alteration and colon cancer

Researchers have discovered a gene alteration that contributes to the growth of colon cancer. The helicase-like transcription factor (HLTF) gene (one of the genes that help stabilize deoxyribonucleic acid and regulate protein production in the cell) is inactivated, which contributes to the transformation of normal colon cells into cancer cells.

When scientists introduced a functional copy of the HLTF gene into the colon cancer cell lines that lacked the gene, the cells stopped growing. This finding suggests that the HLTF gene is itself a tumor suppressor gene that can stop tumors from growing. As a result, scientists have begun drug development that reverses this process.

Now I get it!

Types of colorectal cancer

Colorectal cancer can occur anywhere along the small and large intestine, as well as the rectum.

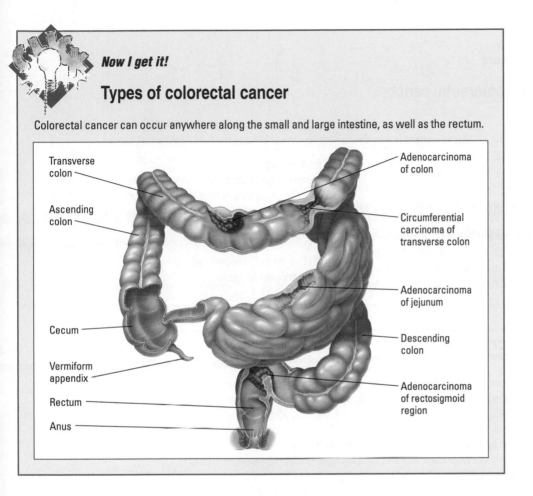

- Transverse colon
- Ascending colon
- Cecum
- Vermiform appendix
- Rectum
- Anus
- Adenocarcinoma of colon
- Circumferential carcinoma of transverse colon
- Adenocarcinoma of jejunum
- Descending colon
- Adenocarcinoma of rectosigmoid region

- Proctoscopy or sigmoidoscopy is used to visualize the lower GI tract and aids detection of two-thirds of all colorectal cancers.
- Colonoscopy is used to visualize and photograph the colon up to the ileocecal valve and provides access for polypectomies and biopsies.
- Barium enema is used to locate lesions not visible or palpable.
- Computed tomography (CT) scan helps to detect cancer spread.
- Carcinoembryonic antigen, a tumor marker, which becomes elevated in about 70% of patients with colorectal cancer, is used to monitor the patient before and after treatment to detect metastasis or recurrence.
- Liver function studies determine whether liver metastasis has occurred.

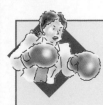

Battling illness

Treating colorectal cancer

Surgery
The most effective treatment for colorectal cancer is surgical removal of the malignant tumor, adjacent tissues, and cancerous lymph nodes. Until recently, laparoscopy wasn't used for colon cancer because of concerns that the cancer was more likely to return after laparoscopy than after standard surgery. However, a recent study has shown that laparoscopic surgery is a viable option for patients with colon cancer who don't require extensive surgery involving organs other than the colon.

The surgical site depends on the location of the tumor. The illustration below shows the different locations in the colon that may be resected for tumor removal. A permanent colostomy is rarely needed in a patient with colorectal cancer.

Chemotherapy
Chemotherapy or chemotherapy in combination with radiation therapy is given before or after surgery to most patients whose cancer has deeply perforated the bowel wall or has spread to the lymph nodes.

Commonly used drugs include oxaliplatin in combination with fluorouracil followed by leucovorin for patients with metastatic carcinoma.

Endometrial cancer

Cancer of the endometrium (also known as uterine cancer) is the most common gynecologic cancer. It typically afflicts postmenopausal females between ages 50 and 60. It's uncommon between ages 30 and 40 and rare before age 30. Most premenopausal females who develop uterine cancer have a history of anovulatory menstrual cycles or other hormonal imbalance. About 33,000 new cases of uterine cancer are reported annually; of these, roughly 5,500 are fatal.

How it happens

Uterine cancer appears linked to several predisposing factors:
• low fertility index and anovulation
• history of infertility or failure of ovulation
• abnormal uterine bleeding
• obesity, hypertension, diabetes, or nulliparity
• familial tendency
• history of uterine polyps or endometrial hyperplasia
• prolonged estrogen therapy with exposure unopposed by progesterone.

In most patients, uterine cancer is an adenocarcinoma that metastasizes late, usually from the endometrium to the cervix, ovaries, fallopian tubes, and other peritoneal structures. It may spread to distant organs, such as the lungs and the brain, by way of the blood or the lymphatic system. Lymph node involvement can also occur. (See *Progression of endometrial cancer.*)

Now I get it!

Progression of endometrial cancer

The illustrations below show the progression of endometrial cancer.

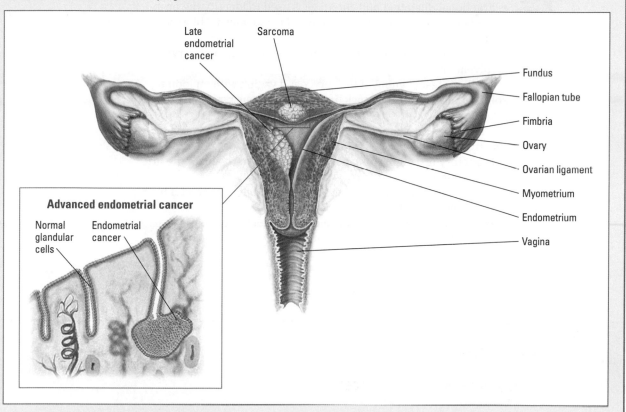

Late endometrial cancer

Sarcoma

Fundus

Fallopian tube

Fimbria

Ovary

Ovarian ligament

Myometrium

Endometrium

Vagina

Advanced endometrial cancer

Normal glandular cells

Endometrial cancer

What to look for

The patient history may reflect one or more predisposing factors.

Pre...

In a younger patient, it may also reveal spotting and protracted, heavy menstrual periods.

...and post

A postmenopausal woman may report that bleeding began 12 or more months after menses had stopped. In either case, the patient may describe the discharge as watery at first, then blood-streaked, and gradually becoming bloodier.

In more advanced stages, palpation may disclose an enlarged uterus.

What tests tell you

- Endometrial, cervical, or endocervical biopsy confirms cancer cells.
- Fractional dilatation and curettage is used to identify the problem when the disease is suspected but the endometrial biopsy is negative.
- Cervical biopsies and endocervical curettage pinpoint cervical involvement.
- Schiller's test staining of the cervix and vagina with an iodine solution turns healthy tissues brown. (Cancerous tissues resist the stain.)
- CT scans or magnetic resonance imaging detect metastasis to the myometrium, cervix, lymph nodes, and other organs.
- Excretory urography and, possibly, cystoscopy evaluate the urinary system.
- Proctoscopy or barium enema studies may be performed if bladder and rectal involvement are suspected.
- Blood studies, urinalysis, and electrocardiography may also help in staging the disease. (See *Treating endometrial cancer.*)

Battling illness

Treating endometrial cancer

Depending on the extent of the disease, the treatment may include one or more of the following:

Surgery
Surgery usually involves total abdominal hysterectomy, bilateral salpingooophorectomy or, possibly, omentectomy with or without pelvic or para-aortic lymphadenectomy. Total pelvic exenteration removes all pelvic organs, including the rectum, bladder, and vagina, and is only performed when the disease is sufficiently contained to allow surgical removal of diseased parts. This surgery seldom is curative, especially in nodal involvement.

Radiation
Radiation therapy is used when the tumor isn't well differentiated. Intracavitary radiation, external radiation, or both may be given 6 weeks before surgery to inhibit recurrence and lengthen survival time.

Hormonal therapy
Hormonal therapy, using tamoxifen (Nolvadex), shows a response rate of 20% to 40%.

Chemotherapy
Chemotherapy, including both cisplatin (Platinol) and doxorubicin (Doxil), is usually tried when other treatments have failed.

Hodgkin's disease

Battling illness

Treating Hodgkin's disease

Depending on the stage of the disease, the patient may receive chemotherapy, radiation therapy, or both. Correct treatment leads to longer survival and may cure many patients.

Other treatments include autologous bone marrow or peripheral stem cell transplantation and immunotherapy, used in conjunction with chemotherapy and radiation therapy.

Chemotherapy combinations

Chemotherapy consists of various combinations of drugs. The well-known MOPP protocol (mechlorethamine, Oncovin [vincristine], procarbazine, and prednisone) was the first to result in significant cures. Another useful combination is doxorubicin, bleomycin, vinblastine, and dacarba-zine. Antiemetics, sedatives, and antidiarrheals may be given with these drugs to prevent adverse GI effects.

Hodgkin's disease causes painless, progressive enlargement of the lymph nodes, spleen, and other lymphoid tissue.

This type of cancer has a higher incidence in men, is slightly more common in whites, and occurs most commonly in two age groups: 15 to 35 and older than age 50. A family history increases the likelihood of acquiring the disease.

Although the disease is fatal if untreated, recent advances have made Hodgkin's disease potentially curable, even in advanced stages. With appropriate treatment, about 90% of patients live at least 5 years. (See *Treating Hodgkin's disease.*)

How it happens

The cause of Hodgkin's disease is unknown. It probably involves a virus. Many patients with Hodgkin's disease have had infectious mononucleosis, so an indirect relationship may exist between the Epstein-Barr virus and Hodgkin's disease. Another possible risk factor is occupational exposure to herbicides and other chemicals.

Enlargement of the lymph nodes, spleen, and other lymphoid tissues results from proliferation of lymphocytes, histiocytes, and, rarely, eosinophils. Patients also have distinct chromosome abnormalities in their lymph node cells. (See *Ann Arbor staging system for Hodgkin's disease*, page 410.)

What to look for

People with Hodgkin's disease can develop signs and symptoms of whole-body involvement, including:
• painless swelling of the lymph nodes, usually beginning in the neck and progressing to the axillary, inguinal, mediastinal, and mesenteric regions
• night sweats
• cancerous masses in the spleen, liver, and bones
• painless swelling of the face and neck
• anemia
• jaundice
• nerve pain
• increased susceptibility to infection
• intermittent fever that can last for several days or weeks

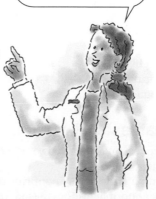

While the cause of Hodgkin's disease is unknown, there are specific signs to look for.

Ann Arbor staging system for Hodgkin's disease

The illustrations below follow the stages of metastasis in the Ann Arbor Staging System.

Stage I
• Involvement of single lymph node region
        or
• Involvement of single extralymphatic site (stage I_E)

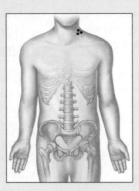

Stage II
• Involvement of two or more lymph node regions on same side of diaphragm
• May include localized extralymphatic involvement on same side of diaphragm (stage II_E)

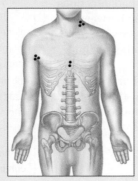

Stage III
• Involvement of lymph node regions on both sides of diaphragm
• May include involvement of spleen (stage III_S), or localized extranodal disease (stage III_E)

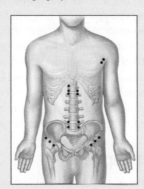

• Hodgkin's disease stage III_1: disease limited to upper abdomen—spleen, splenic hilar, celiac, or portohepatic nodes
• Hodgkin's disease stage III_2: disease limited to lower abdomen—periaortic, pelvic, or inguinal nodes

Stage IV
• Diffuse extralymphatic disease (for example, in liver, bone marrow, lung, skin)

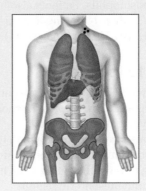

• weight loss
• pruritus
• fatigue.

What tests tell you

These tests may be used to rule out other disorders that enlarge the lymph nodes:
• Lymph node biopsy confirms the presence of Reed-Sternberg cells, abnormal histiocyte (macrophage) proliferation, and nodu-

lar fibrosis and necrosis. It's also used to determine the extent of lymph node involvement.
• Bone marrow, liver, mediastinal, and spleen biopsy are used to determine the extent of lymph node involvement.
• Chest X-ray, abdominal CT scan, lung and bone scans, lymphangiography, and laparoscopy are used to determine the extent and stage of the disease.
• Hematologic tests may show mild to severe normocytic anemia, normochromic anemia (in 50% of patients), and elevated, normal, or reduced white blood cell (WBC) count and differential with neutrophilia, lymphocytopenia, monocytosis, or eosinophilia (in any combination). Elevated serum alkaline phosphatase levels indicate liver or bone involvement.
• Staging laparotomy may be performed for developing a therapeutic care plan.

Leukemia, acute

Acute leukemia is one form of leukemia. Leukemia refers to a group of malignant disorders characterized by abnormal proliferation and maturation of lymphocytes and nonlymphocytic cells, leading to the suppression of normal cells. (See *Facts about leukemia*.)

If untreated, acute leukemia is fatal, usually as a result of complications from leukemic cell infiltration of bone marrow or vital organs. With treatment, the prognosis varies.

Two types of acute leukemia are acute lymphocytic leukemia and acute myeloid leukemia (also known as *acute nonlymphocytic leukemia* or *acute myeloblastic leukemia*).

Acute lymphocytic leukemia

Acute lymphocytic leukemia accounts for 80% of childhood leukemias. Treatment leads to remission in 81% of children, who survive an average of 5 years, and in 65% of adults, who survive an average of 2 years. Children between ages 2 and 8 who receive intensive therapy have the best survival rate.

Acute myeloid leukemia

Acute myeloid leukemia is one of the most common leukemias in adults. Average survival time is only 1 year after diagnosis, even with aggressive treatment. Remissions lasting 2 to 10 months occur in 50% of children.

Facts about leukemia

Classification
Leukemias are classified as:
• chronic or acute
• myeloid or lymphoid.

Statistics
• In the United States, about 30,600 people develop leukemia annually.
• Typically thought of as a childhood disease, leukemia is 10 times more common in adults than in children.
• Leukemia occurs more commonly in males than in females.

The patient's history usually reveals a sudden onset of high fever and abnormal bleeding, such as bruising after minor trauma, nosebleeds, gingival bleeding, and purpura. Fatigue and night sweats may also occur.

How it happens

The exact cause of leukemia isn't known; however, 40% to 50% of patients have mutations in their chromosomes. In addition, individuals with certain chromosomal disorders have a higher risk. People with Down syndrome, trisomy 13, and other heredity disorders have a higher incidence of leukemia.

Other risk factors include cigarette smoking, exposure to certain chemicals (such as benzene, which is present in cigarette smoke and gasoline), and exposure to large doses of ionizing radiation or drugs that depress the bone marrow. Certain viruses, such as HTLV-1, are also associated with an increased risk of leukemia.

What's going on

Here's a description of what probably happens when a patient develops leukemia:

• Immature hematopoietic cells undergo an abnormal transformation, giving rise to leukemic cells.
• Leukemic cells multiply and accumulate, crowding out other types of cells.
• Crowding prevents production of normal red and white blood cells and platelets, leading to pancytopenia—a reduction in the number of all cellular elements of the blood. (See *Histologic findings in acute lymphocytic and acute myeloid leukemia.*)

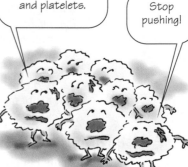

Leukemic cells may crowd out other types of cells, thereby stopping production of normal red and white blood cells and platelets.

Stop pushing!

What to look for

Signs and symptoms of acute lymphocytic and acute myeloid leukemia are similar. Effects of both leukemias are related to suppression of elements of the bone marrow and include:

• infection
• bleeding
• anemia
• malaise
• fever

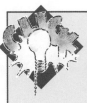

Now I get it!

Histologic findings in acute lymphocytic and acute myeloid leukemia

The illustrations below show the histologic findings in acute lymphocytic and acute myeloid leukemia.

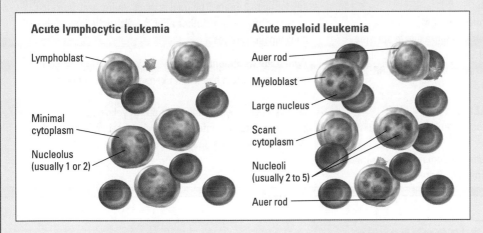

Acute lymphocytic leukemia

- Lymphoblast
- Minimal cytoplasm
- Nucleolus (usually 1 or 2)

Acute myeloid leukemia

- Auer rod
- Myeloblast
- Large nucleus
- Scant cytoplasm
- Nucleoli (usually 2 to 5)
- Auer rod

- lethargy
- paleness
- weight loss
- night sweats. (See *Treating acute leukemia*, page 414.)

What tests tell you

These tests are used to diagnose acute leukemia:
- Blood counts show thrombocytopenia and neutropenia; WBC differential determines cell type.
- Lumbar puncture is used to detect meningeal involvement; cerebrospinal fluid analysis reveals abnormal WBC invasion of the central nervous system (CNS).
- Bone marrow aspiration and biopsy confirms the disease by showing a proliferation of immature WBCs. It's also used to determine whether the leukemia is lymphocytic or myeloid (important because the treatments and prognoses are very different).
- CT scan shows which organs are affected.

Leukemia, chronic lymphocytic

Chronic lymphocytic leukemia is the most benign and slowest progressing form of leukemia. This type of chronic leukemia occurs most commonly in elderly people, and more than one-half of the cases are male. According to the American Cancer Society, this type of leukemia accounts for about one-third of new adult cases annually.

What's the verdict?

The prognosis is poor if anemia, thrombocytopenia, neutropenia, bulky lymphadenopathy, or severe lymphocytosis develops. Gross bone marrow replacement by abnormal lymphocytes is the most common cause of death, usually 4 to 5 years after diagnosis. (See *Treating chronic lymphocytic leukemia*.)

How it happens

Chronic lymphocytic leukemia is a generalized, progressive disease. It causes a proliferation and accumulation of relatively mature looking but immunologically inefficient lymphocytes. After these cells infiltrate, clinical signs appear. (See *Histologic findings in chronic lymphocytic leukemia*.)

Now I get it!

Histologic findings in chronic lymphocytic leukemia

The illustration shows the characteristic histologic findings in chronic lymphocytic leukemia.

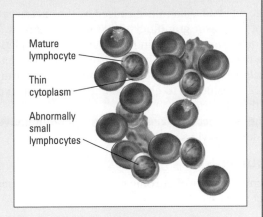

Mature lymphocyte

Thin cytoplasm

Abnormally small lymphocytes

Although the cause of chronic lymphocytic leukemia is unknown, hereditary factors are suspected.

What to look for

Clinical signs may include fever and frequent infections, fatigue, enlargement of lymph nodes, and splenomegaly.

What tests tell you

These tests are used to diagnose chronic lymphocytic leukemia:
• Lymph node biopsy distinguishes between benign and malignant tumors.
• Routine blood tests usually uncover the disease. In the early stages, the lymphocyte count is slightly elevated (greater than 20,000/µl). Although granulocytopenia is generally seen first, the lymphocyte count climbs (greater than 100,000/µl) as the disease progresses. A hemoglobin level lower than 11 g/dl, hypogamma-globulinemia, and depressed serum globulin levels are also evident.
• Bone marrow aspiration and biopsy shows lymphocytic invasion.

Battling illness

Treating chronic lymphocytic leukemia

If the patient is asymptomatic, treatment may begin with close monitoring. When autoimmune hemolytic anemia or thrombocytopenia is present, systemic chemotherapy is administered, using the alkylating agents chlorambucil or cyclophosphamide. The corticosteroid prednisone may be administered when the disease is refractory to treatment.

When obstruction or organ impairment or enlargement occurs, local radiation reduces organ size and helps relieve symptoms. Radiation therapy is also used for enlarged lymph nodes, painful bony lesions, or massive splenomegaly. Allopurinol can prevent hyperuricemia.

Leukemia, chronic myeloid

Also called *chronic myologenous leukemia*, chronic myeloid leukemia is characterized by myeloproliferation in bone marrow, peripheral blood, and body tissues. It's most common in middle age but may affect any age-group, and it affects both sexes equally. In the United States, 4,300 cases are diagnosed annually, accounting for about 20% of all cases of leukemia.

How it happens

Chronic myeloid leukemia is caused by the excessive development of neoplastic granulocytes in the bone marrow. The neoplastic granulocytes circulate into the peripheral circulation, infiltrating the liver and spleen. These cells contain a distinct abnormality, the *Philadelphia chromosome*, in which the long arm of chromosome 22 translocates to chromosome 9. Radiation exposure may cause this abnormality.

Other suspected causes include myeloproliferative diseases or an unidentified virus.

An unyielding course

The clinical course of chronic myeloid leukemia proceeds in two distinct phases:

☞ the chronic phase, characterized by anemia and bleeding abnormalities

✌ the terminal or *blastic phase*, in which myeloblasts, the most primitive granulocytic precursors, proliferate rapidly. (See *Histologic findings in chronic myeloid leukemia*.)

Now I get it!

Histologic findings in chronic myeloid leukemia

The illustration shows the histologic findings in chronic myeloid leukemia.

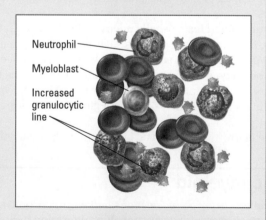

Neutrophil

Myeloblast

Increased granulocytic line

Battling illness

Treating chronic myeloid leukemia

In chronic myeloid leu-kemia, the treatment goal is to control leukocytosis and thrombocytosis. Imatinib mesylate is a highly specific new anticancer drug that has recently been approved by the Food and Drug Administration for treating the disorder.

Other commonly used drugs are busulfan and hydroxyurea. Aspirin may help prevent a stroke if the patient's platelet count exceeds 1 million/µl. Bone marrow transplantation may be effective. Antibiotics and blood transfusions are supportive treatments.

Supplemental therapy
• Local splenic radiation or splenectomy to increase the platelet count and decrease effects of splenomegaly
• Leukapheresis (selective leukocyte removal) to reduce white blood cell count
• Allopurinol to prevent secondary hyperuricemia and colchicine to relieve gouty attacks.

Chronic myeloid leukemia is a deadly disease. The average survival time is 3 to 4 years after onset of the chronic phase and 3 to 6 months after onset of the terminal phase. (See *Treating chronic myeloid leukemia.*)

What to look for

Common signs and symptoms of chronic myeloid leukemia include:
• fatigue
• weight loss
• heat intolerance
• fever
• splenomegaly with abdominal fullness
• bruising
• joint pain
• weakness.

What tests tell you

These tests are used to diagnose chronic myeloid leukemia:
• Chromosomal studies of peripheral blood or bone marrow confirm the disease.
• Serum analysis shows WBC abnormalities, such as leukocytosis (WBC count greater than 50,000/µl to as high as 250,000/µl), leukopenia (WBC count less than 5,000/µl), neutropenia (neutrophil count lower than 1,500/µl) despite high WBC count, and increased circulating myeloblasts. Other blood abnormalities may include a decreased hemoglobin level (below 10 g/dl), low hematocrit (less than 30%), and thrombocytosis (more than 1 million thrombocytes/µl). The serum uric acid level may exceed 8 mg/dl.

- Bone marrow biopsy may be hypercellular, showing bone marrow infiltration by a high number of myeloid elements. In the acute phase, myeloblasts predominate.
- CT scan may be used to identify the affected organs.

Lung cancer

Although lung cancer is largely preventable, it remains the most common cause of cancer death in men and women.

Lung cancer is divided into two major classes: small-cell and non–small-cell cancer. The most common type of lung cancer, accounting for almost 80% of cases, is non–small-cell cancer. Types of non–small-cell cancer include:
- adenocarcinoma
- squamous cell
- large-cell.

Small-cell lung cancer accounts for 20% of all lung cancers. It starts in the hormonal cells in the lungs. Small-cell lung cancers include:
- oat cell
- intermediate
- combined (small-cell combined with squamous or adenocarcinoma).

The prognosis for lung cancer is generally poor, depending on the extent of the cancer and the cells' growth rate. Only about 13% of patients survive 5 years after diagnosis.

How it happens

Lung cancer most commonly results from repeated tissue trauma from inhalation of irritants or carcinogens. These substances include tobacco smoke, air pollution, arsenic, asbestos, nickel, and radon.

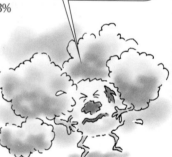

See what happens to us lung cells when we're exposed to irritants or carcinogens.

All choked up

Almost all lung cancers start in the epithelium of the lungs.
- In normal lungs, the epithelium lines and protects the tissue below it. However, when exposed to irritants or carcinogens, the epithelium continually replaces itself until the cells develop chromosomal changes and become dysplastic (altered in size, shape, and organization).
- Dysplastic cells don't function well as protectors, so underlying tissue gets exposed to irritants and carcinogens.
- Eventually, the dysplastic cells turn into neoplastic carcinoma and start invading deeper tissues. (See *Tumor infiltration in lung cancer*.)

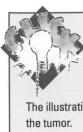

Now I get it!

Tumor infiltration in lung cancer

The illustrations below show tumor infiltration in lung cancer as well as a bronchoscopic view of the tumor.

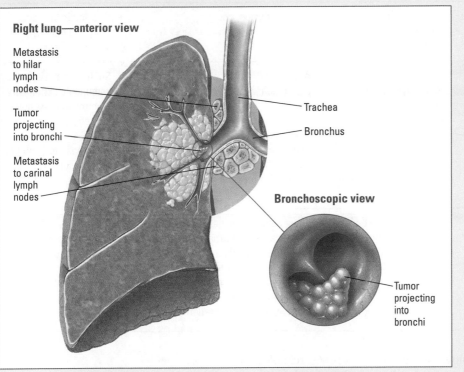

Right lung—anterior view

Metastasis to hilar lymph nodes

Tumor projecting into bronchi

Metastasis to carinal lymph nodes

Trachea

Bronchus

Bronchoscopic view

Tumor projecting into bronchi

What to look for

For information on the signs and symptoms of different types of lung cancers, see *Common lung cancers*, page 420.

What tests tell you

These tests are used to diagnose lung cancer:
• Chest X-ray usually shows an advanced lesion but can reveal damage 2 years before signs and symptoms appear. This test may be used to determine tumor size and location. (See *Treating lung cancer*, page 421.)

Common lung cancers

The table below describes the growth rate, metastasis sites, diagnostic tests, and signs and symptoms of four common lung cancers.

Type of cancer	Rate of growth	Metastasis	Signs and symptoms	Diagnostic tests
Adenocarcinoma	Moderate	Early metastasis to hilar nodes, chest wall, and mediastinum	Pleural effusion, cough	Fiber-optic bronchoscopy, radiography, electron microscopy
Squamous cell	Slow	Late metastasis mainly to hilar lymph nodes, chest wall, and mediastinum	Airway obstruction, cough, sputum production	Sputum analysis, biopsy, immunohistochemistry, electron microscopy, bronchoscopy
Large-cell	Fast	Early, extensive metastasis to other thoracic structures and other organs	Cough, hemoptysis, chest wall pain, pleural effusion, sputum production, pneumonia-induced airway obstruction	Bronchoscopy, sputum analysis, electron microscopy
Small-cell	Very fast	Very early metastasis to mediastinum, hilar lymph nodes, and other organ sites	Chest pain, cough, hemoptysis, dyspnea, localized wheezing, pneumonia-induced airway obstruction, muscle weakness, facial edema, hypokalemia, hyperglycemia, hypertension, and other signs and symptoms related to excessive hormone secretion	Sputum analysis, immunohistochemistry, electron microscopy, radiography, bronchoscopy

• Cytologic sputum analysis is 80% reliable and requires a specimen expectorated from the lungs and tracheobronchial tree.
• Bronchoscopy may reveal the tumor site; bronchoscopic washings provide material for cytologic and histologic study.
• Needle biopsy is used to locate peripheral tumors in the lungs and to collect tissue specimens for analysis; it confirms the diagnosis in 80% of patients.
• Tissue biopsy of metastatic sites is used to assess the extent (stage) of the disease and determine prognosis and treatment.
• Thoracentesis allows chemical and cytologic examination of pleural fluid.
• CT scan may help to evaluate mediastinal and hilar lymph node involvement and the extent of the disease.
• Bone scan, CT brain scan, liver function studies, and gallium scans of the liver and spleen are used to detect metastasis.

Battling illness

Treating lung cancer

Various combinations of surgery, radiation therapy, and chemotherapy may improve the patient's prognosis and prolong survival. Treatment depends on the stage of illness. Unfortunately, lung cancer is usually advanced at diagnosis.

Surgery

Surgery may involve partial lung removal (wedge resection, segmental resection, lobectomy, or radical lobectomy) or total lung removal (pneumonectomy). Complete surgical resection is the only chance for a cure, but fewer than 25% of patients have disease that's responsive to surgery.

Radiation

Preoperative radiation therapy may reduce the tumor's bulk, allowing surgical resection and improving the patient's response.

Radiation therapy is also generally recommended for stage I and stage II lesions if surgery is contraindicated and for stage III disease confined to the involved hemithorax and the ipsilateral supraclavicular lymph nodes.

Chemotherapy

Chemotherapy has caused dramatic, although temporary, responses in patients with small-cell carcinoma. The other types of lung cancer are fairly resistant to it. Drug combinations include cyclophosphamide, doxorubicin, and vincristine; cyclo-phosphamide, doxorubicin, vincristine, and etoposide; and etoposide, cisplatin, cyclophosphamide, and doxorubicin. Unfortunately, patients usually relapse in 7 to 14 months.

Other treatments

Gefitinib, a drug that blocks growth factor receptor activity, was approved for advanced non–small-cell lung cancer. It's administered as monotherapy when chemotherapeutic agents fail.

Malignant melanoma

Malignant melanoma is the most lethal skin cancer. It accounts for 1% to 2% of all malignant tumors, is slightly more common in women, is unusual in children, and occurs most commonly between ages 40 and 50. The incidence in younger age-groups is increasing because of increased sun exposure or, possibly, a decrease in the ozone layer.

How it happens

This disease arises from *melanocytes* (cells that synthesize the pigment melanin). In addition to the skin, melanocytes are also found in the meninges, alimentary canal, respiratory tract, and lymph nodes.

Melanoma spreads through the lymphatic and vascular systems and metastasizes to the regional lymph nodes, skin, liver, lungs, and CNS. In most patients, superficial le-

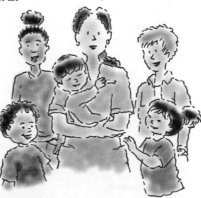

Limiting sun exposure and using sunscreen now can keep your skin healthy!

sions are curable, but deeper lesions are more likely to metastasize. (See *Looking at malignant melanoma.*)

Common sites are the head and neck in men, the legs in women, and the backs of people exposed to excessive sunlight. Up to 70% of malignant melanomas arise from a preexisting nevus (circumscribed malformation of the skin) or mole. (See *Treating malignant melanoma.*)

Rundown on risk factors

Risk factors for developing melanoma are:
- excessive exposure to sunlight
- increased nevi
- tendency to freckle from the sun
- hormonal factors such as pregnancy
- a family history of melanoma
- a past history of melanoma
- red hair, fair skin, blue eyes, susceptibility to sunburn, and Celtic or Scandinavian ancestry. (Melanoma is rare in Blacks.) (See *Shedding light on melanoma.*)

An organelle in the melanocyte called a *melanosome* is responsible for producing melanin. One theory proposes that melanoma arises because the melanosome is abnormal or absent.

What to look for

Suspect malignant melanoma when any preexisting skin lesion or nevus enlarges, changes color, becomes inflamed or sore, itches, ulcerates, bleeds, changes texture, or shows signs of surrounding

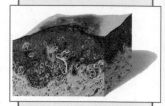

Looking at malignant melanoma

Malignant melanoma can arise on normal skin or from an existing mole. If not treated promptly, it can spread to other areas of skin, lymph nodes, or internal organs.

Battling illness

Treating malignant melanoma

Treatment always involves surgical resection of the tumor and a 3- to 5-cm margin. The extent of resection depends on the size and location of the primary lesion. If a skin graft is needed to close a wide resection, plastic surgery provides excellent cosmetic repair. Surgical treatment may also include regional lymphadenectomy.

Other treatments

In addition to surgery, five other treatments are available:

Deep primary lesions may require chemotherapy, usually with dacarbazine.

Immunotherapy with bacille Calmette-Guérin vaccine is used in advanced melanoma. In theory, this treatment combats cancer by boosting the body's disease-fighting systems.

For metastatic disease, chemotherapy with dacarbazine has been used with some success.

Radiation therapy, usually reserved for metastatic disease, doesn't prolong survival but may reduce pain and tumor size.

 Gene therapy.

The genetic link

Shedding light on melanoma

Ultraviolet light

During the past few years, scientists have gained an understanding about how ultraviolet light damages DNA and how DNA changes cause normal skin to become cancerous. Scientists have also found that DNA damage affecting certain genes causes melanocytes to change into melanoma. Typically, this damage is caused by sun exposure.

Inherited genes

On the other hand, some people may inherit mutated genes from their parents. The p16 gene, recently discovered by scientists, causes some melanomas that run in certain families.

Possible treatments

These discoveries have led to new treatment options. One approach is to add a specific gene to melanoma cells. This gene makes the melanoma sensitive to oblimersen, a gene-blocker drug that's made up of short strands of DNA and neutralizes the melanoma cell's ability to make certain proteins. This drug prevents the cells from making the BCL2 protein, which is found in high levels in most melanoma cells and prevents the cancer cells from dying.

In preliminary studies, the combination of this drug plus chemotherapy with dacarbazine caused some metastatic melanoma tumors to shrink.

ABCDEs of malignant melanoma

Use the ABCDE rule to assess a mole's malignant potential.

1. Asymmetry: Is the mole irregular in shape?

2. Border: Is the border irregular, notched, or poorly defined?

3. Color: Does the color vary, for example, between shades of brown, red, white, blue, or black?

4. Diameter: Is the diameter more than 6mm?

5. Elevation: Is the lesion elevated or enlarged?

pigment regression. When seeking to assess the malignant potential of a mole, look for asymmetry, an irregular border, color variation, and a diameter greater than 6 mm. (See *ABCDEs of malignant melanoma.*)

What tests tell you

Diagnostic tests for malignant melanoma include the following:
• Excisional biopsy and full-depth punch biopsy with histologic examination are used to distinguish malignant melanoma from a benign nevus, seborrheic keratosis, or pigmented basal cell epi-thelioma; they're also used to determine tumor thickness and disease stage.
• Chest X-ray, gallium scan, bone scan, magnetic resonance imaging (MRI), and CT scans of the chest, abdomen, or brain may be used to diagnose or detect metastasis, depending on the depth of tumor invasion.

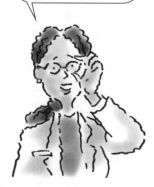

Keep your eyes alert for changes to skin lesions or moles.

Multiple myeloma

Multiple myeloma is a disseminated cancer of marrow plasma cells that infiltrates bone to produce lesions throughout the flat bones, vertebrae, skull, pelvis, and ribs. In late stages, it infiltrates the liver, spleen, lymph nodes, lungs, adrenal glands, kidneys, skin, and GI tract. (See *Treating multiple myeloma*.)

The best hope: An early diagnosis

Multiple myeloma strikes about 12,300 people yearly, is slightly more common in men, and strikes between the ages of 50 and 80. The prognosis is poor because, by the time it's diagnosed, the vertebrae, pelvis, skull, ribs, clavicles, and sternum are infiltrated and skeletal destruction is widespread. More than 50% of patients die within 3 months of diagnosis; 90% die within 2 years. However, if

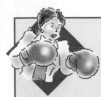

Battling illness

Treating multiple myeloma

Long-term treatment of multiple myeloma consists mainly of chemotherapy to suppress plasma cell growth and control pain. The most common regimen uses vincristine, doxorubicin, and dexamethasone for induction. Other chemotherapy drugs that may be used but are less suitable for induction include melphalan and carmustine.

A new drug, bortezomib, a proteasome inhibitor, is used in patients who have had two prior therapies and have demonstrated disease progression with the last therapy. This type of treatment is sometimes referred to as *salvage therapy*. Local radiation reduces acute lesions and relieves the pain of collapsed vertebrae.

Survival rates have improved by using high-dose chemotherapy and stem-cell transplantation. However, adverse effects make this option available only to patients who were healthy before acquiring the disease.

Thalidomide, an immunomodulatory drug, has been effective in treating multiple myeloma but it causes sleepiness and nerve damage, limiting its use.

Other treatment includes analgesics for pain, laminectomy for vertebral compression, and dialysis for renal complications. Interferon may prolong the plateau phase after the initial chemo-therapy is completed.

Calcium surplus

Because patients may have bone demineralization and may lose large amounts of calcium into blood and urine, they're prime candidates for renal calculi and renal failure from hypercalcemia. Hypercalcemia is treated with hydration, diuretics, corticosteroids, pamidronate, and inorganic phosphates. Plasmapheresis temporarily removes the Bence Jones protein from withdrawn blood and retransfuses the cells to the patient.

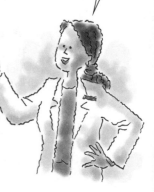

Here's a description of normal cell activity and how things go awry in multiple myeloma.

Now I get it!

Bone marrow aspirate in multiple myeloma

This illustration shows the abnormal plasma cells found in multiple myeloma.

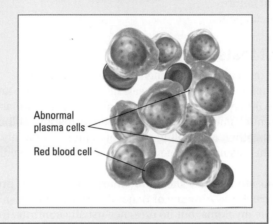

Abnormal plasma cells

Red blood cell

the disease is diagnosed early, treatment may prolong life by 3 to 5 years. (See *Bone marrow aspirate in multiple myeloma*.)

How it happens

The cause of multiple myeloma isn't known. The disorder has been linked to genetic factors, viral infection, and occupational exposure to certain chemicals and radiation.

In normal cell activity, stem cells within the bone marrow can self-replicate or differentiate (mature into specific cell types). The lymphoid stem cell can differentiate into T lymphocytes, which participate in cell-mediated immunity, or B lymphocytes, which participate in humoral immunity. B lymphocytes eventually become plasma cells that produce and release immunoglobulins. Immunoglobulin G (IgG) is the most common immunoglobulin in humans.

In multiple myeloma, an unknown factor stimulates the B lymphocytes to turn into malignant plasma cells, which produce huge amounts of IgG, IgA, or Bence Jones proteins. This leads to a hyperviscosity syndrome commonly seen in myeloma patients.

What to look for

Infection is a common complication of multiple myeloma. However, patients may exhibit various symptoms, including:
• vision disturbances

- headaches
- somnolence
- irritability
- confusion
- intolerance to cold
- renal failure
- skeletal pain.

What tests tell you

These tests are used to diagnose multiple myeloma:
- Complete blood count reveals moderate to severe anemia, with 40% to 50% lymphocytes but seldom more than 3% plasma cells. A differential smear also shows rouleau formations (blood cells that stick together, resembling stacks of coins). Commonly the first clue, this results from elevation of the erythrocyte sedimentation rate.
- Urine studies may show proteinuria, Bence Jones protein, and hypercalciuria. Absence of Bence Jones protein doesn't rule out multiple myeloma, but its presence usually confirms the disease.
- Bone marrow aspiration is used to detect an abnormal number of immature plasma cells (10% to 95% instead of 3% to 5%).
- Serum electrophoresis shows the characteristic M band containing paraprotein.
- X-rays during the early stages may reveal only diffuse osteoporosis; later, they show multiple, sharply circumscribed osteolytic (punched out) lesions, particularly on the skull, pelvis, and spine.
- Serum calcium levels are elevated because calcium lost from the bone is reabsorbed into the serum.

Prostate cancer

Prostate cancer is the most common cancer affecting men and the second cause of cancer death. Death rates in Black men are more than twice as high as rates in White men. About 85% of these cancers originate in the posterior prostate gland; the rest grow near the urethra. Adenocarcinoma is the most common form. (See *Treating prostate cancer.*)

How it happens

Risk factors for prostate cancer include:
- age (more than 70% of all prostate cancer cases are diagnosed in men older than age 65)
- diet high in saturated fats (see *Looking at prostate cancer,* page 428)

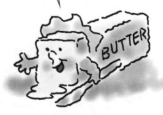

A diet high in saturated fat is a risk factor for prostate cancer.

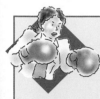

Battling illness

Treating prostate cancer

Therapy varies depending on the stage of the cancer and may include radiation, prostatectomy, and hormone therapy. Because most prostate cancers are androgen- or hormone-dependent, the main treatments are antiandrogens to suppress adrenal function or medical castration with estrogen or gonadotropin-releasing hormone analogs.

The Food and Drug Administration recently approved docetaxel, a chemotherapy agent, for men with advanced prostate cancer that doesn't respond to hormone therapy. The drug is administered along with the steroid prednisone. Docetaxel is the first drug shown to improve the survival rate in men with the advanced stage of the disease.

Radical prostatectomy usually works for localized lesions without metastasis.

Transurethral resection of the prostate may be used to relieve an obstruction.

Nonsurgical treatments

Radiation therapy may cure locally invasive lesions in early disease and may relieve bone pain from metastatic skeletal involvement. It's also used prophylactically to prevent tumor growth for patients with tumors in regional lymph nodes. Radioactive "seeds" may also be implanted into the prostate. This treatment increases radiation to the area while minimizing exposure to surrounding tissues.

Chemotherapy with combinations of cyclophosphamide, doxorubicin, fluorouracil, methotrexate, estramustine, vinblastine, and cisplatin reduce pain from metastasis but hasn't helped patients live longer.

* ethnicity. (Black men have the highest prostate cancer incidence in the world. The disease is common in North America and northwestern Europe and is rare in Asia and South America.)

A slow progress

Prostate cancer grows slowly. When primary lesions spread beyond the prostate gland, they invade the prostatic capsule and then spread along the ejaculatory ducts in the space between the seminal vesicles or perivesicular fascia. (See *Pathway for metastasis of prostate cancer*, page 429.)

Again, early detection is key

When prostate cancer is treated in its localized form, the 5-year survival rate is 70%; after metastasis, it's lower than 35%. Fatal prostate cancer usually results from widespread bone metastasis.

What to look for

Prostate cancer seldom produces signs and symptoms until it's advanced. Signs of advanced disease include a slow urinary stream,

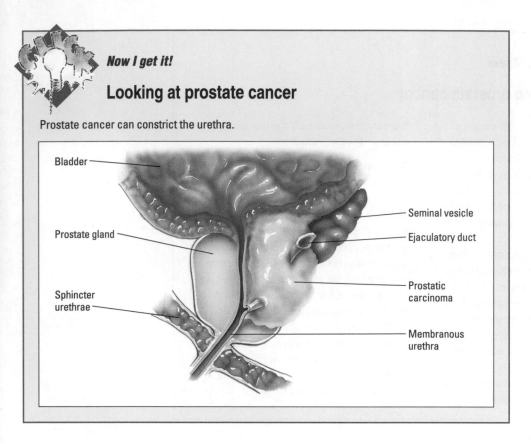

Looking at prostate cancer

Prostate cancer can constrict the urethra.

Bladder

Prostate gland

Sphincter urethrae

Seminal vesicle

Ejaculatory duct

Prostatic carcinoma

Membranous urethra

hematuria, urinary hesitancy, incomplete bladder emptying, and dysuria. These symptoms are due to obstruction caused by tumor progression.

What tests tell you

These tests and results are common in prostate cancer:
• DRE is performed to determine prostate location, size, and the presence of nodules.
• Biopsy of the prostate may distinguish between a benign or malignant mass.
• Blood tests may show elevated levels of prostate-specific antigen (PSA). Although an elevated PSA level occurs with metastasis, it also occurs with other prostate diseases.
• Transrectal prostatic ultrasonography may be used for patients with abnormal DRE and PSA findings.
• Bone scan and excretory urography determine the extent of the disease.
• MRI and CT scans help define the tumor's extent.

Now I get it!

Pathway for metastasis of prostate cancer

When primary prostatic lesions metastasize, they typically invade the prostatic capsule, spreading along the ejaculatory ducts in the space between the seminal vesicles or perivesicular fascia.

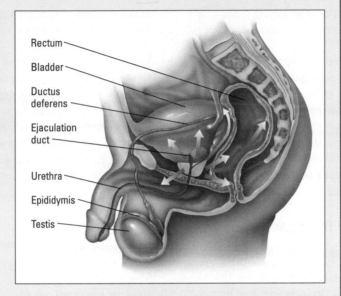

Rectum
Bladder
Ductus deferens
Ejaculation duct
Urethra
Epididymis
Testis

Testicular cancer

Malignant testicular tumors are the most prevalent solid tumors in males ages 20 to 40. Testicular cancer is rare in nonwhite males and accounts for less than 1% of all male cancer deaths. Rarely, testicular cancer occurs in children.

With few exceptions, testicular tumors originate from germinal cells. About 40% become *seminomas*. These tumors, which are characterized by uniform, undifferentiated cells, resemble primitive gonadal cells. Other tumors—*nonseminomas*—show various degrees of differentiation.

The prognosis depends on the cancer cell type and stage. When treated with surgery, chemotherapy, and radiation therapy, almost all patients with localized disease survive beyond 5 years. Typically, when testicular cancer extends beyond the testes, it spreads through the lymphatic system to the iliac, para-aortic, and mediastinal nodes. Metastases affect the lungs, liver, viscera, and bone. (See *Treating testicular cancer*, page 430.)

Treating testicular cancer

In testicular cancer, treatment includes surgery, radiation therapy, and chemotherapy. Treatment intensity varies with the tumor cell type and stage.

Surgical options include orchiectomy and retroperitoneal node dissection to prevent disease extension and assess its stage. Most surgeons remove just the testis, not the scrotum. The patient may need hormonal replacement therapy after bilateral orchiectomy.

Treatment of seminomas involves postoperative radiation to the retroperitoneal and homolateral iliac nodes. Patients whose disease extends to retroperitoneal structures may be given prophylactic radiation to the mediastinal and supraclavicular nodes. Treatment of nonseminoma includes radiation directed to all cancerous lymph nodes.

Chemotherapy is most effective for late-stage seminomas and most nonseminomas when used for recurrent cancer after orchiectomy and removal of the retroperitoneal lymph nodes.

Autologous bone marrow transplantation is usually reserved for patients who don't respond to standard therapy. It involves giving high-dose chemotherapy, removing and treating the patient's bone marrow to kill remaining cancer cells, and returning the processed bone marrow to the patient.

How it happens

Although researchers don't know the immediate cause of testicular cancer, they suspect that cryptorchidism (even when surgically corrected) plays a role in the developing disease. A history of mumps orchitis, inguinal hernia in childhood, or maternal use of diethylstilbestrol (DES) or other estrogen-progestin combinations during pregnancy also increases the risk for this disease. (See *Looking at testicular cancer.*)

What to look for

The patient history may disclose previous injuries to the scrotum, viral infections (such as mumps), or the use of DES or other estrogen-progestin drugs by the patient's mother during pregnancy. The patient may describe a feeling of heaviness or a dragging sensation in the scrotum. He may also report swollen testes or a painless lump found while performing testicular self-examination. In late disease stages, the patient may complain of weight loss, a cough, hemoptysis, shortness of breath, lethargy, and fatigue.

Looking

On inspection, you may notice that the patient has enlarged testes. Gynecomastia, a sign that the tumor produces chorionic gonadotropins or estrogen, may be obvious also. In later stages of testicular cancer, the patient may appear lethargic, thin, and pallid.

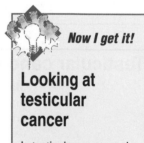

Now I get it!

Looking at testicular cancer

In testicular cancer, palpation may reveal a firm, smooth testicular mass.

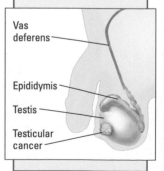

Vas deferens

Epididymis

Testis

Testicular cancer

Feeling

Palpation findings include a firm, smooth testicular mass and enlarged lymph nodes in surrounding areas. In later disease stages, palpation may disclose an abdominal mass as well.

Listening

On auscultation you may hear decreased breath sounds. (See *Staging testicular cancer.*)

What tests tell you

• Serum analyses may be done to evaluate beta subunit human chorionic gonadotropin (HCG) and alpha-fetoprotein (AFP) levels. Elevated levels of these proteins (tumor markers) suggest testicu-

Now I get it!

Staging testicular cancer

The illustration below shows the usual metastatic sites of testicular cancer.

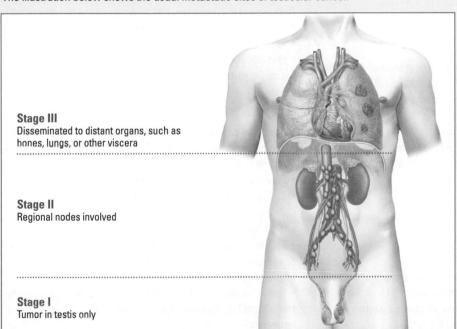

Stage III
Disseminated to distant organs, such as bones, lungs, or other viscera

Stage II
Regional nodes involved

Stage I
Tumor in testis only

lar cancer and can differentiate a seminoma from a nonseminoma: elevated HCG and AFP levels point to a nonseminoma; elevated HCG and normal AFP levels indicate a seminoma.

• CT scanning can detect metastasis. Chest X-rays may demonstrate pulmonary metastases. Lymphangiography, ultrasonography, and magnetic resonance imaging may disclose additional metastases.

• Excretory urography may detect ureteral displacement, which is caused by metastasis to a para-aortic lymph node.

• Biopsy can confirm the diagnosis, help stage the disease, and plan treatment.

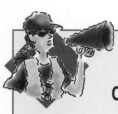

That's a wrap!

Cancer review

Cancer facts
• Second leading cause of death
• Classified by tissues or blood cells of origin
• No single cause identified

Understanding cancer
Abnormal cell growth
Cancer is characterized by the abnormal growth of cells that develop from tissues or blood. Most cancers develop from epithelial tissues and are called *carcinomas*. Others arise from these tissues and cells:
• glandular tissues (adenocarcinoma)
• connective, muscle, and bone tissues (sarcomas)
• tissue of the brain and spinal cord (gliomas)
• pigment cells (melanomas)
• plasma cells (myelomas)
• lymphatic tissue (lymphomas)
• leukocytes (leukemia)
• erythrocytes (erythroleukemia).
Uncontrolled cell growth
Cancer cells develop without the control that normal cells have, and they spread from the site of origin in three ways:
• circulating through the blood and lymphatic system
• accidentally transplanted during surgery
• spreading to adjacent organs and tissues.

Causes
All cancers involve malfunction of genes that control growth and division of cells. Carcinogenesis, the cell's transformation from normal to cancerous, has no single cause but may result from complex interactions between:
• viruses
• physical and chemical carcinogens
• genetic, dietary, immunologic, metabolic, and hormonal factors.

Types
• *Basal cell carcinoma*—undifferentiated basal cells become carcinomatous instead of differentiating into sweat glands, sebum and hair
• *Breast cancer*—genetic link BRCA1 and BRCA2
• *Cervical cancer*—linked to human papilloma virus
• *Colorectal cancer*—genetic link deletion on chromosomes 17 and 18 may promote malignancy
• *Endometrial cancer*—usually adenocarcinoma that metastasizes from the endometrium to the cervix, ovaries, fallopian tubes, and other peritoneal structures
• *Hodgkin's disease*—virus may have indirect relationship; proliferation of lymphocytes and histiocytes cause lymph node enlargement

Cancer review *(continued)*

• *Acute leukemia*—immature cells transform to leukemia cells, multiply, crowd out other cells
• *Chronic lymphocytic leukemia*—proliferation and accumulation of immunodeficient lymphocytes
• *Chronic myeloid leukemia*—excessive development of neoplastic granulocytes
• *Lung cancer*—epithelial cells of the lung develop chromosomal changes, dysplastic cells arise, cells turn into cancer and invade deeper tissues

• *Malignant melanoma*—arises from melanocytes, spreads through lymph and vascular systems, metastasizes in skin, liver, lungs, CNS
• *Multiple myeloma*—B lymphocytes stimulated to turn into malignant plasma cells; leads to hyperviscosity
• *Prostate cancer*—age, diet high in saturated fats, and hormones play a role; cancer grows slowly
• *Testicular cancer*—associated with cryptorchidism (even when surgically repaired).

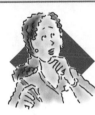

Quick quiz

1. Lymphedema occurs in the patient with breast cancer because the:
    A.   breast tissue causes the patient to retain fluid.
    B.   lymphatic system is swollen with immune-response factors to fight the cancer.
    C.   area is traumatized, which causes it to swell.
    D.   tumor has metastasized.

Answer: B. The lymphatic system brings immune response factors to the area to fight the cancer, which causes lymphedema.

2. The presence of Reed-Sternberg cells is associated with:
    A.   prostate cancer.
    B.   malignant melanoma.
    C.   lung cancer.
    D.   Hodgkin's disease.

Answer: D. Reed-Sternberg cells must be present before a diagnosis of Hodgkin's disease can be made.

3. Bone marrow aspiration is performed on a patient with leukemia to:
    A.   examine the platelets.
    B.   determine if the cancer is lymphocytic or myeloid.
    C.   measure the amount of marrow in the bone.
    D.   measure the WBC count.

Answer: B. Bone marrow aspiration determines what type of immature WBC is involved, which directs the type of treatment.

4.   A change in the shape, color, and texture of a nevus may indicate:
   A.   multiple myeloma.
   B.   malignant melanoma.
   C.   healing of the nevus.
   D.   leukemia.

Answer: B. An obvious change in a wart or mole is a sign of malignant melanoma and is one of the seven warning signs of cancer identified by the American Cancer Society.

5.   Multiple myeloma is related to the immunity factor:
   A.   histamine.
   B.   serotonin.
   C.   IgG.
   D.   IgA.

Answer: C. In multiple myeloma, plasma cells secrete an unusually large amount of IgG.

6.   A risk factor for prostate cancer is:
   A.   being older than age 40.
   B.   a history of infertility.
   C.   poverty.
   D.   low-fat diet.

Answer: A. Prostate cancer seldom develops in men younger than age 40. Socioeconomic status and infertility don't appear to affect the risk of prostate cancer.

Scoring

☆☆☆   If you answered all six items correctly, amazing! Your knowledge of pathophysiology is proliferating with remarkable speed and efficiency.

☆☆   If you answered four or five items correctly, good work! Your skill at learning is due to a remarkable combination of environmental, genetic, dietary, and other unspecified factors.

☆   If you answered fewer than four items correctly, never fear. Remember that early detection is key, and you still have time to assess your learning skills, review the chapter again, and improve your prognosis.

13

Genetics

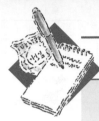

Just the facts

In this chapter, you'll learn:

♦ the role of genes and chromosomes and how cells divide

♦ the types of genetic abnormalities and how they're inherited

♦ the causes, pathophysiology, diagnostic tests, and treatments for several common genetic disorders.

Understanding genetics

Genetics is the study of heredity, the passing of traits from parents to their children. Physical traits such as eye color are inherited as well as biochemical and physiologic traits, including the tendency to develop certain diseases.

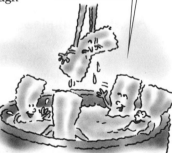

Hop on in the gene pool and learn about genetics!

Transmitting an inheritance

Inherited traits are transmitted from parents to offspring through genes in germ cells, or gametes. Human gametes are eggs, or ova, and sperm. A person's genetic makeup is determined at fertilization, when ovum and sperm are united.

In the nucleus of each germ cell are structures called *chromosomes*. Each chromosome contains a strand of genetic material called *deoxyribonucleic acid (DNA)*. DNA is a long molecule that's made up of thousands of segments called *genes*. Each of the traits that a person inherits— from blood type to toe shape and a myriad of others in between—is coded in their genes.

Counting chromosomes

A human ovum contains 23 chromosomes. A sperm also contains 23 chromosomes, each similar in size and shape to a chromosome in the ovum. When ovum and sperm unite, the corresponding chromosomes pair up. The result is a fertilized cell with 46 chromosomes (23 pairs) in the nucleus.

The fertilized cell soon undergoes cell division (*mitosis*). In mitosis, each of the 46 chromosomes produces an exact duplicate of itself. The cell then divides, and each new cell receives one set of 46 chromosomes. Each of the two cells that result likewise divides, and so on, eventually forming a many-celled human body. Therefore, each cell in a person's body (except the ova or sperm) contains 46 identical chromosomes.

A different division

The ova and sperm are formed by a different cell-division process called *meiosis*. In meiosis, there are two cell divisions, and each new cell (an ovum or sperm) receives one set of 23 chromosomes.

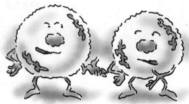

In mitosis, DNA duplicates; then the cell divides into two equal cells.

Location, location, location

The location of a gene on a chromosome is called a *locus*. The locus of each gene is specific and doesn't vary from person to person. This allows each of the thousands of genes in an ovum to join the corresponding genes from a sperm when the chromosomes pair up at fertilization.

Pass it on

A person receives one set of chromosomes and genes from each parent. This means there are two genes for each trait that a person inherits. One gene may be more influential than the other in developing a specific trait. The more influential gene is said to be dominant, and the less influential gene is recessive.

For example, a child may receive a gene for brown eyes from one parent and a gene for blue eyes from the other parent. The gene for brown eyes is dominant; the gene for blue eyes is recessive. The dominant gene is more likely to be expressed. Therefore, the child is more likely to have brown eyes.

All about alleles

A variation of a gene and the trait it controls—such as brown, green, or blue eye color—is called an *allele*. When two different alleles are inherited, they're said to be *heterozygous*. When the alleles are identical, they're termed *homozygous*.

A dominant allele may be expressed when it's carried by only one of the chromosomes in a pair. A recessive allele is incapable of expression unless recessive alleles are carried by both chromosomes in a pair.

Gen XX (or XY)

Of the 23 pairs of chromosomes in each living human cell, 22 pairs are *not* involved in controlling a person's gender; they're called *autosomes*.

The two sex chromosomes of the 23rd pair determine a person's gender. In a female, both chromosomes are relatively large, and each is designated by the letter X; females have two X chromosomes. In a male, one sex chromosome is an X chromosome, and one is a smaller chromosome, designated by the letter Y.

Each gamete produced by a male contains either an X or a Y chromosome. When a sperm with an X chromosome fertilizes an ovum, the offspring is female. When a sperm with a Y chromosome fertilizes an ovum, the offspring is male.

An explanation of mutation

A mutation is a permanent change in genetic material. When a gene mutates, it may produce a trait that's different from its original trait. Gene mutations in a gamete may be transmitted during reproduction. Some mutations cause serious or deadly disorders that occur in three different forms:
- single-gene disorders
- chromosomal disorders
- multifactorial disorders.

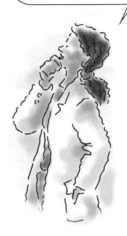

Let me see if I've got this right—of the 23 pairs of chromosomes in each living human cell, 22 pairs are not involved in controlling a person's gender.

Single-gene disorders

Single-gene disorders are inherited in clearly identifiable patterns. Two important inheritance patterns are called *autosomal dominant* and *autosomal recessive*. Because there are 22 pairs of autosomes and only 1 pair of sex chromosomes, most hereditary disorders are caused by autosomal defects.

In a third inheritance pattern, sex-linked inheritance, single-gene disorders are passed through the X chromosome.

Parent patterns

Keep the definitions of the terms *dominant* and *recessive* in mind. Dominant genes produce abnormal traits in offspring even if only one parent has the gene; recessive genes don't produce abnormal traits unless both parents have the gene and pass them to their offspring.

Autosomal dominant inheritance

The autosomal dominant inheritance pattern has these characteristics:
- Male and female offspring are affected equally.
- One of the parents is also usually affected.
- If one parent is affected, the children have a 50% chance of being affected.
- If both parents are affected, all of their children will be affected.

Marfan syndrome is an example of an autosomal dominant disorder. (See *Understanding autosomal dominant inheritance,* page 438.)

Memory jogger

Remember: **Dominant** genes **dominate** any situation—even if only one parent carries the gene.

Recessive genes **recede** into the background, unless both parents carry the gene.

Now I get it!

Understanding autosomal dominant inheritance

This diagram shows the possible offspring of a parent with recessive normal genes (aa) and a parent with an altered dominant gene (Aa). Note that with each pregnancy there is a 50% chance that the offspring will be affected.

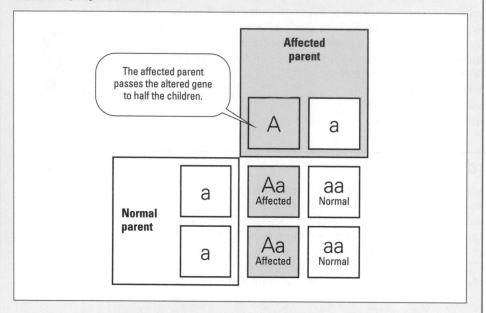

Autosomal recessive inheritance

The autosomal recessive inheritance pattern has these characteristics:

• Male and female offspring are affected equally.

• If both parents are unaffected but heterozygous for the trait (carriers), each of their offspring has a one in four chance of being affected.

• If both parents are affected, all of their offspring will be affected.

• If one parent is affected and the other is not a carrier, all of the parents' offspring will be unaffected but will carry the altered gene.

• If one parent is affected and the other is a carrier, each of the offspring will have a one in two chance of being affected and a one in two chance of being a carrier.

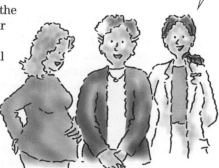

Most genetic disorders are caused by changes in the autosomes.

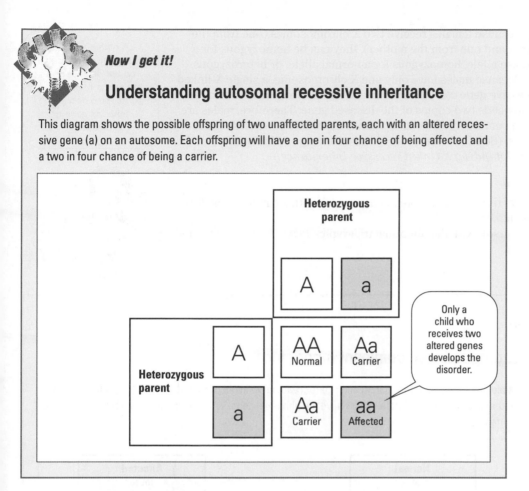

Now I get it!

Understanding autosomal recessive inheritance

This diagram shows the possible offspring of two unaffected parents, each with an altered recessive gene (a) on an autosome. Each offspring will have a one in four chance of being affected and a two in four chance of being a carrier.

- Certain autosomal recessive conditions are more common in specific ethnic groups; for example, cystic fibrosis is more common in Whites and sickle cell anemia is more common in Blacks. (See *Understanding autosomal recessive inheritance*.)

Negative history

In many cases, no evidence of the trait appears in past generations. If you enjoy clinical jargon, you can say the patient has a "negative family history."

Sex-linked inheritance

Some genetic disorders are caused by genes located on the sex chromosomes and are termed *sex-linked*. Because the Y chromosome isn't known to carry disease-causing genes, the terms *X-linked* and *sex-linked* are interchangeable.

Because females receive two X chromosomes (one from the father and one from the mother), they can be homozygous for a disease allele, homozygous for a normal allele, or heterozygous.

Because males have only one X chromosome, a single X-linked recessive gene can cause disease in a male. In comparison, a female needs two copies of the diseased gene. Therefore, males are more commonly affected by X-linked recessive diseases than females. (See *Understanding X-linked dominant inheritance* and *Understanding X-linked recessive inheritance.*)

> A single X-linked recessive gene can cause disease in a male. In a female, two copies of the diseased gene are needed.

Dominant facts

Characteristics of X-linked dominant inheritance include the following:

• A person with the abnormal trait typically will have one affected parent.

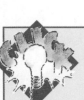

Now I get it!

Understanding X-linked dominant inheritance

This diagram shows the possible offspring of a normal parent and a parent with an X-linked dominant gene on the X chromosome (shown by a dot). When the father is affected, only his daughters have the abnormal gene. When the mother is affected, both male and female offspring may be affected.

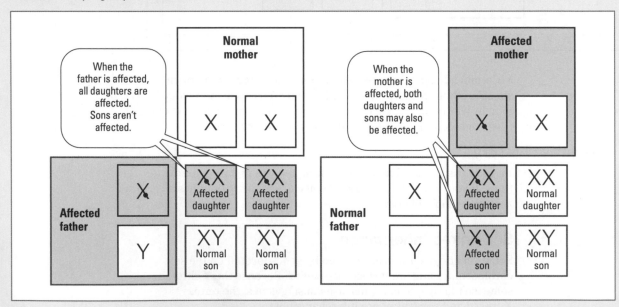

Now I get it!

Understanding X-linked recessive inheritance

This diagram shows the possible offspring of a normal parent and a parent with a recessive gene on the X chromosome (shown by an open dot). All of the female offspring of an affected male will be carriers. The son of a female carrier may inherit a recessive gene on the X chromosome and be affected by the disease.

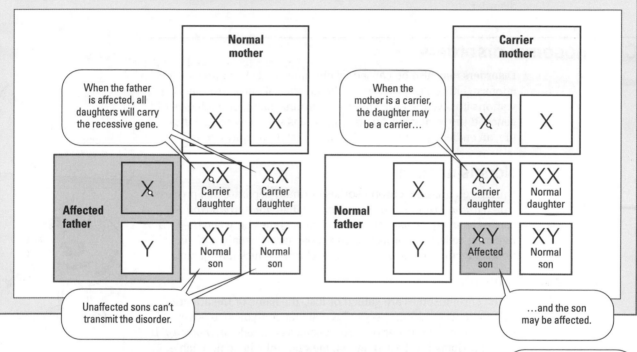

• If a father has an X-linked dominant disorder, all of his daughters and none of his sons will be affected.

• If a mother has an X-linked dominant disorder, there's a 50% chance that each of her children will be affected.

• Evidence of the inherited trait most commonly appears in the family history.

• X-linked dominant disorders are commonly lethal in males (prenatal or neonatal deaths). The family history may show miscarriages and the predominance of female offspring.

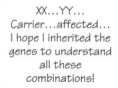

XX...YY... Carrier...affected... I hope I inherited the genes to understand all these combinations!

A recessive reading

Here are the basic facts about the X-linked recessive inheritance pattern:

• In most cases, affected people are males with unaffected parents. In rare cases, the father is affected and the mother is a carrier.
• All of the daughters of an affected male will be carriers.
• Sons of an affected male are unaffected. Unaffected sons can't transmit the disorder.
• The unaffected male children of a female carrier don't transmit the disorder.

Hemophilia is an example of an X-linked recessive inheritance disorder.

Chromosomal disorders

Disorders may also be caused by chromosomal aberrations—deviations in either the structure or the number of chromosomes. Deviations involve the loss, addition, rearrangement, or exchange of genes. If the remaining genetic material is sufficient to maintain life, an endless variety of clinical manifestations may occur.

Nondisjunction

During cell division, chromosomes normally separate in a process called *disjunction*. Failure to do so—called *nondisjunction*—causes an unequal distribution of chromosomes between the two resulting cells. Gain or loss of chromosomes is usually due to nondisjunction of autosomes or sex chromosomes during meiosis.

One fewer or more

When chromosomes are gained or lost, the name of the affected cell contains the suffix "-somy." A cell that contains one fewer than the normal number of chromosomes is called a *monosomy*. If the monosomy involves an autosome, the cell will be nonviable. However, monosomy X can be viable and result in a female who has Turner's syndrome. A cell that contains one extra chromosome is called a *trisomy*. (See *Understanding nondisjunction of chromosomes*.)

Mixed results

Nondisjunction may occur during very early cell divisions after fertilization and may or may not involve all the resulting cells. A mixture of cells, some with a specific chromosome aberration and some with normal cells, results in *mosaicism*. The effect on the offspring depends on the percentage of normal cells.

The incidence of nondisjunction increases with parental age, especially maternal age. Miscarriages can also result from chromosomal aberrations. Fertilization of an ovum with a chromosome aberration by a sperm with a chromosome aberration usually doesn't occur.

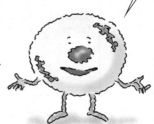

Nondisjunction is a malfunction in which some of my chromosomes fail to separate as they should.

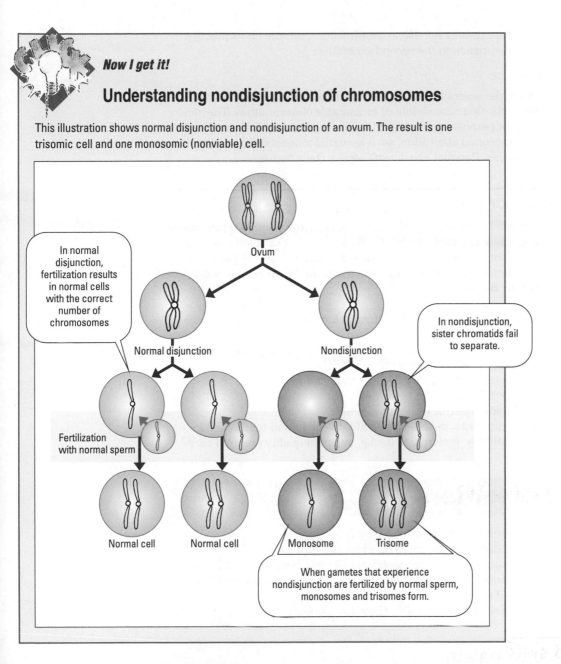

Now I get it!

Understanding nondisjunction of chromosomes

This illustration shows normal disjunction and nondisjunction of an ovum. The result is one trisomic cell and one monosomic (nonviable) cell.

Ovum

In normal disjunction, fertilization results in normal cells with the correct number of chromosomes

Normal disjunction

Nondisjunction

In nondisjunction, sister chromatids fail to separate.

Fertilization with normal sperm

Normal cell

Normal cell

Monosome

Trisome

When gametes that experience nondisjunction are fertilized by normal sperm, monosomes and trisomes form.

Translocation

Another aberration, *translocation*, is the shifting or moving of a chromosome. It occurs when chromosomes break and rejoin in an abnormal arrangement. When the rearrangements preserve the normal amount of genetic material (balanced translocations), there are usually no visible abnormalities, but the abnormalities may be present in the second generation.

A shift in balance

When the rearrangements alter the amount of genetic material, typically, there are visible or measurable abnormalities. The children of parents with balanced translocations may have serious chromosomal aberration, such as partial monosomies or partial trisomies. Parental age doesn't seem to be a factor.

Multifactorial disorders

Disorders caused by both genetic and environmental factors are classified as multifactorial. Examples are cleft lip, cleft palate, and myelomeningocele (spina bifida with a portion of the spinal cord and membranes protruding). Environmental factors that contribute include:
- maternal age
- use of chemicals (such as drugs, alcohol, or hormones) by the mother or father
- maternal infections during pregnancy or existing diseases in the mother
- maternal or paternal exposure to radiation
- maternal nutritional factors
- general maternal or paternal health
- other factors, including high altitude, maternal-fetal blood incompatibility, maternal smoking, and poor-quality prenatal care.

Genetic disorders

This section describes:
- multifactorial disorders (cleft lip and cleft palate)
- six single-gene disorders (cystic fibrosis, hemophilia, Marfan syndrome, phenylketonuria [PKU], sickle cell anemia, and Tay-Sachs disease)
- a chromosomal disorder (Down syndrome).

Cleft lip and cleft palate

Cleft lip and cleft palate malformations occur in about 1 in 800 births. Cleft lip with or without cleft palate is more common in males, and cleft palate alone is more common in females. Nutritional intake is affected by an abnormal lip and palate. Furthermore, children with cleft palates commonly have hearing problems caused by middle ear damage or infection.

How it happens

Cleft lip and cleft palate is a multifactorial genetic disorder. It originates in the second month of gestation when the front and sides of the face and the shelves of the palate fuse imperfectly. These malformations fall into four categories:

- clefts of the lip (unilateral or bilateral)
- clefts of the palate (along the midline)
- unilateral clefts of the lip, alveolus (gum pad), and palate
- bilateral clefts of the lip, alveolus, and palate. (See *Types of cleft lip and cleft palate.*)

Now I get it!

Types of cleft lip and cleft palate

The illustrations below show four variations of cleft lip and cleft palate.

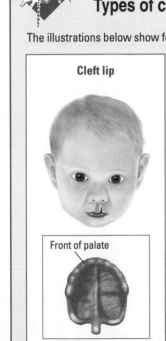

Cleft lip

Front of palate

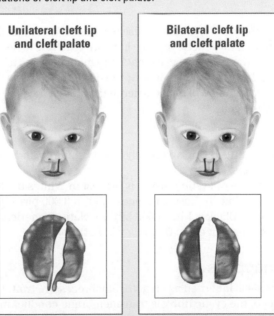

Unilateral cleft lip and cleft palate

Bilateral cleft lip and cleft palate

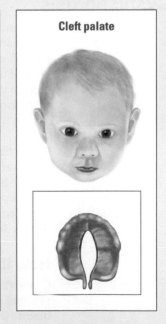

Cleft palate

What to look for

The malformation may range from a simple notch to a complete cleft that extends from the lip through the floor of the nostril on either side of the midline. A complete cleft palate may involve the soft palate, the bones of the maxilla (upper jawbone), and the cavity on one or both sides of the premaxilla (front of the upper jawbone).

In a bilateral cleft, the most severe of all cleft malformation, the cleft runs from the soft palate forward to either side of the nose, separating the maxilla and the premaxilla into free-moving segments. The tongue and other muscles can displace these segments, enlarging the cleft.

Another cleft malformation, Pierre Robin malformation sequence, occurs when abnormal smallness of the jaw (micrognathia) and downward dropping of the tongue (glossoptosis) accompany cleft palate.

Because the palate is essential to speech, structural changes can permanently affect speech, even after surgical repair. (See *Treating cleft lip and cleft palate*.)

What tests tell you

Cleft lip may be detected prenatally using a level 2 ultrasound.

Battling illness

Treating cleft lip and cleft palate

Cleft malformations must be treated with a combination of speech therapy and surgery. The timing of surgery varies.

Infants with Pierre Robin malformation sequence should never be placed on their backs because the tongue can fall back and obstruct the airway.

Special bottles and nipples designed for infants with cleft palate should be used for feedings.

Cystic fibrosis

A chronic, progressive, inherited disease, cystic fibrosis is the most common fatal genetic disease in white children. When both parents carry the recessive gene, each pregnancy brings a 25% chance that the offspring will inherit the disease. There's a 50% chance that the child will be a carrier and a 25% chance the child won't carry the gene.

The odds are...

Cystic fibrosis affects approximately 30,000 children and adults in the United States.

The incidence of cystic fibrosis is highest in Whites of Northern European (Danish, Russian) ancestry (1 in 3,300 births). It's less common in Blacks (1 in 15,300 births), Native Americans, and Asians. It occurs with equal frequency in both sexes.

How it happens

Cystic fibrosis is inherited as an autosomal recessive trait. One implicated gene, the cystic fibrosis transmembrane conductance regulator (CFTR) gene, is located on chromosome 7. Research now suggests that there may be more than 900 CFTR mutations that code for cystic fibrosis.

Most cases arise from a mutation that affects the genetic coding for a single amino acid, resulting in a protein that doesn't function properly. The abnormal protein resembles other transmembrane transport proteins. However, it lacks a phenylalanine (an essential amino acid) that's usually produced by normal genes. This abnormal protein may interfere with chloride transport by preventing adenosine triphosphate from binding to the protein or by interfering with activation by protein kinase. The lack of an essential amino acid leads to dehydration and mucosal thickening in the respiratory and intestinal tracts.

What to look for

Cystic fibrosis increases the viscosity of bronchial, pancreatic, and other mucous gland secretions, obstructing glandular ducts.

Respiratory results

The accumulation of thick, tenacious secretions in the bronchioles and alveoli causes these respiratory changes:
- frequent upper respiratory tract infections
- dyspnea
- paroxysmal (sudden) cough
- frequent bouts of pneumonia.

Respiratory effects may eventually lead to collapsed lungs (atelectasis) or emphyscma.

Gastrointestinal issues

Cystic fibrosis also affects the intestines, pancreas, and liver:
- Diabetes and pancreatitis may result from insult to the pancreas.
- Hepatic failure and cholecystitis may result from blockage of pancreatic ducts.
- Deficiency of the enzymes trypsin, amylase, and lipase (also a result of obstruction of pancreatic ducts) may prevent the conversion and absorption of fat and protein in the intestinal tract, which interferes with food digestion and absorption of the fat-soluble vitamins A, D, E, and K. Patients typically have greasy, bulky stools and poor weight gain (despite an excessive appetite).

Reproductive repercussions

Males may experience lack of sperm in the semen (azoospermia); females may experience secondary amenorrhea and increased mucus in the reproductive tracts that blocks passage of the ovum.

Battling illness

Treating cystic fibrosis

Cystic fibrosis has no cure, so treatment aims to help the patient lead as normal a life as possible. Specific treatments depend on the organ systems involved.

Salt supplements are used to combat electrolyte loss through sweat, and oral pancreatic enzymes taken with meals and snacks offset deficiencies. Broad-spectrum antibiotics and oxygen therapy are used as needed. To man-

age pulmonary dysfunction, chest physiotherapy, including postural drainage and chest percussion over all lobes, is usually performed several times per day.

Dornase alfa, a mucus-thinning drug, is given to improve lung function and reduce the number of lung infections. Lung, heart, and pancreas transplantation may also be needed.

The genetic link

Gene therapy and cystic fibrosis

Researchers believe that gene therapy can correct the basic genetic defect that causes cystic fibrosis. Therapy would include adding enough normal genes to the patient's airway to correct the defective cells with the goal of retaining existing lung function and preventing further damage.

Clinical trials have shown that normal genes can be safely transferred to a cystic fibrosis–affected airway, but scientists are currently working on developing efficient delivery methods.

Child watch

A child with cystic fibrosis may have a barrel chest, cyanosis, clubbing of the fingers and toes, and a distended abdomen. He may cough and expectorate tenacious, yellow-green sputum and have wheezy respirations and crackles on auscultation. (See *Treating cystic fibrosis.*)

Although scientists have not yet found a cure for this disease, medical research has greatly increased life expectancy. (See *Gene therapy and cystic fibrosis.*)

What tests tell you

According to the Cystic Fibrosis Foundation, a diagnosis of cystic fibrosis should be based on:
• the presence of one or more of the clinical findings typically associated with cystic fibrosis
• a history of cystic fibrosis in a sibling
• two elevated sweat chloride tests obtained on separate days
• identification of mutations in each CFTR gene.
    Several tests may support the diagnosis:
• If a patient's sweat chloride concentrations are normal or borderline, a nasal potential difference measurement is obtained. This test measures salt transport in the nasal cavity; an abnormality obtained on two separate days indicates cystic fibrosis.
• Chest X-rays will show early signs of lung obstruction.
• Stool specimen analysis will show the absence of trypsin, suggesting pancreatic insufficiency.
• DNA testing can detect CFTR mutations that cause cystic fibrosis. This test can also be used to detect carriers and for prenatal diagnosis in families with an affected child.

Down syndrome

The first disorder attributed to a chromosomal aberration, Down syndrome produces mental retardation, characteristic facial features, and distinctive physical abnormalities. It's also associated with heart defects and other congenital disorders.

Life expectancy and quality of life for patients with Down syndrome have increased significantly because of improved treatment of related complications and better developmental education programs. Nevertheless, up to 44% of patients with congenital heart disease die before they reach age 1.

Breaking down the stats

Overall, Down syndrome occurs in 1 per 800 to 1,000 births, but the risk of having a child with Down syndrome increases with maternal age. For instance, at age 20, a mother has about 1 chance in 2,000 of having a child with Down syndrome; by age 49, she has 1 chance in 12. Although women older than age 35 account for fewer than 8% of all births, they bear 20% of all children with Down syndrome. The prevalence of Down syndrome has decreased with the widespread use of prenatal testing such as amniocentesis.

How it happens

Also called *trisomy 21*, Down syndrome is caused by an aberration in which chromosome 21 has three copies instead of two. The most common cause of this extra chromosome 21 is nondisjunction. Although the incidence of nondisjunction increases with maternal age, the extra chromosome originates from the mother more than 90% of the time. About 4% of the time, Down syndrome results from translocation and infusion of the long arm of chromosome 21 and 14. This phenomenon is known as *Robertsonian translocation*. (See *Understanding Down syndrome*, page 450.)

Studies suggest that in some cases, the abnormality results from deterioration of the oocyte (primitive egg), which can be caused by age or the cumulative effects of environmental factors, such as radiation and viruses.

47, not 46

Patients with Down syndrome exhibit a karyotype (chromosomal arrangement) of 47 chromosomes instead of the normal 46. Mortality rates are high in both the fetus and neonate. If the patient survives to adulthood, premature senile dementia, similar to Alzheimer's disease, usually occurs in the fourth decade. Patients are also prone to leukemia, acute and chronic infections, diabetes mellitus, and thyroid disorders. (See *Treating Down syndrome*, page 451.)

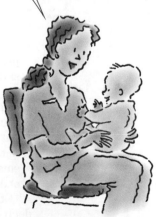

Children with Down syndrome can be extremely engaging and loving!

Now I get it!

Understanding Down syndrome

Human chromosomes are arranged in seven groups, designated by the letters A through G. These illustrations show the arrangement of chromosomes (karyotype) in a normal person and a person with Down syndrome. In most cases of Down syndrome, there's an extra chromosome.

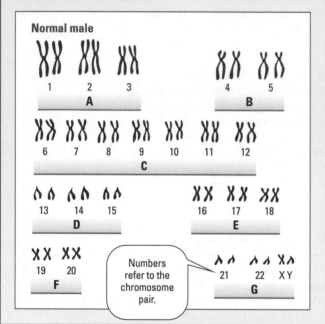

Normal male

Numbers refer to the chromosome pair.

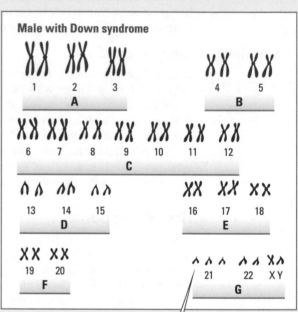

Male with Down syndrome

In Down syndrome, there are three number 21 chromosomes. This is called *trisomy 21*.

What to look for

The physical signs of Down syndrome are apparent at birth. The infant is lethargic, with one or more of these anomalies:
- slanting, almond-shaped eyes
- protruding tongue
- small, open mouth
- single, transverse crease on the palm (called a *simian crease*)
- small white spots on the iris (Brushfield's spots)
- small skull
- flat nose bridge
- flattened face
- small ears
- short neck with excess skin.

Other characteristic findings include dry, sensitive skin with decreased elasticity, umbilical hernia, short stature, and short extremities. The hands and feet are broad, flat, and squarish, and the feet have a wide space between the first and second toes. Decreased muscle tone in limbs impairs reflex development.

Many infants have congenital heart disease, duodenal obstruction, clubfoot, imperforate anus, cleft lip and cleft palate, Hirschsprung's disease (congenital colon enlargement), myelomeningocele, and pelvic bone abnormalities.

In the later years

As the child grows, dental development is slow, with abnormal or absent teeth. Strabismus and, occasionally, cataracts occur. The genitalia develop poorly, and puberty is delayed. While significant impairments in fertility are present in both sexes, males and females with Down syndrome can produce children, and not all of the children are affected with Down syndrome. Women with Down syndrome who become pregnant have a significantly higher risk of preterm birth and low-birth-weight neonates.

Patients may have an IQ as low as 30, although most can be educated. Some have IQs approaching 80. Social performance is usually beyond that expected for their mental age. However, intellectual development slows with age.

What tests tell you

A karyotype showing the chromosomal abnormality confirms the diagnosis of Down syndrome. These tests reveal Down syndrome before birth:
• Prenatal ultrasonography suggests Down syndrome if a duodenal obstruction or an atrioventricular canal defect is seen.
• Maternal blood tests during pregnancy show low alpha-fetoprotein levels, low unconjugated estriol levels, and high human chorionic gonadotropin levels, all indicative of Down syndrome.
• Amniocentesis or chorionic villi sampling is recommended for pregnant women older than age 35 and for a pregnant woman of any age when she or the father is a known carrier of a translocated chromosome.

Battling illness

Treating Down syndrome

Treatment for Down syndrome includes surgery to correct cardiac defects and other congenital abnormalities, antibiotic therapy for recurrent infections, and thyroid hormone replacement for hypothyroidism. Plastic surgery is performed to correct protruding tongue, cleft lip, and cleft palate. These measures improve the patient's appearance and speech and reduce susceptibility to cavities and orthodontic problems.

Special education programs, mandated in most communities, promote self-esteem and help children to achieve their potential.

Hemophilia

A hereditary bleeding disorder, hemophilia most commonly affects males. Female cases are extremely rare. Hemophilia is the most common X-linked genetic disease, occurring in about 125 of 1 million male births.

Two types of hemophilia may occur:
• hemophilia A, or classic hemophilia, which affects more than 80% of all hemophiliacs
• hemophilia B, or *Christmas disease*, which affects 15% of all hemophiliacs. (In 1952, researchers studying a 10-year-old boy

named Stephen Christmas discovered that the boy's hemophilia was different from the other forms they studied, and they named the form *Christmas disease*.)

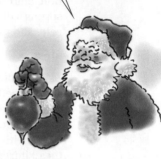

One type of hemophilia is known as *Christmas* disease.

A matter of degree

The severity and prognosis of the disease vary with the degree of deficiency or nonfunction and the site of bleeding. Advances in treatment have greatly improved the prognosis, and many patients live normal life spans.

How it happens

Hemophilia A is caused by deficiency or nonfunction of factor VIII; hemophilia B is caused by deficiency or nonfunction of factor IX. Both are inherited as X-linked recessive traits. This means that female carriers have a 50% chance of transmitting the gene to each daughter, making her a carrier, and a 50% chance of transmitting the gene to each son, who would be born with hemophilia.

Hemophilia produces mild to severe abnormal bleeding. After a platelet plug develops at a bleeding site, the lack of clotting factor prevents a stable fibrin clot from forming. Although hemorrhaging doesn't usually happen immediately, delayed bleeding is common.

Effects of increased bleeding

Bleeding into joints and muscles causes severe pain, swelling, extreme tenderness, limited range of motion and, sometimes, permanent deformity.

Bleeding near peripheral nerves may cause peripheral neuropathies, pain, paresthesia, and muscle atrophy.

If bleeding impairs blood flow through a major vessel, it can cause ischemia and gangrene.

What to look for

Signs and symptoms vary, depending on the severity of the patient's condition:

- Severe hemophilia causes spontaneous bleeding. Commonly, the first sign is excessive bleeding after circumcision. Later, spontaneous or severe bleeding after minor trauma may produce large subcutaneous and deep intramuscular hematomas.
- Moderate hemophilia causes symptoms similar to severe hemophilia, but spontaneous bleeding occurs only occasionally.
- Mild hemophilia commonly goes undiagnosed until adulthood because the patient doesn't bleed spontaneously or after minor trauma. However, major trauma or surgery can cause prolonged

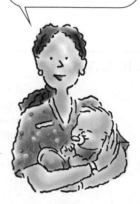

Commonly, the first sign of hemophilia is excessive bleeding after circumcision.

bleeding. Blood may ooze slowly or stop and start for up to 8 days after surgery. Patients with mild hemophilia have the best prognosis.

Warning! Warning! Warning!

Patients with undiagnosed hemophilia usually complain of pain and swelling in a weight-bearing joint, such as the hip, knee, or ankle. The history may reveal prolonged bleeding after surgery, dental extractions, or trauma. The patient may also have signs and symptoms of internal bleeding, such as abdominal, chest, or flank pain; hematuria (bloody urine) or hematemesis (bloody vomit); and tarry stools. Inspection may reveal hematomas on the extremities, torso, or both, and joint swelling if bleeding has occurred there.

The perils of poor perfusion

Signs and symptoms of decreased tissue perfusion may occur, including restlessness, anxiety, confusion, pallor, cool and clammy skin, chest pain, decreased urine output, hypotension, and tachycardia. (See *Treating hemophilia.*)

Battling illness

Treating hemophilia

Hemophilia isn't curable, but treatment can prevent crippling deformities and prolong life. Increasing plasma levels of deficient clotting factors helps prevent disabling deformities caused by repeated bleeding into muscles, joints, and organs.

Clotting factor

In hemophilia A, administration of cryoprecipitate antihemophilic factor (AHF) and lyophilized AHF (AHF that's been frozen and dehydrated under high vacuum) can result in normal hemostasis (arrest of bleeding). In hemophilia B, administration of recombinant factor VIII and purified factor IX promotes hemostasis. Doses should be large enough to raise clotting factor levels, which must be kept within the desired range until the wound heals. Fresh frozen plasma can also be given, but it has drawbacks, such as the potential for volume overload and a transfusion reaction.

A hemophiliac who undergoes surgery needs factor replacement before and after the procedure. This may be necessary even for minor surgery such as a dental extraction.

Other treatments

Joint pain may be controlled with an analgesic. However, don't give the drug by I.M. injection because hematomas may form at the site. Also, never give aspirin or aspirin-containing drugs because they decrease platelet adherence and may increase bleeding.

To help avoid injury, young children should wear clothing with padded patches on the knees and elbows. Older children should avoid contact sports such as football. Warn parents to notify the doctor immediately after even a minor injury, especially to the head, neck, or abdomen. Early recognition is the key to stopping bleeding.

What tests tell you

Specific coagulation factor assays can diagnose the type and severity of hemophilia. A family history can also aid in diagnosis.

These tests help diagnose hemophilia A:
• Factor VIII assay reveals 0% to 25% of normal factor VIII.
• Partial thromboplastin time is prolonged.
• Platelet count and function, bleeding time, prothrombin time, and International Normalized Ratio are normal.

These tests help diagnose hemophilia B:
• Factor IX assay shows deficiency.
• Baseline coagulation result is similar to that of hemophilia A, with normal factor VIII.

Marfan syndrome

Marfan syndrome is an inherited disease of the connective tissue that primarily causes ocular, skeletal, and cardiovascular anomalies. Signs and symptoms range from mild to severe. The disorder affects men and women equally, with an incidence of about 1 in 5,000 people in the United States.

How it happens

Marfan syndrome is inherited as an autosomal dominant trait. Patients are heterozygous for the mutation. This means that patients have one gene with the mutation and one normal gene.

This genetic disorder has been mapped to a specific chromosome location: chromosome 15 (of the 22 autosomes in the human cell). On this chromosome, more than 20 mutations have been identified that can occur in a gene that codes for fibrillin, a component of connective tissue. These small fibers are abundant in the large blood vessels and the suspensory ligaments of the ocular lenses. The exact function of fibrillin, however, is unknown.

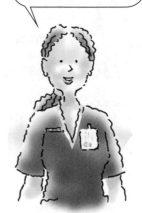

Patients with Marfan syndrome are heterozygous for the mutation—one gene with, one gene without.

What to look for

Genetic mutations may result in functional and structural changes.

Skeletal effects

Skeletal malformations include:
• increased height (patients are usually taller than family members)
• unusually long extremities
• arachnodactyly—a spiderlike appearance of the hands and fingers
• chest depression (pectus excavatum)

- chest protrusion (pectus carinatum)
- chest asymmetry
- scoliosis and kyphosis
- arched palate
- joint hypermobility.

Ocular outcomes

Lens displacement usually isn't progressive, but it may contribute to cataract formation. An elongated ocular globe causes nearsightedness in most patients. Retinal detachments may also develop, as well as retinal tears. However, most patients have adequate vision with corrective lenses.

Cardiac consequences

Cardiovascular abnormalities are the most serious consequences of Marfan syndrome. These abnormalities may occur in the valves and aorta.

Valvular abnormalities result from anatomic defects, such as redundancy to the leaflets, stretching of the chordae tendineae, and calcification of the mitral annulus. Mitral valve prolapse (dropping down of the cusps of the mitral valve into the left atrium during systole) develops early in life. It can progress to severe mitral valve regurgitation (backflow of blood from the left ventricle into the left atrium).

Dilation of the aortic root and ascending aorta may cause aortic regurgitation (backflow of blood into the left ventricle), dissection (separation of the layers of the aortic wall), and rupture. In adults, dilation may be accelerated by physical and emotional stress as well as by pregnancy.

And there's more...

Marfan syndrome may also cause:
- thin body build with little subcutaneous fat
- striae over the shoulders and buttocks
- spontaneous pneumothorax
- inguinal and incisional hernias
- dilation of the dural sac.

No established treatment exists for Marfan syndrome. (See *Treating Marfan syndrome.*)

What tests tell you

To date, no laboratory tests exist to diagnose Marfan syndrome. Diagnostic tests based on detection of fibrillin defects in cultured skin fibroblasts or DNA analysis of the gene may be available in the near future.

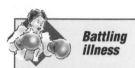

Battling illness

Treating Marfan syndrome

No established treatment exists for Marfan syndrome. Propranolol (Inderal) or other beta-adrenergic blocking agents may delay or prevent aortic dilation. Surgery to repair the aorta may be necessary. Surgical replacement of the aortic valve and mitral valve has been successful in some patients.

Scoliosis is progressive and should be treated by mechanical bracing and physical therapy if the curvature is greater than 20 degrees. Surgery may be required if the curvature progresses beyond 45 degrees.

Getting physical

Currently, a diagnosis may be made through physical examination and medical and family history. Diagnosis may be made if skeletal system involvement is found and at least two other systems are affected.

Diagnosis may also be made if only two body systems are involved and there's a documented family history of Marfan syndrome. Diagnosis of ectopia lentis is made by pupillary dilation and slit lamp examination. Cardiac problems may be discovered by an echocardiogram.

Phenylketonuria

PKU is an inborn error in metabolism of the amino acid phenylalanine. It causes high serum levels of phenylalanine and increased urine concentrations of phenylalanine and its by-products. It results in cerebral damage and mental retardation.

The disorder occurs in about 1 of 14,000 births in the United States, and about 1 person in 60 is an asymptomatic carrier. PKU has a low incidence among Blacks and Ashkenazic Jews and a higher incidence among Whites and Native Americans.

How it happens

PKU is transmitted through an autosomal recessive gene. Patients with classic PKU have almost no activity of phenylalanine hydroxylase, an enzyme that helps convert phenylalanine to tyrosine. As a result, phenylalanine accumulates in the blood and urine, and tyrosine levels are low.

All in the family

Patients may have a family history of PKU. Usually, no abnormalities are apparent at birth, when blood phenylalanine levels are essentially normal. But levels begin to rise within a few days, and by the time they reach about 30 mg/dl, cerebral damage has begun. Irreversible damage is probably complete by age 2 or 3, although early detection and treatment can minimize it. (See *Treating PKU*.)

What to look for

By age 4 months, the untreated child begins to show signs of arrested brain development, including mental retardation. Later, personality disturbances occur, such as schizoid and antisocial behavior and uncontrollable temper. About one-third of patients have seizures, which usually begin between ages 6 and 12 months. Many patients also show a precipitous decrease in IQ.

Battling illness

Treating PKU

To prevent or minimize brain damage from phenylketonuria (PKU), phenylalanine blood levels are kept between 3 and 15 mg/dl by restricting dietary intake of phenylalanine. Dietary restrictions with supplementation will be necessary for the patient's entire life. A special, low-phenylalanine amino acid mixture is substituted for most dietary protein, supplemented with a small amount of natural foods.

Dietary restrictions
Patients must avoid bread, cheese, eggs, flour, meat, poultry, fish, nuts, milk, legumes, and aspartame. Even with this diet, central nervous system dysfunction may occur. Frequent tests for urine phenylpyruvic acid and blood phenylalanine levels evaluate the diet's effectiveness. Patients need careful monitoring because overzealous dietary restrictions can induce phenylalanine deficiency, causing lethargy, anorexia, anemia, rashes, diarrhea, and death.

Other signs include macrocephaly; eczematous skin lesions or dry, rough skin; hyperactivity; irritability; purposeless, repetitive motions; and an awkward gait. You may also note a musty odor from skin and urine excretion of phenylacetic acid.

What tests tell you

Several tests are used to diagnose PKU:
- The Guthrie screening test on a capillary blood sample reliably detects PKU and is required by most states at birth. However, because phenylalanine levels may be normal at birth, infants should be reevaluated 24 to 48 hours after they begin protein feedings.
- Fluorometric or chromatographic assays provide additional diagnostic information.
- Electroencephalography is abnormal in about 80% of untreated affected children.
- DNA-based tests are used in prenatal diagnosis of PKU.

Sickle cell anemia

Sickle cell anemia is a congenital hematologic disease that causes impaired circulation, chronic ill health, and premature death. In the United States, it's estimated that more than 70,000 people have sickle cell disease. It's most common in people of African descent, but it also occurs in Puerto Rico, Turkey, India, the Middle East, and the Mediterranean. If two carriers have offspring, each child has a one in four chance of developing the disease. About 1 in 10 Blacks carries the abnormal gene, and 1 in every 400 to 600 Black children has sickle cell anemia.

A trend toward the better

In the past, many people with this disease died in their early 20s. Today, however, the average life expectancy is age 45, with 40% to 50% of patients living into their 40s and 50s.

How it happens

Sickle cell anemia results from homozygous inheritance of an autosomal recessive gene mutation that produces a defective hemoglobin molecule (hemoglobin S). Hemoglobin S causes red blood cells (RBCs) to become sickle shaped. Sickle cell trait, which results from heterozygous inheritance of this gene mutation, causes few or no symptoms. However, these people are carriers and can pass the gene to their offspring. This gene mutation may have persisted because the heterozygous sickle cell trait provides resistance to malaria.

Sickle cell anemia occurs as a result of a mutation in the gene that encodes the beta chain of hemoglobin. This mutation causes a structural change in hemoglobin. A single amino acid change from glutamic acid to valine occurs in the sixth position of the beta-hemoglobin chain. (See *Distinguishing between sickled cells and normal cells.*)

Rigid and rough

When hypoxia (oxygen deficiency) occurs, the hemoglobin S in the RBCs becomes insoluble. As a result, the blood cells get rigid and rough, forming an elongated crescent, or *sickle*, shape. Sickling can cause hemolysis (cell destruction).

Sickle cells also accumulate in capillaries and smaller blood vessels, causing occlusions and increasing blood viscosity. This impairs normal circulation, causing pain, tissue infarctions (tissue death), swelling, and anoxic changes that lead to further sickling and obstruction.

Triggering a crisis

Each patient with sickle cell anemia has a different hypoxic threshold and different factors that trigger a sickle cell crisis. Illness, cold exposure, stress, anything that induces an acidotic state, or any pathophysiologic process that pulls water out of sick-

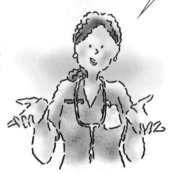

In sickle cell anemia, the RBCs become rigid and rough, forming an elongated crescent, or sickle, shape.

Now I get it!

Distinguishing between sickled cells and normal cells

Normal red blood cells (RBCs) and sickled cells vary in more ways than shape. They also differ in life span, oxygen-carrying capacity, and the rate at which they're destroyed.

Normal RBCs
- 120-day life span
- Normal oxygen-carrying capacity
- 12 to 14 g of hemoglobin per milliliter
- RBCs destroyed at a normal rate

Sickled cells
- 30- to 40-day life span
- Decreased oxygen-carrying capacity
- 6 to 9 g of hemoglobin per milliliter
- RBCs destroyed at an accelerated rate

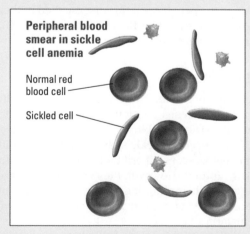

Peripheral blood smear in sickle cell anemia

Normal red blood cell

Sickled cell

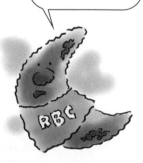

Look at the shape I'm in! This disease impairs my circulation and really cramps my style.

Now I get it!

Understanding sickle cell crisis

Sickle cell crisis is triggered by infection, cold exposure, high altitudes, overexertion, and other conditions that cause cellular oxygen deprivation. Here's what happens:

• Deoxygenated, sickle-shaped erythrocytes adhere to the capillary wall and to one another, blocking blood flow and causing cellular hypoxia.

• The crisis worsens as tissue hypoxia and acidic waste products cause more sickling and cell damage.

• With each new crisis, organs and tissues are destroyed and areas of tissue die slowly—especially in the spleen and kidneys.

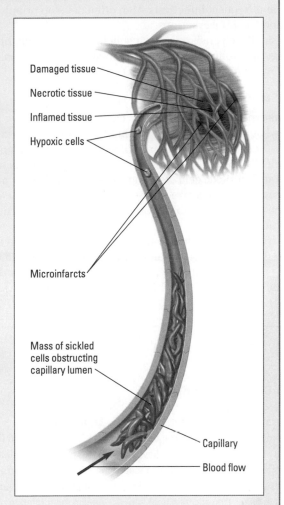

Damaged tissue
Necrotic tissue
Inflamed tissue
Hypoxic cells
Microinfarcts
Mass of sickled cells obstructing capillary lumen
Capillary
Blood flow

le cells will precipitate a crisis in most patients. (See *Understanding sickle cell crisis.*)

What to look for

Signs and symptoms of sickle cell anemia usually don't develop until after age 6 months because large amounts of fetal hemoglo-

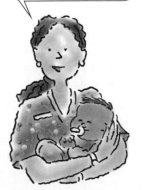

Neonates are protected from the signs and symptoms of sickle cell anemia by fetal hemoglobin for up to 6 months.

bin protect infants until then. Fetal hemoglobin has a higher oxygen concentration and inhibits sickling.

The patient's history includes chronic fatigue, unexplained dyspnea or dyspnea on exertion, joint swelling, aching bones, severe localized and generalized pain, leg ulcers (especially on the ankles), and frequent infections. Men often develop priapism, or unexplained, painful erections.

In sickle cell crisis, symptoms include severe pain, hematuria, lethargy, irritability, and pale lips, tongue, palms, and nail beds. (See *Treating sickle cell anemia*.)

One crisis after another

Various types of sickle cell crises can occur. Here's how to determine what type the patient is having:

• *Painful crisis* is the hallmark of sickle cell anemia, appearing periodically after age 5. It results from blood vessel obstruction by rigid, tangled sickle cells, leading to tissue anoxia and, possibly, necrosis. It's characterized by severe abdominal, thoracic, muscle, or bone pain and, possibly, worsened jaundice, dark urine, or a low-grade fever.

• *Aplastic crisis* results from bone marrow depression and is associated with infection (usually viral). It's characterized by pallor, lethargy, sleepiness, dyspnea, possible coma, markedly decreased bone marrow activity, and RBC hemolysis (destruction).

Now I get it!

Treating sickle cell anemia

Treatment for sickle cell anemia aims to alleviate symptoms and prevent painful crises. Analgesics, such as hydromorphone or morphine, and warm compresses may help relieve the pain from vasoocclusive crises. I.V. therapy may be needed to prevent dehydration and vessel occlusion. Patients should be encouraged to drink plenty of fluids. Iron and folic acid supplements may help prevent anemia. If the patient's hemoglobin level drops, blood transfusions may be needed.

Reducing complications
Complications resulting from the disease and from transfusion therapy may be reduced using certain vaccines, antiinfectives such as low-dose penicillin, or chelating agents such as deferoxamine.

Easing pain
In 1998, the Food and Drug Administration approved the drug hydroxyurea, an antitumor drug, for reducing painful episodes in adults with a severe form of sickle cell anemia (at least three painful crises in the previous year). Hydroxyurea works by inducing the formation of fetal hemaglobin—a hemoglobin normally found in the fetus or neonate. When present in patients with sickle cell anemia, fetal hemoglobin prevents sickling. Patients receiving hydroxyurea must be monitored closely to make sure their blood count isn't depressed to a level that places them at risk for bleeding or infection.

• *Acute sequestration crisis* (rare) occurs in infants between ages 8 months and 2 years and may cause sudden, massive entrapment of RBCs in the spleen and liver. Lethargy and pallor progress to hypovolemic shock and death if untreated.

• *Hemolytic crisis* (rare) usually affects patients who have glucose-6-phosphate dehydrogenase deficiency along with sickle cell anemia. It probably results from complications of sickle cell anemia, such as infection, rather than from the disease itself. In this crisis, degenerative changes cause liver congestion and enlargement, and chronic jaundice worsens.

What tests tell you

A family history and typical clinical features suggest sickle cell anemia. These tests are also performed:

• Stained blood smear shows sickle cells, and hemoglobin electrophoresis shows hemoglobin S. These tests confirm the disease.

• Additional blood tests show low RBC counts, elevated white blood cell and platelet counts, decreased erythrocyte sedimentation rate, increased serum iron levels, decreased RBC survival, and reticulocytosis. Hemoglobin levels may be low or normal.

• Lateral chest X-ray detects the "Lincoln log" deformity in the vertebrae of many adults and some adolescents.

Tay-Sachs disease

Tay-Sachs disease results from a congenital enzyme deficiency. It causes progressive mental and motor deterioration and is always fatal, usually before age 5. It occurs in fewer than 100 infants born each year in the United States and strikes people of Ashkenazic Jewish ancestry about 100 times more often than the general population.

In this ethnic group, it occurs in about 1 of 3,600 live births. About 1 in 30 are heterozygous carriers of the defective gene. If two carriers have children, each of their offspring has a 25% chance of having Tay-Sachs disease.

How it happens

Tay-Sachs disease is an autosomal recessive disorder in which the enzyme hexosaminidase A is deficient. Hexosaminidase A is necessary for metabolism of gangliosides, water-soluble glycolipids found primarily in tissues of the central nervous system (CNS). Without hexosaminidase A, accumulating lipid pigments distend and progressively demyelinate (remove the protective myelin sheath) and destroy CNS cells.

What to look for

The child usually looks normal at birth; abnormal clinical signs appear between ages 5 and 6 months. Progressive weakness of the neck, trunk, arm, and leg muscles prevents him from sitting up or lifting his head. He has trouble turning over, can't grasp objects, and has vision loss progressing to blindness. He is also easily startled by loud sounds.

By age 18 months, the patient may have seizures, generalized paralysis, and spasticity. His pupils are always dilated and, although blind, he may hold his eyes wide open and roll his eyeballs. Decerebrate rigidity and a complete vegetative state follow. Around age 2, the patient contracts recurrent bronchopneumonia, which is usually fatal before age 5.

Other findings include an enlarged head circumference, optic nerve atrophy, and a distinctive cherry red spot on the retina.

Most children with Tay-Sachs disease are treated at home with the aid of hospice care. (See *Treating Tay-Sachs disease*.)

What tests tell you

Serum analysis shows deficient hexosaminidase A in affected infants.

A simple blood test can identify carriers. Carrier screening is offered to all couples in which one or both are of Ashkenazic Jewish ancestry and for others with a family history of the disease.

Battling illness

Treating Tay-Sachs disease

Tay-Sachs disease has no known cure, so all treatment is supportive. Treatment includes tube feedings with nutritional supplements, suctioning and postural drainage to remove secretions, skin care to prevent pressure ulcers when the child becomes bedridden, and mild laxatives to relieve neurogenic constipation. Anticonvulsants usually don't prevent seizures.

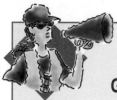

That's a wrap!

Genetics review

Genetic facts
• Ova and sperm each contain 23 chromosomes
• A fertilized cell has 46 chromosomes
• Each chromosome contains DNA
• DNA contains genes
• A person receives one set of chromosomes and genes from each parent
• More influential gene is dominant
• Less influential gene is recessive

Types of disorders
• Single-gene—inherited in clearly identifiable patterns; two important inheritance patterns are:
  – autosomal dominant
  – autosomal recessive
• Chromosomal—deviations in either the structure or the number of chromosomes involving the loss, addition, rearrangement, or exchange of genes
• Multifactoral—caused by genetic and environmental factors

Genetics review *(continued)*

Genetic disorders

• *Cleft lip and cleft palate*—arise from interaction of several genes that originates in the second gestational month
• *Cystic fibrosis*—inherited as an autosomal recessive trait; protein doesn't function properly, which leads to dehydration and mucosal thickening
• *Down syndrome*—caused by aberration of chromosome 21
• *Hemophilia*—inherited as an X-linked recessive trait; two types include:
  – *hemophilia A*—factor VIII deficiency
  – *hemophilia B*—factor IX deficiency

• *Marfan syndrome*—inherited as an autosomal dominant trait that causes connective tissue disease
• *Phenylketonuria*—inherited as an autosomal recessive gene that leads to brain damage due to phenylalanine accumulating in blood
• *Sickle cell anemia*—inherited as an autosomal recessive gene mutation, which impairs normal blood circulation
• *Tay-Sachs disease*—inherited as an autosomal recessive disorder that causes lipid pigments to accumulate, destroying central nervous system cells

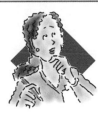

Quick quiz

1. A patient with an aortic aneurysm at the base of the aorta, spiderlike extremities, and a displaced ocular lens is likely to have:
    A.   an autosomal recessive inheritance disorder.
    B.   Marfan syndrome.
    C.   Down syndrome.
    D.   Tay-Sachs disease.

Answer: B. Marfan syndrome is an autosomal dominant disorder caused by a mutation in the gene that codes for fibrillin.

2. Cystic fibrosis affects the exocrine glands, causing:
    A.   increased viscosity of bronchial, pancreatic, and other mucous gland secretions, leading to atelectasis and emphysema.
    B.   increased sperm in males.
    C.   overhydration.
    D.   sodium retention.

Answer: A. Cystic fibrosis also causes dehydration and absence of sperm in the semen.

3. If PKU isn't diagnosed and treated early, it can cause:
    A. frequent bouts of pneumonia.
    B. spontaneous hemorrhaging and hypovolemic shock.
    C. thick, tenacious secretions of bronchial ducts, atelectasis, and respiratory distress.
    D. cerebral damage and mental retardation.

Answer: D. Untreated infants show signs of arrested brain development by age 4 months, but early detection and treatment can minimize cerebral damage.

4. Sickle-cell anemia is caused by:
    A. an autosomal recessive gene mutation.
    B. an autosomal dominant trait.
    C. a chromosomal aberration.
    D. genetic and environmental factors.

Answer: A. Sickle cell anemia results from homozygous inheritance of an autosomal recessive gene mutation.

Scoring

☆☆☆ If you answered all four items correctly, outasight! You display such a brilliant grasp of genetic concepts, we're thinking of having you cloned!

☆☆ If you answered three items correctly, that's terrific! You've inherited the right stuff to be a genetic genius.

☆ If you answered fewer than three items correctly, don't worry! Your performance on the Quick quiz is just a mutation.

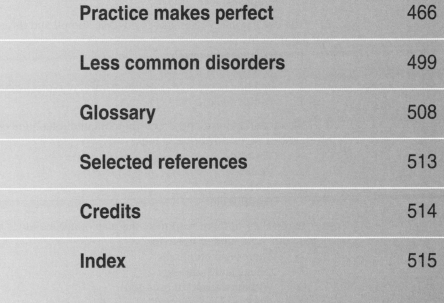

Appendices and index

Practice makes perfect	466
Less common disorders	499
Glossary	508
Selected references	513
Credits	514
Index	515

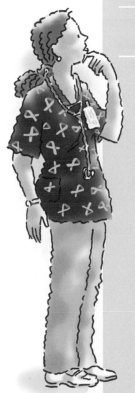

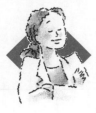

Practice makes perfect

1. What intracellular structure (organelle) is responsible for producing cellular energy?
    1. Ribosome
    2. Mitochondrion
    3. Golgi apparatus
    4. Nucleus

2. The cell's primary response to adverse stimuli and threats to cellular integrity is:
    1. cellular adaptation.
    2. cellular regeneration.
    3. sending nerve signals to the central nervous system.
    4. cellular death.

3. Which endocrine gland is central to maintaining homeostasis by means of regulating other glands?
    1. Thyroid
    2. Pituitary
    3. Adrenal
    4. Parathyroid

4. In the fight-or-flight response, the rush of adrenaline is associated with what kind of behavior?
    1. Aggression and panic
    2. Crying and sadness
    3. Withdrawal and depression
    4. Panic and withdrawal

5. The prodromal stage of a disease is when:
    1. the disease reaches its full intensity.
    2. the body regains health and homeostasis.
    3. signs and symptoms are mild and nonspecific.
    4. the patient progresses toward recovery.

6. A 63-year-old patient is diagnosed with carcinoma. A carcinoma is a cancer that derives from what kind of tissue?
    1. Glandular
    2. Liver
    3. Bone marrow
    4. Epithelium

7. When instructing a patient on performing breast self-examination, which area of the breast should you point out as the one in which the majority of tumors arise?

1. Upper outer quadrant
2. Lower inner quadrant
3. Areolar area
4. Upper inner quadrant

8. A 60-year-old patient tells you that she hates the rectal examination portion of her annual gynecologic check-up. Which statement will help her understand the importance of the rectal examination?

1. Colorectal cancer is the most common cause of death in women older than age 60.
2. The rectal examination is important for identifying most polyps.
3. The rectal examination is a way to check for occult blood in feces.
4. The rectal examination is the best way to detect colon cancer.

9. A patient of Celtic ancestry knows that he's at increased risk for developing malignant melanoma and asks you how he can check himself for this disease. Which recommendation would be the most accurate?

1. He should check existing moles for changes, such as enlargement or discoloration.
2. He should have yearly examinations by his family practitioner.
3. He should be especially concerned about new moles on his abdomen.
4. He should be concerned if a nevus develops.

10. Which cancer should you be on the lookout for in a patient with a history of infectious mononucleosis?

1. Multiple myeloma
2. Leukemia
3. Malignant melanoma
4. Hodgkin's disease

11. Which term indicates cell-damaging proteins derived from bacteria?

1. Erythrogenic toxins
2. Exotoxins
3. Neurotoxins
4. Endotoxins

12. A patient arrives for her annual gynecologic examination and mentions to you that she's pregnant. You know from previous visits that she has pets. What should you warn her about with regard to her cats?

1. She should be sure that they're tested and vaccinated against feline leukemia.
2. She should have someone else change the litter.
3. She should avoid contact with the cats during the summer flea season.
4. She should avoid being scratched by the cats.

13. What's the most likely cause of diarrhea in an 84-year-old patient who, 3 to 4 days earlier, was given a supplemental drink to which a raw egg had been added for protein supplementation?

1. Toxoplasmosis
2. Typhoid fever
3. Salmonellosis
4. Botulism

14. A patient has a history of cold sores and she's upset because her significant other has contracted a genital herpes infection, thinking that there has been infidelity. What can you tell her to help her understand more about her situation?

1. The virus that causes cold sores is unlikely to have caused the genital herpes.
2. The virus that caused her partner's infection can also infect her.
3. The virus that caused her partner's infection could have come from her cold sore.
4. The virus that caused her partner's infection won't infect her.

15. A student comes to the student health clinic complaining of a terrible sore throat and fever. The prescribed antibiotics haven't helped after 1 week. What other disease should he be tested for?

1. Hodgkin's disease
2. Rubella
3. Infectious mononucleosis
4. Leukemia

16. A 12-year-old patient's mother mentions she's worried that her son isn't getting enough sleep because he has dark circles under his eyes. This should alert you to inquire about:

1. bruises and darkened areas elsewhere on his body.
2. periods of altered states of consciousness such as staring off into space.
3. drug use.
4. headaches and nasal congestion.

17. A hospital employee comes to the emergency department after being stung by a bee while working outside on the hospital grounds. He tells you that he has a history of severe reactions to bee stings. Which medication should he receive immediately?

1. Epinephrine
2. Aminophylline
3. Diphenhydramine
4. Methylprednisolone

18. In an effort to determine the presence of human immunodeficiency virus (HIV) infection, which test would be most useful if ordered initially for a 26-year-old female presenting with a history of I.V. drug use, recurrent vaginal candidiasis, and herpes simplex infections?

1. White blood cell (WBC) count
2. Erythrocyte sedimentation rate
3. Enzyme-linked immunosorbent assay (ELISA)
4. Serum beta microglobulin

19. A 38-year-old woman comes to the office complaining of morning stiffness and pain affecting the small joints of her hands and feet. The symptoms have progressively worsened over several months, and she isn't aware of having fever, rash, or other symptoms. Which disorder is the most likely cause of her symptoms?

1. Systemic lupus erythematosis (SLE)
2. Rheumatoid arthritis (RA)
3. Osteoarthritis
4. Lyme disease

20. A patient with a kidney transplant is taking steroids to suppress rejection of the transplanted organ. Which part of the immune system is responsible for rejecting organ transplants?

1. Humoral
2. Complement system
3. Autoimmunity
4. Cell-mediated

21. Two fair-haired persons are planning to marry. They come to you for advice because the male has mild cystic fibrosis. They ask what the chances are that one of their children would have cystic fibrosis. What can you tell them?

1. If he has a mild case, they may have a child with a mild case although it isn't likely.
2. They should both be tested.
3. Each male child would have a 25% chance of having the disease.
4. There's no chance their child will have the disease.

22. The caretaker of a 24-year-old patient with Down syndrome notices that the patient has begun to urinate frequently and in large amounts. You're alerted to the development of which disease that's common in adults with Down syndrome?

1. Diabetes mellitus (DM)
2. Diabetes insipidus (DI)
3. Rheumatoid arthritis (RA)
4. Syndrome of inappropriate antidiuretic hormone (SIADH)

23. A patient whose son has hemophilia is pregnant. The fetus has been determined to be female. What can you tell the patient about the chances that the child will be born with the disease?

1. There is a 25% chance that the child will have hemophilia.
2. The child isn't at risk for the disease.
3. It's unusual for two children of the same parents to develop the disease.
4. The child will most likely have hemophilia.

24. Your patient with sickle cell trait is married to someone who has just learned that he has the trait, too. He asks you what the chances are that one of their children will have sickle cell anemia. What do you tell him?

1. Each child has a 1 in 2 chance.
2. Each child has a 1 in 4 chance.
3. Each child has a 1 in 8 chance.
4. Each child will have sickle cell disease.

25. A pregnant black woman has learned that a neonate is given a blood test that requires taking blood from the heel. She complains that she doesn't want this done to her baby. What can you tell her about the purpose of the test for phenylketonuria (PKU) that may alleviate her anxiety?

1. PKU is most common in people of African descent.
2. The test shows whether the child will contract the disease later in life.
3. Testing for PKU is mandatory in the state.
4. PKU affects infants in the first few months of life, causing devastating irreversible damage.

26. A patient has been diagnosed with Addison's disease. Which signs and symptoms probably tipped off the practitioners to the diagnosis?

1. Darkening skin and a craving for salty food
2. A craving for sweet foods and other carbohydrates
3. Weakness and weight loss
4. Buffalo hump and thinning scalp hair

27. A 49-year-old patient comes to the clinic complaining of nervousness, weight loss despite an increased appetite, and excessive sweating. You're immediately alert to the possibility of Graves' disease. Which assessment would be most informative in making an accurate diagnosis in this case?

1. Checking the patient's reflexes
2. Doing a urinalysis
3. Checking for Romberg's sign
4. Checking urine specific gravity

28. What's the most likely diagnosis for a woman who takes prednisone for her chronic asthma, complains of fragile skin that bruises easily and doesn't heal well, displays a lump on the back of her neck, and has a round, swollen face?

1. Cushing's syndrome
2. Addison's disease
3. Hyperthyroidism
4. Graves' disease

29. A patient has been diagnosed with a simple goiter. The enlargement of her thyroid gland is the result of:

1. inflammation or neoplasm of the thyroid gland.
2. overproduction of estrogen.
3. increased thyroid cell activity and overall thyroid mass.
4. overproduction of thyroid hormone.

30. A patient presents with complaints of burning pain in her feet and lower legs. Which disease should you ask about when you take her history?

1. Hashimoto's disease
2. Diabetes insipidus
3. Cushing's disease
4. Diabetes mellitus

31. A 73-year-old patient with a history of chronic obstructive pulmonary disease (COPD) is admitted with respiratory failure. The patient is intubated and placed on mechanical ventilation. Which process is interrupted when oxygen is delivered directly to the lower airways?

1. Gas exchange
2. Humidifying and warming of air
3. Conversion of oxygen to carbon dioxide
4. Reflex bronchospasm

32. A ventilation-perfusion ($\dot{V}/\dot{Q}$) scan is done on your patient and the result indicates a high $\dot{V}/\dot{Q}$ ratio. This indicates a problem with which process?
1.   Decreased alveolar perfusion
2.   Increased alveolar perfusion
3.   Pulmonary edema
4.   Decreased ventilation

33. A 65-year-old patient with chronic obstructive pulmonary disease (COPD) has a sudden onset of unilateral pleuritic chest pain that worsens when he coughs and severe shortness of breath. You also note that his chest wall movement is asymmetrical. When you listen to his lungs, which finding is most significant in establishing the diagnosis?
1.   Crackles in both lung bases
2.   Significantly decreased breath sounds on the symptomatic side
3.   Expiratory wheezing
4.   Rhonchi scattered throughout both lung fields

34. A patient, who has a 40-pack-per-year history of smoking, is found to have cor pulmonale. Cor pulmonale is best described as:
1.   left-sided heart failure.
2.   pulmonary hypertension.
3.   ventilation-perfusion ($\dot{V}/\dot{Q}$) mismatch.
4.   hypertrophy of the right ventricle.

35. A 76-year-old patient is admitted with a history of heart failure and now presents with pulmonary edema. What pathophysiologic process is occurring?
1.   Perfusion to the lungs is interrupted by a pulmonary embolus.
2.   Increased hydrostatic pressure in the capillaries causes fluid to leak into the alveoli, collapsing them.
3.   Increased hydrostatic pressure in the capillaries causes fluid to leak into the interstitial spaces.
4.   Fluid accumulates in the lung interstitium, alveolar spaces, and small airways.

36. A patient with a history of chronic renal failure is admitted in respiratory distress. The practitioner suspects cardiac tamponade. The best method of assessing this patient for associated pulsus paradoxus is:
1.   checking to see if his central venous pressure is elevated more than 15 mm Hg above normal.
2.   auscultating for muffled heart sounds on inspiration.
3.   measuring his blood pressure at rest and again while he slowly inspires to check if the systolic pressure drops more than 15 mm Hg during inspiration.
4.   checking the electrocardiogram (ECG) for reduced amplitude.

37. When myocardial cells are hypoxic, they signal the body to produce epinephrine and norepinephrine, which cause the heart to beat stronger and faster (thus increasing blood flow to the cells). Why is this compensatory mechanism sometimes harmful?
1. It actually increases oxygen demand in the heart.
2. It depletes the myocardial cells of calcium.
3. It diverts blood to the extremities.
4. It decreases contractility of the heart.

38. You must obtain a throat culture on an 8-year-old child who presents with fever, purulent drainage on the tonsils, and difficulty swallowing. Which bacteria are you most concerned about identifying?
1. *Staphylococcus aureus*
2. Group A beta-hemolytic streptococci
3. *Clostridium perfringens*
4. *Pseudomonas aeruginosa*

39. A patient with chronic heart failure caused by aortic stenosis begins to have symptoms of abdominal pain and distention. On examination he's found to have an enlarged liver. What's the most likely cause of these new signs and symptoms?
1. Cirrhosis
2. Hepatic vein engorgement
3. Hepatitis
4. Ascites

40. A patient with a history of chronic renal failure develops left-sided chest pain that begins in his sternum and radiates to his neck. It worsens with deep inspiration and eases when he sits up and leans forward. As you perform your assessment, you note that heart sounds are diminished. Which condition is most likely causing his symptoms?
1. Pneumonia
2. Cardiac tamponade
3. Myocardial infarction
4. Pericarditis

41. A 30-year-old female presents with a recent onset of blurred vision, loss of sensation in her lower legs, and difficulty speaking clearly. The symptoms come and go unpredictably, but they have been occurring for several months. What's the most likely cause of these symptoms?
1. Multiple sclerosis
2. Myasthenia gravis
3. Aneurysm
4. Guillain-Barré syndrome

42. You're walking down a forest path when you suddenly see a bear in front of you. Your heart begins to pound and your mouth becomes dry. Which portion of the neurologic system causes this response?
1. Somatic
2. Extrapyramidal
3. Pyramidal
4. Autonomic

43. Which neurotransmitter is deficient in the brains of patients with Alzheimer's disease?
1. Dopamine
2. Serotonin
3. Norepinephrine
4. Acetylcholine

44. What's the most common cause of stroke in middle-age and elderly patients?
1. Aneurysm
2. Thrombosis
3. Embolism
4. Hypertension

45. A patient with a history of hallucinations and vertigo isn't psychotic or mentally impaired. He's diagnosed with a seizure disorder. Based on the patient's history, which type of seizure disorder does he have?
1. Absence seizure
2. Parietal lobe sensory seizure
3. Jacksonian seizure
4. Grand mal seizure

46. A 72-year-old patient with chronic renal failure also has anemia. The most likely cause of his anemia is:
1. loss of albumin through impaired renal tubular filtration.
2. bleeding from damaged tubules.
3. lack of erythropoietin.
4. blood loss from hemodialysis.

47. A patient has been found to have an increase in white blood cell (WBC) precursor cells in the bone marrow. Which condition is the most likely cause?
1. Leukemia
2. Polycythemia
3. Thrombocytopenia
4. Multiple myeloma

48. A patient who suffered an acute myocardial infarction has an intra-aortic balloon pump in place. His platelet count reveals thrombocytopenia. Which condition is the most likely cause?
1. Malnutrition
2. Platelet destruction
3. Internal hemorrhage
4. Disseminated intravascular coagulation (DIC)

49. A patient develops petechiae and a blood blister in his mouth. Thrombocytopenia is suspected and a platelet count is obtained. Which platelet count confirms the diagnosis?
1. $400,000/mm^3$
2. $90,000/mm^3$
3. $500,000/mm^3$
4. $150,000/mm^3$

50. A patient diagnosed with disseminated intravascular coagulation (DIC) is receiving anticoagulants. This is done to:
1. prevent emboli formation that may occur as a result of increased clotting factors seen in DIC.
2. combat clot formation in the small blood vessels.
3. prevent clot formation that may develop as blood pools beneath the skin.
4. prevent thrombus formation that may occur because the patient requires bed rest.

51. An obese woman, who consumes a high-cholesterol diet, is receiving hormone replacement therapy (HRT). This patient carries an increased risk for what disorder?
1. Appendicitis
2. Cirrhosis
3. Pancreatitis
4. Cholecystitis

52. What hepatic tissue changes have taken place in a patient newly diagnosed with cirrhosis?
1. Hepatic cells are distended and misshapen.
2. Hepatic blood vessels are destroyed.
3. Fibrous tissue replaces normal hepatic cells.
4. Hepatic cells begin to die.

53. A man with a history of alcohol abuse and gastric ulcers comes to the emergency department with severe, persistent, piercing abdominal pain in his left upper quadrant, which began after consuming a large meal. What's the most likely cause of this patient's pain?
1. Perforated gastric ulcer
2. Pancreatitis
3. Appendicitis
4. Cholecystitis

54. A 44-year-old patient presents to the emergency department complaining of severe midepigastric pain. Pancreatitis is suspected. Which laboratory tests help to confirm the diagnosis?

1. White blood cell (WBC) count and hemoglobin level
2. Serum amylase and lipase levels
3. Serum lipid and trypsin levels
4. Total serum bilirubin and indirect bilirubin levels

55. A 52-year-old patient is diagnosed with peptic ulcer disease caused by *Helicobacter pylori* infection. Infection with this bacteria leads to ulceration because:

1. bacteria colonize the mucous lining.
2. bacteria cause regurgitation of duodenal contents into the stomach.
3. bacteria release a toxin that destroys the stomach's mucous lining.
4. bacteria cause persistent inflammation of the stomach.

56. A patient has been diagnosed with chronic renal failure. What percent of his renal tissue is probably nonfunctional?

1. Less than 25%
2. 25% to 50%
3. 50% to 75%
4. Greater than 75%

57. A 67-year-old patient who underwent bowel resection for a ruptured diverticulum is recovering from septic shock. His blood pressure is stable and he's receiving I.V. antibiotics and fluid replacement. His urine output for the past 8 hours totals 100 ml. Why is his urine output inadequate?

1. He now has an acid-base imbalance.
2. He's experiencing blood loss.
3. He's experiencing acute tubular necrosis.
4. He's dehydrated.

58. A 55-year-old male patient has been diagnosed with acute bacterial prostatitis. This is commonly caused by:

1. an ascending infection of the urinary tract.
2. lymphatic migration of pathogenic bacteria.
3. prostatic hyperplasia.
4. an infection in the patient's blood.

59. A patient presents with acute, severe pain in his lower back, radiating to the side and pubic region. Renal calculi are suspected. What test is most likely performed to confirm the diagnosis?

    1.   Computed tomography (CT) scan of the abdomen
    2.   Magnetic resonance imaging (MRI) of the pelvis
    3.   Cystoscopy of the bladder
    4.   Kidney-ureter-bladder (KUB) radiography

60. An athlete is most likely to experience injury in which type of joint?

    1.   Synarthrosis
    2.   Amphiarthrosis
    3.   Diarthrosis
    4.   Synovial

61. A 62-year-old patient who takes furosemide twice per day complains of pain in her right great toe. Gout is diagnosed. The pain she experiences is caused by deposition of which substance in her great toe?

    1.   Calcium pyrophosphate
    2.   Sodium urate
    3.   Ammonia sulfate
    4.   Sodium bicarbonate

62. An elderly woman complains of progressively worsening pain in one knee that's more severe in the morning when she arises. This pain is most likely caused by which disorder?

    1.   Rheumatoid arthritis (RA)
    2.   Systemic lupus erythematosus (SLE)
    3.   Gouty arthritis
    4.   Osteoarthritis

63. A 73-year-old patient is admitted with difficulty breathing. His admission arterial blood gas (ABG) results are pH 7.25, $Paco_2$ 70 mm Hg, Pao_2 52 mm Hg, and HCO_3^- 32 mEq/L. Which acid-base imbalance is this patient exhibiting?

    1.   Metabolic acidosis
    2.   Metabolic alkalosis
    3.   Respiratory acidosis
    4.   Respiratory alkalosis

64. A patient comes to the emergency department with a history of vomiting for the past 5 days. An arterial blood gas (ABG) analysis obtained on admission reveals the following:

FLOWSHEET	
02/01/08	Laboratory called with ABG results: pH = 7.5,
0530	$Paco_2$ = 48 mm Hg, HCO_3^- = 39 mEq/L, and Pao_2 =
	110 mm Hg. Dr. Riggins notified of ABG results.
	⎯⎯⎯⎯⎯⎯⎯⎯⎯ Louise Reynolds, RN

These ABG results reveal which acidbase imbalance?
1. Respiratory acidosis
2. Respiratory alkalosis
3. Metabolic acidosis
4. Metabolic alkalosis

65. What's a cause of metabolic acidosis?
1. Central nervous system (CNS) depression from drugs
2. Renal disease
3. Gram-negative bacteremia
4. Asphyxia

66. Which disorder presents with partial pressure of arterial carbon dioxide ($Paco_2$) above 50 mm Hg and partial pressure of arterial oxygen (Pao_2) below 50 mm Hg in patients with essentially normal lung tissue?
1. Acute respiratory failure
2. Severe acute respiratory syndrome
3. Asthma
4. Cor pulmonale

67. Diverticular disease is more prevalent in developed countries. One factor may be:
1. low intake of dietary protein.
2. high intake of dietary fiber.
3. high dietary intake of saturated fat.
4. low intake of dietary fiber.

68. Which type of diverticular disease causes constipation, ribbonlike stools, intermittent diarrhea, and abdominal distention?
1. Diverticulosis
2. Mild diverticulitis
3. Severe diverticulitis
4. Chronic diverticulitis

69. Which statement best describes the pathophysiology behind gastroesophageal reflux disease (GERD)?
1. The sphincter doesn't remain closed and the pressure in the stomach pushes the stomach contents into the esophagus.
2. The mucosa takes on a "cobblestone" appearance.
3. A defect in the diaphragm permits a portion of the stomach to pass through the esophageal hiatus into the chest cavity.
4. *Helicobacter pylori* bacteria release a toxin that destroys the stomach's mucous lining.

70. Which laboratory test helps distinguish esophagitis from cardiac disorders?
1. Esophageal manometry
2. Barium swallow
3. Acid-perfusion test
4. Upper GI series

71. Which disorder occurs more commonly in children than adults?
1. Osteoarthritis
2. Osteomyelitis
3. Osteomalacia
4. Osteoporosis

72. What's the most common causative organism in osteomyelitis?
1. *Staphylococcus aureus*
2. *Streptococcus pyogenes*
3. *Pseudomonas aeruginosa*
4. *Proteus vulgaris*

73. Pulmonary embolism generally results from an obstruction of the pulmonary arterial bed caused by:

1. sickle cell disease.
2. foreign substance.
3. heart valve growth.
4. dislodged thrombi originating in the leg veins or pelvis.

74. Which signs and symptoms are associated with severe acute respiratory syndrome (SARS)? Select all that apply.

1. High fever
2. Chills
3. Sudden onset of chest pain
4. Dry cough
5. Shortness of breath
6. Neck stiffness

75. A 72-year-old patient is admitted to the emergency department with a stroke. The patient was believed to be lying on the floor for more than 24 hours. Rhabdomyolysis is also suspected. When rhabdomyolysis occurs, which substances are released from necrotic muscle fibers into the circulation? Select all that apply.

1. Myoglobin
2. Potassium
3. Creatine kinase (CK)
4. Urate
5. Sodium
6. Calcium

76. Which test findings help to confirm the diagnosis of rhabdomyolysis? Select all that apply.

1. Elevated cardiac troponin level
2. Severely elevated creatine kinase (CK) level
3. Hypercalcemia (in early stages)
4. Elevated serum creatinine level
5. Elevated intracompartmental venous pressure
6. Urine myoglobin level greater than 0.5 mg/dl

77. Rank in order the pathological progression of rhabdomyolysis. Use all of the options.

1.	Local edema increases compartment pressure and tamponade.

2.	Pressure from severe swelling causes blood vessels to collapse.

3.	Substances are released from the necrotic muscle fibers into the circulation.

4.	Muscle trauma compresses tissue.

5.	Tissue ischemia and necrosis occur.

78. In gastroesophageal reflux disease, the lower esophageal sphincter (LES) doesn't remain closed because of deficient lower esophageal pressure. Place an "X" over the LES.

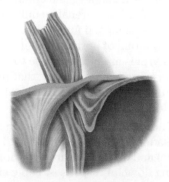

79. A patient is hospitalized for observation after a head injury. He's now having tonic-clonic seizures and has been ordered an immediate injection of 15 mg/kg phenytoin I.V. The patient's weight on admission was 176 lb. In grams, what total dose of phenytoin should be administered by slow I.V. infusion? Record your answer using one decimal place.

_____ grams

Answers

1. 2. Adenosine triphosphate, which is the energy that fuels cellular activity, is made in the mitochondria. The ribosome is a submicroscopic ribonucleic acid-containing particle in the cytoplasm of a cell, sometimes closely associated with endoplasmic reticulum and the site of cellular protein synthesis. The Golgi apparatus is a lamellar membranous structure near the nucleus of almost all cells. It contains a curved parallel series of flattened saccules that are often expanded at their ends. In secretory cells, the apparatus concentrates and packages the secretory product. The nucleus is the structure within a cell that contains the chromosomes. It's responsible for the cell's metabolism, growth, and reproduction. CN: Physiological integrity; CNS: Physiological adaptation; CL: Knowledge

2. 1. When cellular integrity is threatened, the cell reacts by drawing on its reserves to keep functioning and adapting through changes. Cellular regeneration pertains to cellular repair or regrowth. Sending nerve signals to the central nervous system is the responsibility of an afferent sensory nerve. Cellular death is cessation of cellular function. CN: Physiological integrity; CNS: Physiological adaptation; CL: Knowledge

3. 2. The pituitary gland regulates the function of other glands and is commonly referred to as the "master" gland. The thyroid gland contains active substances such as thyroxine and triiodothyronine. The adrenal gland is a double gland composed of the outer cortex and an inner medulla. The adrenal medulla is controlled by the sympathetic nervous system and functions in conjunction with it. The cortex secretes a group of hormones that vary in quantity and quality. The parathyroids are located close to the thyroid gland and secrete a hormone, parathormone, that regulates calcium and phosphorus metabolism. CN: Physiological integrity; CNS: Physiological adaptation; CL: Knowledge

4. 1. The release of adrenaline is associated with panic and aggression. Crying and sadness aren't associated with the rush of adrenaline. Withdrawal and depression are behaviors that are associated with a slowing down of responses. Panic and withdrawal is incorrect because withdrawal doesn't correlate with an automatic fight-or-flight response. CN: Physiological integrity; CNS: Physiological adaptation; CL: Comprehension

5. 3. The prodromal stage is an early phase of disease, when signs and symptoms have begun to appear but are mild and not fully expressed. Thus, the disease hasn't reached its full intensity, the body hasn't regained health and homeostasis, nor has the patient begun to recover from illness. CN: Physiological integrity; CNS: Physiological adaptation; CL: Knowledge

6. 4. Most cancers derive from epithelial cells and are called *carcinomas. Glandular* pertains to or of the nature of a gland. The liver is the largest organ in the body. Bone marrow is the soft tissue occupying the medullary cavities of the sternum, long bones, some haversian canals, and spaces between the trabeculae of cancellous or spongy bone. CN: Physiological integrity; CNS: Physiological adaptation; CL: Knowledge

7. 1. About 50% of breast cancers are located in the upper outer quadrant of the breast (not the lower inner quadrant or the upper inner quadrant). The areolar area and nipple area are the second most common sites for tumors to arise. CN: Physiological integrity; CNS: Reduction of risk potential; CL: Application

8. 3. The rectal examination provides a stool sample for performing an occult blood test of feces, which is the simplest and most important screening examination for colorectal cancer. Colorectal cancer is the second most common cause of death from cancer in the U.S. The rectal examination helps in determining whether there are masses in the pelvic region. More extensive examinations are needed for diagnosis of polyps. Proctoscopy is necessary to detect colon cancer. CN: Physiological integrity; CNS: Physiological adaptation; CL: Comprehension

9. 1. Because most melanomas arise from existing moles, he should be most concerned about checking these moles for enlargement or discoloration. Yearly examinations by his family practitioner isn't the best answer, as existing moles can change any time. This would delay diagnosis and intervention, which could lead to a poor outcome. All moles should be monitored for changes in appearance or size, scaliness, oozing, bleeding, itchiness, tenderness, or pain. Development of a nevus (mole) doesn't increase the risk for developing malignant melanoma. CN: Physiological integrity; CNS: Reduction of risk potential; CL: Application

10. 4. Although the exact cause of Hodgkin's disease is unknown, it's believed to involve a virus because many patients with Hodgkin's disease have had infectious mononucleosis. Multiple myeloma is a neoplastic disease characterized by the infiltration of bone and bone marrow by myeloma cells forming multiple tumor masses that lead to pathological fractures. The condition is usually progressive and fatal. It's common in the sixth decade of life. Leukemia is a malignancy of the blood-forming cells in the bone marrow. In most patients, the cause is unknown. Malignant melanoma is a malignant, darkly pigmented mole, or tumor of the skin. Etiology includes excessive exposure to the sun; heredity may also be important. CN: Health promotion and maintenance; CNS: None; CL: Analysis

11. 4. Endotoxins are released when the bacterial cell wall decomposes. Erythrogenic toxins pertain to the development of red blood cells. Exotoxins are poisonous substances produced by certain bacteria, including staphylococci, streptococci, and tetanus bacteria. Neurotoxins are substances that attack nerve cells. CN: Physiological integrity; CNS: Physiological adaptation; CL: Knowledge

12. 2. *Toxoplasma gondii* is commonly found in cat feces and therefore the cat litter; it can cause serious birth defects if the disease is contracted by the mother early in pregnancy. Feline leukemia, contact with cats during the summer flea season, and scratches from cats won't affect the developing human fetus. CN: Physiological integrity; CNS: Reduction of risk potential; CL: Application

13. 3. Salmonellosis commonly follows ingestion of inadequately processed foods, especially chicken, turkey, and duck. Toxoplasmosis is a disease caused by infection with the protozoan *Toxoplasma gondii*. The organism is found in many mammals and birds. Diarrhea isn't a symptom. Typhoid fever is an acute infectious disease caused by *Salmonella typhi* found in infected water or milk supplies. Early symptoms are headache, weakness, indefinite pains, and nosebleed. Botulism is a severe form of food poisoning from foods containing the botulinus toxins produced by *Clostridium botulinum* bacteria, which is found in soil and in the intestinal tract of domestic animals. It's usually associated with improperly canned or preserved foods, especially meats (as ham and sausage) and nonacid vegetables (as string beans). CN: Physiological integrity; CNS: Reduction of risk potential; CL: Analysis

14. 3. Although Type 1 herpes infections usually occur in the skin and mucous membranes around the mouth (or eyes), they can also occur in the genital area. Type 2 herpes infections can occur in either location as well, although more commonly in the genital area. There are two types of herpes simplex virus (HSV): Type 1 and Type 2 (genital herpes). HSV Type 2, usually spread by sexual contact, is classified as a sexually transmitted disease. However, HSV Type 1 can be spread to the genitalia through oral sex. HSV lesions are highly contagious, therefore contact with exudates must be avoided. CN: Physiological integrity; CNS: Reduction of risk potential; CL: Application

15. 3. Infectious mononucleosis usually presents as a sore throat and fever along with fatigue in young adults. Hodgkin's disease is a malignancy that usually begins in lymph nodes of the supraclavicular, high cervical, or mediastinal area. Rubella is a highly infectious, febrile, viral disease common in children; slight sore throat, lymphadenopathy, and rash are the main symptoms. Clinical findings of leukemia include fatigue, lethargy, and fever; bone and joint pain may also be present. CN: Safe, effective care environment; CNS: Reduction of risk potential; CL: Analysis

16. 4. Allergic shiners, headaches, and nasal congestion are typical symptoms of allergic rhinitis and are common in young children and adolescents. Bruises and darkened areas other than near the eyes aren't symptoms of allergic rhinitis. Periods of altered states of consciousness, such as staring off into space, are symptomatic of seizure activity, specifically petit mal seizures. Drug use would likely produce physiologic and behavioral changes well beyond those discussed in this case. CN: Physiological integrity; CNS: Reduction of risk potential; CL: Analysis

17. 1. The single most important medication for this patient is I.M. or subcutaneous epinephrine in a 1:1,000 aqueous solution, 0.1 to 0.5 ml. Aminophylline is used to treat asthma that hasn't responded to epinephrine. It's also used as a stimulant to the respiratory center and heart muscle and as a diuretic. Diphenhydramine is an antihistamine. Methylprednisolone is an adrenal corticosteroid. CN: Physiological integrity; CNS: Reduction of risk potential; CL: Knowledge

18. 3. ELISA is ordered because it's highly sensitive to viral antibodies. However, the test is nonspecific, and it's necessary to follow-up with additional, more specific tests to make sure that the infection is caused by HIV. WBC count measures the number of white blood cells; white cells are leukocytes. Erythrocyte sedimentation rate measures the rate at which erythrocytes settle out of unclotted blood in an hour. The test is based on the fact that inflammatory processes cause an alteration in blood proteins. Serum beta microglobulin measures beta globulins present in blood plasma or serum, the fraction of the blood serum with which antibodies are associated. CN: Physiological integrity; CNS: Reduction of risk potential; CL: Analysis

19. 2. RA usually attacks small, peripheral joints in women ages 35 to 50. Patients with SLE present with a wide diversity of symptoms, but polyarthralgia, polyarthritis, glomerulonephritis, fever, malaise, normocytic anemia, and vasculitis of the hands and feet causing peripheral neuropathy are most common. Osteoarthritis is a type of arthritis marked by progressive cartilage deterioration in synovial joints and vertebrae. Lyme disease is a multisystem disorder caused by the tick-transmitted spirochete *Borrelia burgdor-*

feri. The patient has a skin lesion, flulike symptoms, and headache. CN: Physiological integrity; CNS: Reduction of risk potential; CL: Analysis

20. 4. Cell-mediated immunity is responsible for destroying cells targeted as foreign to the body. Humoral immunity is acquired immunity in which the role of circulating antibody is predominant. Complement system pertains to a group of proteins in the blood that play a vital role in the body's immune defenses through a cascade of alterations. Autoimmunity is the body's tolerance of the antigens present on its own cells. CN: Physiological integrity; CNS: Reduction of risk potential; CL: Knowledge

21. 2. They should both be tested. People of northern European ancestry are more likely to carry the gene and, because the gene is autosomal recessive, the female may carry the gene but not the disease. Cystic fibrosis is a single-gene defect manifesting in multiple body systems. The etiology and primary defect of cystic fibrosis are unknown. There's no way of knowing when the defect will occur. CN: Health promotion and maintenance; CNS: None; CL: Application

22. 1. Adults with Down syndrome have a high incidence of DM. DI is characterized by polyuria and polydipsia caused by inadequate secretion of antidiuretic hormone from the hypothalamus or its release by the posterior pituitary gland. RA is a form of arthritis, the cause of which is unknown, although infection, hypersensitivity, hormone imbalance, and psychological stress have been suggested as possible causes. SIADH isn't associated with Down syndrome. CN: Physiological integrity; CNS: Reduction of risk potential; CL: Analysis

23. 2. The child isn't at risk for hemophilia because an X-linked chromosomal abnormality causes it. The daughter may carry the trait but won't have the disease; classic hemophilia is hereditary and is limited to males. It's always transmitted through the female to the second generation. CN: Physiological integrity; CNS: Reduction of risk potential; CL: Analysis

24. 2. Because sickle cell trait is an autosomal recessive gene, one normal gene will suppress the trait. Thus, there's a 1 in 4 chance that each parent's sickle cell gene will be passed on to the child, who would then have the disease. CN: Physiological integrity; CNS: Reduction of risk potential; CL: Knowledge

25. 4. PKU affects infants in the first few months of life, causing devastating irreversible cerebral damage very quickly. By the time an untreated child begins to show signs of arrested brain development, usually at about 4 months, the damage is significant. Persons with PKU are usually blue-eyed and blond, the skin being excessively sensitive to light. The disorder can be detected at or shortly after birth. The test is required by law in several (not all) states, and the facts presented in this question didn't address where the patient lived. CN: Physiological integrity; CNS: Reduction of risk potential; CL: Application

26. 1. Darkening skin coloration and a craving for salty foods are most specific to Addison's disease. A craving for sweet foods and other carbohydrates would suggest premenstrual syndrome. Weakness and weight loss suggest hyperthyroidism. Buffalo hump and thinning scalp hair are more indicative of Cushing's syndrome. CN: Physiological integrity; CNS: Physiological adaptation; CL: Comprehension

27. 1. A patient with hyperthyroidism has hyperactive reflexes; therefore, you should check the patient's reflexes. Urinalysis isn't a diagnostic test for Graves' disease. Romberg's sign is used to test for sensory ataxia. Checking urine specific gravity won't be diagnostic for Graves' disease. CN: Physiological integrity; CNS: Reduction of risk potential; CL: Analysis

28. 1. The symptoms the patient is exhibiting are those associated with Cushing's syndrome and result from the presence of excess glucocorticoid. Addison's disease results from deficiency in the secretion of adrenocortical hormones. The symptoms are increased pigmentation of skin and mucous membranes, black freckles over the head and neck, fatigue, nausea, vomiting, diarrhea, abdominal discomfort and hypoglycemia. Hyperthyroidism is marked by overactivity of the thyroid gland, which causes tachycardia, nervousness, weight loss, and anxiety. Graves' disease is the most common cause of hyperthyroidism. CN: Physiological integrity; CNS: Physiological adaptation; CL: Analysis

29. 3. A simple goiter is the result of the thyroid gland's increased metabolic activity in response to low levels of iodine or certain types of drugs or food. Inflammation or neoplasm of the thyroid gland is much more serious than a simple goiter. Overproduction of estrogen isn't the hormone that's causing the simple goiter. Overproduction of thyroid hormone isn't likely; the most likely cause is a lack of iodine in the diet. CN: Physiological integrity; CNS: Physiological adaptation; CL: Knowledge

30. 4. Diabetes mellitus produces damage to peripheral nerve fibers, causing the patient to lose sensation in her extremities and making her susceptible to unrecognized trauma and infections. Hashimoto's thyroiditis is a form of autoimmune thyroiditis that affects women eight times more often than men. Diabetes insipidus is exhibited by poluria and polydipsia caused by inadequate secretion of antidiuretic hormone from the hypothalamus or its release by the posterior pituitary gland. Cushing's disease results from hypersecetion of the adrenal cortex in which there's excessive production of glucocorticoids. CN: Physiological integrity; CNS: Reduction of risk potential; CL: Analysis

31. 2. Normal humidifying and warming that take place in the upper airways are interrupted by mechanical ventilation. Therefore, air is warmed and humidified artificially by the ventilator. Gas exchange occurs with exchange of oxygen and carbon dioxide with inspiration and expiration at the alveolar-capillary membrane. Conversion of oxygen to carbon dioxide occurs in the lung tissues. Reflex bronchospasm occurs sometimes during intubation. CN: Physiological integrity; CNS: Physiological adaptation; CL: Knowledge

32. 1. When ventilation is greater than perfusion, the blood supply to the alveoli is decreased. Increased alveolar perfusion indicates increased perfusion of air in the pulmonary alveoli that's involved in the pulmonary exchange of gases. Pulmonary edema occurs when blood backs up from the left atrium of the heart into the lungs. Decreased ventilation indicates decreased, inadequate, or ineffective respiratory exchange. CN: Physiological integrity; CNS: Reduction of risk potential; CL: Analysis

33. 2. Significantly decreased breath sounds on one side aren't typical of COPD and should alert you to the possibility of spontaneous pneumothorax. Crackles in both lung bases indicate fluid in the lung bases. Expiratory wheezing results from constriction or obstruction of the throat, pharynx, trachea, or bronchi. Rhonchi scattered throughout both lung fields result in a coarse, dry crackle in the bronchial tubes. CN: Physiological integrity; CNS: Reduction of risk potential; CL: Analysis

34. 4. Cor pulmonale is defined as hypertrophy and dilation of the right ventricle caused by disease affecting the lungs or pulmonary vasculature. Left-sided heart failure would indicate congestive heart failure, which is the inability of the heart to pump sufficient blood to ensure normal flow through the circulation. Pulmonary hypertension is hypertension in the pulmonary arteries. $\dot{V}/\dot{Q}$ mismatch occurs when there's a pathologic problem that inhibits normal exchange of oxygen and carbon dioxide in the pulmonary alveoli. CN: Physiological integrity; CNS: Physiological adaptation; CL: Knowledge

35. 3. There's increased hydrostatic pressure in the pulmonary capillaries, causing fluid to leak into the interstitial spaces, thus collapsing the alveoli. Perfusion to the lungs that's interrupted by an obstruction of the pulmonary artery or one of its branches is usually caused by an embolus from the thrombosis in a lower extremity. Increased hydrostatic pressure in the capillaries that causes fluid to leak into the alveoli, collapsing them, indicates heart failure. Fluid that accumulates in the lung interstitium, alveolar spaces, and small airways indicates severe refractory heart failure. CN: Physiological integrity; CNS: Physiological adaptation; CL: Comprehension

36. 3. You would measure his blood pressure at rest and again while he slowly inspires to check if the systolic pressure drops more than 15 mm Hg during inspiration. Although the other options are signs of cardiac tamponade, pulsus paradoxus occurs when negative intrathoracic pressure reduces left ventricular filling and stroke volume. Checking to see if his central venous pressure is elevated more that 15 mm Hg above normal would indicate congestive heart failure. Auscultating for muffled heart sounds on inspiration isn't the best method of assessment at this time because a quiet heart with faint sounds usually accompanies only severe tamponade and occurs within minutes of the tamponade. Checking the ECG for reduced amplitude is diagnostic of cardiac tamponade, but may not always be apparent. CN: Physiological integrity; CNS: Reduction of risk potential; CL: Application

37. 1. The compensatory mechanism can be harmful because, as epinephrine and norepinephrine make the heart work harder to beat stronger and faster, the heart's oxygen demand increases. Myocardial cells are depleted of potassium (not calcium), due to use of diuretics. The blood isn't diverted to the extremities, the heart perfuses during diastole, so less volume is ejected to the extremities. The contractility of the heart would hopefully be increased. CN: Physiological integrity; CNS: Physiological adaptation; CL: Analysis

38. 2. Group A beta-hemolytic streptococcal infections can become systemic, causing rheumatic fever. *Staphylococcus aureus* causes suppurative conditions such as boils, carbuncles, and internal abscesses in humans. *Clostridium perfringens* causes gas gangrene. *Pseudomonas aeruginosa* may cause urinary tract infections, otitis externa, or folliculitis, including inflammation that may follow use of a "hot tub." CN: Physiological integrity; CNS: Reduction of risk potential; CL: Knowledge

39. 2. Patients with chronic heart failure frequently develop symptoms of liver failure as venous congestion develops from right-sided heart failure. Cirrhosis is a chronic disease. Symptoms include anorexia; chronic dyspepsia; indigestion; nausea and vomiting; dull, aching abdominal pain; acites; and jaundice. Hepatitis is marked by gradual onset of general malaise, low-grade fever, anorexia, nausea and vomiting, muscle and joint pain, fatigue, headache, dark urine, and clay-colored stools. Acites refers to abdominal distention that occurs from cirrhosis. CN: Physiological integrity; CNS: Reduction of risk potential; CL: Comprehension

40. 4. Chest pain that increases with deep inspiration and is relieved when the patient sits up and leans forward is typically associated with pericarditis. Pneumonia would have decreased or absent breath sounds. In cardiac tamponade, inspiratory heart sounds would be muffled. The chest pain experienced with myocardial infarction isn't positional. CN: Physiological integrity; CNS: Reduction of risk potential; CL: Analysis

41. 1. Signs and symptoms of multiple sclerosis may be transient, or they may last for hours or weeks. They may wax and wane with no predictable pattern. In most patients, vision problems and sensory impairment, such as burning, pins and needles, and electrical sensations, are the first signs that something may be wrong. Associated signs and symptoms include poorly articulated or scanning speech and dysphagia. The average age of onset is 18 to 40, and it occurs most commonly in women from higher socioeconomic classes from northern urban areas. Patients with myasthenia gravis find that certain muscles feel weak and tire quickly on exertion. Muscles frequently affected are those of the face, eyelids, larynx, and throat. Drooping of the eyelids and difficulty chewing or swallowing may be the first symptoms. Symptoms of an aneurysm include generalized abdominal pain, low back pain unaffected by movement, and systolic bruit over the aorta. In Guillain-Barré syndrome, paresthesia usually occurs first, followed by muscle weakness and flaccid paralysis that most commonly ascends from the extremities to the head. CN: Physiological integrity; CNS: Reduction of risk potential; CL: Analysis

42. 4. The autonomic nervous system controls involuntary body functions, including the fight-or-flight response, which causes the mouth to become dry and the heart to beat faster. Somatic pertains to nonreproductive cells or tissues. Extrapyramidal is outside the pyramidal tracts of the central nervous system. Pyramidal is any part of the body resembling a pyramid. CN: Physiological integrity; CNS: Physiological adaptation; CL: Knowledge

43. 4. The brains of patients with Alzheimer's disease may contain as little as 10% of the normal amount of acetylcholine. Dopamine is altered in Parkinson's disease. Serotonin is altered in depression. A disturbance in norepinephrine's metabolism at important brain sites has been implicated in affective disorders. CN: Physiological integrity; CNS: Physiological adaptation; CL: Knowledge

44. 2. Thrombosis is the most common cause of stroke in middle-age and elderly patients. Aneurysm refers to an abnormal dilation of a blood vessel, usually an artery, due to a congenital defect or weakness in the vessel wall. Embolism refers to a mass of undissolved matter present in a blood or lymphatic vessel, brought there by the blood or lymph current. Emboli may be solid, liquid, or gaseous. Hypertension is rarely a direct cause of death. It's more often an indication that there's something wrong, either physically or emotionally, that must be corrected. CN: Physiological integrity; CNS: Reduction of risk potential; CL: Knowledge

45. 2. Sensory type seizures cause hallucinations and vertigo, along with the sensations of seeing flashing lights, experiencing déjà vu, and smelling a particular odor. In absence (petit mal) seizure, activity ceases for a few seconds to several minutes. In Jacksonian seizure, movement "marches" from one part of the body to another. Grand mal seizures involve the whole body. CN: Physiological integrity; CNS: Physiological adaptation; CL: Analysis

46. 3. In response to tissue oxygen deprivation, the kidneys typically release erythropoietin. Patients with chronic renal failure typically lack erythropoietin because of the kidney's inability to respond. Loss of albumin through impaired renal tubular filtration wouldn't cause anemia. Bleeding from damaged tubules would result in gross hematuria, which would also be recognized quickly. Blood loss from hemodialysis would be recognized quickly. CN: Physiological integrity; CNS: Physiological adaptation; CL: Comprehension

47. 1. In leukemia, immature WBCs are overproduced. The immature WBCs crowd normal WBCs and interfere with their production. Polycythemia is an abnormal increase in the erythrocyte count or in hemoglobin concentration. Thrombocytopenia is a decrease in the number of platelets in circulating blood. Multiple myeloma is a primary malignant tumor of bone marrow. CN: Physiological integrity; CNS: Physiological adaptation; CL: Knowledge

48. 2. Platelet destruction caused by the intra-aortic balloon pump most likely caused this patient's thrombocytopenia. Malnutrition would have occurred over a long time. Internal hemorrhage would cause a decrease in the complete red blood cell count. DIC involves bleeding from surgical or invasive procedure sites and bleeding gums, cutaneous oozing, petechia, ecchymoses, and hematomas. CN: Physiological integrity; CNS: Reduction of risk potential; CL: Analysis

49. 2. A platelet count below $150,000/mm^3$ indicates thrombocytopenia. $400,000/mm^3$ is within the normal range. $500,000/mm^3$ is too high. $150,000/mm^3$ is within the normal range. CN: Physiological integrity; CNS: Reduction of risk potential; CL: Knowledge

50. 2. Anticoagulants are administered to combat clot formation in the small blood vessels, which occurs with DIC. Anticoagulants won't prevent emboli formation that may occur as a result of increased clotting factors seen in DIC. Anticoagulants won't prevent clot formation that may develop as blood pools beneath the skin.

Anticoagulants won't prevent thrombus formation that may occur due to bed rest. CN: Physiological integrity; CNS: Reduction of risk potential; CL: Application

51. 4. This patient is at risk for developing cholecystitis. These risk factors predispose a person to gallstones: obesity and a high-calorie, high-cholesterol diet; increased estrogen levels from hormonal contraceptives, HRT, or pregnancy; use of clofibrate, an antilipemic drug; diabetes mellitus; ileal disease; blood disorders; liver disease; or pancreatitis. HRT doesn't increase risk for appendicitis, cirrhosis, or pancreatitis. CN: Physiological integrity; CNS: Reduction of risk potential; CL: Analysis

52. 3. In a patient with newly diagnosed cirrhosis, normal hepatic cells are typically replaced by fibrous, nonfunctional tissue. In later stages of cirrhosis, hepatic cells become distended and misshapen, blood vessels become destroyed, and the cells begin to die. CN: Physiological integrity; CNS: Physiological adaptation; CL: Knowledge

53. 2. Acute pancreatitis causes severe, persistent, piercing abdominal pain, usually in the midepigastric region, although it may be generalized or occur in the left upper quadrant radiating to the back. The pain usually begins suddenly after eating a large meal or drinking alcohol. It increases when the patient lies on his back and is relieved when he rests on his knees and upper chest. Perforated gastric ulcer causes peritonitis, in which the abdomen becomes rigid and sensitive to touch. Fever, vomiting, and extreme weakness is observed. Appendicitis causes right lower quadrant pain. Cholecystitis causes right upper quadrant pain. CN: Physiological integrity; CNS: Physiological adaptation; CL: Analysis

54. 2. Elevated serum amylase and lipase levels are the diagnostic hallmarks that confirm acute pancreatitis. A WBC count usually is ordered to see if infection is present. Hemoglobin measures red blood cell count, which may indicate anemia. Elevated lipid and trypsin levels would appear in stool samples, not serum samples. Total serum bilirubin and indirect bilirubin levels measure liver dysfunction. CN: Physiological integrity; CNS: Reduction of risk potential; CL: Knowledge

55. 3. *H. pylori* releases a toxin that destroys the stomach's mucous lining, reducing the epithelium's resistance to acid digestion and causing gastritis and ulcer disease. *H. pylori* doesn't cause bacteria to colonize the mucous lining, regurgitation of duodenal contents into the stomach, or persistent inflammation of the stomach. CN: Physiological integrity; CNS: Physiological adaptation; CL: Knowledge

56. 4. The kidneys can usually maintain homeostasis with just 25% of their normal functioning capacity. When greater than 75%

of the functioning capacity is destroyed, signs and symptoms of chronic renal failure occur. CN: Physiological integrity; CNS: Physiological adaptation; CL: Knowledge

57. 3. Because the patient suffered a lack of blood flow to the kidneys while in septic shock, he's now experiencing acute tubular necrosis. Early-stage acute tubular necrosis may be difficult to identify because the patient's primary disease may obscure the signs and symptoms. The first recognizable effect may be decreased urine output, usually less than 400 ml/24 hours. An acid-base imbalance is associated with acidosis or alkalosis imbalance and isn't the etiology of septic shock. Blood loss leads to anemia and hypovolemia, but isn't the etiology of septic shock. Dehydration leads to hypovolemia and isn't the etiology of septic shock. CN: Physiological integrity; CNS: Physiological adaptation; CL: Analysis

58. 1. Acute bacterial prostatitis is usually caused by an ascending infection of the urinary tract. Lymphatic migration of pathologic bacteria would circulate in the bloodstream. Prostatic hyperplasia is excessive proliferation of normal cells in the normal tissues of the prostate. An infection in the patient's blood wouldn't be specific to prostatitis. CN: Physiological integrity; CNS: Reduction of risk potential; CL: Comprehension

59. 4. KUB radiography confirms the diagnosis of most renal calculi. CT scan of the abdomen would produce a precise reconstructed image of the abdomen and would show the relationship of structures. MRI of the pelvis provides soft-tissue images of the central nervous and musculoskeltal systems. Cystoscopy of the bladder would examine the bladder only with a cystoscope. CN: Physiological integrity; CNS: Reduction of risk potential; CL: Knowledge

60. 3. Athletes are prone to injury of the diarthroses. These joints include the ankle, wrist, knee, hip, and shoulder. Synarthrosis is a type of joint in which the skeletal elements are united by a continuous intervening substance. Movement is absent or limited. Amphiarthrosis is a form of articulation in which the body surfaces are connected by cartilage; mobility is slight but may be exerted in all directions. Synovial pertains to the lubricating fluid of the joints. CN: Physiological integrity; CNS: Reduction of risk potential; CL: Knowledge

61. 2. Sodium urate forms crystalline deposits in the affected joints. Calcium pyrophosphate, called *pseudogout*, is deposition of calcium phosphate crystals in the joints. Ammonia sulfate is an inorganic chemical compound. Sodium bicarbonate is a white odorless powder, used to treat acidosis. CN: Physiological integrity; CNS: Physiological adaptation; CL: Knowledge

62. 4. Osteoarthritis pain is worse on initial movement and is commonly most exaggerated in an isolated weight-bearing joint. RA is a generalized disease characterized by a persistent synovitis of peripheral joints. SLE is an idiopathic autoimmune disease characterized primarily by fatigue, fever, migratory arthralgia, weight loss, and sicca syndrome. Gouty arthritis presents with acute painful attacks of swelling joints. CN: Physiological integrity; CNS: Physiological adaptation; CL: Analysis

63. 3. This patient is exhibiting signs of respiratory acidosis (excess carbon dioxide retention). It's present when ABG values are pH less than 7.35, HCO_3^- greater than 26 mEq/L (if compensating), and $Paco_2$ greater than 45 mm Hg. Metabolic acidosis is a state in which the blood pH is low (under 7.35), due to increased production of H by the body or the inability of the body to form bicarbonate (HCO) in the kidney. Metabolic alkalosis depletes the body of hydrogen (H) ions leading to an increase of bicarbonate in the body. The pH is high (greater than 7.35). Respiratory alkalosis is a state in which the blood pH is high (greater than 7.35) due to increased levels of carbon dioxide "blown" off by the lungs, which are hyperventilating. CN: Physiological integrity; CNS: Reduction of risk potential; CL: Analysis

64. 4. These ABG results reveal metabolic alkalosis. Metabolic acidosis is present when ABG results show pH greater than 7.45, HCO_3^- greater than 26 mEq/L, and $Paco_2$ greater than 45 mm Hg (if compensating). Respiratory acidosis is diagnosed when pH is less than 7.35 with a $Paco_2$ greater than 45 mm Hg. Respiratory alkalosis is diagnosed when the pH is greater than 7.45 with a $Paco_2$ less than 35 mm Hg. Metabolic acidosis is diagnosed when pH is less than 7.35 and the bicarbonate level (HCO_3^-) is less than 22 mEq/L. CN: Physiological integrity; CNS: Reduction of risk potential; CL: Analysis

65. 2. Inadequate excretion of acids as a result of renal disease can cause metabolic acidosis. CNS depression from drugs would cause respiratory acidosis. Gram-negative bacteremia would be associated with respiratory alkalosis. Asphyxia would cause respiratory acidosis. CN: Physiological integrity; CNS: Reduction of risk potential; CL: Analysis

66. 1. In patients with essentially normal lung tissue, acute respiratory failure usually presents with $Paco_2$ above 50 mm Hg and Pao_2 below 50 mm Hg. These limits, however, don't apply to patients with chronic obstructive pulmonary disease (COPD), who usually have a consistently high $Paco_2$. In patients with COPD, only acute deterioration in arterial blood gas values, with corresponding clinical deterioration, indicates acute respiratory failure. A patient with severe acute respiratory syndrome would have a $Paco_2$ above 50 mm Hg and a $Paco_2$ below 50 mm Hg but the lung tissue wouldn't be essentially normal. A patient with asthma would have a $Paco_2$ greater than 50 mm Hg and a $Paco_2$ less than 50 mm Hg, but the lung tissue wouldn't be normal. A patient with cor pulmonale would have decreased perfusion of the heart, which could lead to a $Paco_2$ below 50 mm Hg, but the lungs are compromised. CN: Physiological integrity; CNS: Physiological adaptation; CL: Analysis

67. 4. One factor may be low intake of dietary fiber. High-fiber diets increase stool bulk, thereby decreasing the wall tension in the colon. High wall tension is thought to increase the risk of developing diverticula. Low intake of dietary protein is associated with lower bone mineral density and greater risk of fractures. High intake of dietary fiber increases risk of kidney abnormalities. High dietary intake of saturated fat increases cholesterol. CN: Physiological integrity; CNS: Reduction of risk potential; CL: Analysis

68. 4. In chronic diverticulitis, signs and symptoms include constipation, ribbonlike stools, intermittent diarrhea, abdominal distention, abdominal rigidity and pain, diminishing or absent bowel sounds, nausea, and vomiting. Diverticulosis is associated with abdominal cramps, bloating, and constipation. Mild diverticulitis is characterized by abdominal pain, vomiting, chills, and constipation. In severe diverticulitis the symptoms depend on the extent of infection and complications. Symptoms include severe abdominal pain, vomiting, chills, and constipation. CN: Physiological integrity; CNS: Physiological adaptation; CL: Knowledge

69. 1. In GERD, the sphincter doesn't remain closed (usually due to deficient lower esophageal sphincter [LES] pressure or pressure within the stomach that exceeds LES pressure), and the pressure in the stomach pushes the stomach contents into the esophagus. The high acidity of the stomach contents causes pain and irritation when it enters the esophagus. Mucosa that takes on a "cobblestone" appearance could be related to many conditions other than GERD. A defect in the diaphragm that permits a portion of the stomach to pass through the esophageal hiatus into the chest cavity is a hiatal hernia. Destruction of the stomach's mucous lining by *H. pylori* is diagnostic of an ulcer. CN: Physiological integrity; CNS: Physiological adaptation; CL: Comprehension

70. 3. The acid-perfusion test confirms esophagitis and distinguishes it from cardiac disorders. Esophageal manometry measures pressure within the esophagus. Barium swallow is used to determine the cause of painful swallowing. Upper GI series is used to diagnose problems in the esophagus. CN: Physiological integrity; CNS: Reduction of risk potential; CL: Knowledge

71. 2. Osteomyelitis occurs more commonly in children (particularly boys) than in adults—usually as a complication of an acute localized infection. Osteoarthritis occurs more commonly in adults. Osteomalacia is the adult equivalent of the disease rickets. Osteoporosis occurs more commonly in older adults. CN: Physiological integrity; CNS: Reduction of risk potential; CL: Knowledge

72. 1. While each of these organisms causes osteomyelitis, the most common causative organism is *S. aureus. Streptococcus pyogenes* is a common bacterium of the skin. *Pseudomonas aeruginosa* is the most common organism in urinary tract, respiratory, skin, bone, and joint infections. *Proteus vulgaris* commonly causes urinary and hospital-acquired infections. CN: Physiological integrity; CNS: Reduction of risk potential; CL: Knowledge

73. 4. Pulmonary embolism generally results from dislodged thrombi originating in the leg veins or pelvis. In sickle cell disease, the red blood cell changes shape upon deoxygenation. A foreign substance is the "invader" into the body system. A heart valve growth would be "attached" to the heart valve. CN: Physiological integrity; CNS: Reduction of risk potential; CL: Knowledge

74. 1, 2, 4, 5. SARS begins with a high fever (usually a temperature greater than 100.4° F [38° C]), chills, and achiness. Patients develop respiratory symptoms 4 to 7 days after the onset of fever. Respiratory symptoms can be mild to severe and include dry cough, shortness of breath, hypoxemia, and pneumonia. As many as 20% of patients develop diarrhea. A sudden onset of chest pain wouldn't be associated with SARS, but is associated with cardiovascular etiology. Neck stiffness is associated with infection or musculoskeletal conditions. CN: Physiological integrity; CNS: Physiological adaptation; CL: Analysis

75. 1, 2, 3, 4. With rhabdomyolysis, myoglobin, potassium, CK, and urate are released from the necrotic muscle fibers into the circulation. Sodium is located in the blood and the space surrounding the cells. Calcium is located mostly in the teeth and bones. CN: Physiological integrity; CNS: Physiological adaptation; CL: Application

76. 2, 4, 5, 6. Severely elevated CK level, hypocalcemia (in early stages), elevated serum creatinine level, elevated intracompartmental venous pressure, and urine myoglobin level greater than 0.5 mg/dl are all findings that help to confirm the diagnosis of rhabdomyolysis. Elevated cardiac troponin level indicates myocardial tissue damage. Hypercalcemia (in early stages) primarily indicates hyperparathyroidism and malignancy. CN: Physiological integrity; CNS: Physiological adaptation; CL: Knowledge

77.

4.	Muscle trauma compresses tissue.

5.	Tissue ischemia and necrosis occur.

1.	Local edema increases compartment pressure and tamponade.

2.	Pressure from severe swelling causes blood vessels to collapse.

3.	Substances are released from the necrotic muscle fibers into the circulation.

Muscle trauma that compresses tissue causes ischemia and necrosis. The ensuing local edema further increases compartment pressure and tamponade; pressure from severe swelling causes blood vessels to collapse, leading to tissue hypoxia, muscle infarction, and neural damage in the area of the fracture. Myoglobin, potassium, creatine kinase, and urate are released from the necrotic muscle fibers into the circulation. Local edema increases compartment pressure and tamponade. Pressure from severe swelling causes blood vessels to collapse. Substances are released from the necrotic muscle fibers into the circulation. CN: Physiological integrity; CNS: Physiological adaptation; CL: Analysis

78. The LES is located under the diaphragm. CN: Physiological integrity; CNS: Physiological adaptation; CL: Analysis

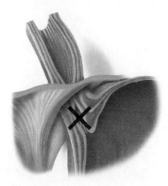

79. 1.2

First, calculate the patient's weight in kilograms by using the conversion factor 1 kg = 2.2 lb:

$$\frac{1\text{ kg}}{2.2\text{ lb}} = \frac{X\text{ kg}}{176\text{ lb}}$$

Cross multiply and divide both sides by 2.2:

$$2.2X = 176$$

$$X = 80$$

Next, determine how many milligrams of phenytoin would be given:

$$15\text{ mg} \times 80\text{ kg} = 1,200\text{ mg}$$

Finally, convert milligrams to grams:

$$1,200\text{ mg} \div 1,000 = 1.2\text{ g}$$

CN: Physiological integrity; CNS: Pharmacological and parenteral therapies; CL: Application

Less common disorders

Disease and causes	Pathophysiology	Signs and symptoms
Amyloidosis • Pressure caused by accumulation and infiltration of amyloid that leads to atrophy of nearby cells; abnormal immunoglobulin synthesis and reticuloendothelial cell dysfunction may occur • Familial inheritance in persons with Portuguese ancestry	A rare, chronic disease of abnormal fibrillar scleroprotein accumulation that infiltrates body organs and soft tissues. Perireticular type affects the inner coats of blood vessels whereas pericollagen type affects the outer coats. Amyloidosis can result in permanent, even life-threatening, organ damage.	• Proteinuria, leading to nephrotic syndrome and eventually to renal failure • Heart failure caused by cardiomegaly, arrhythmias, and amyloid deposits in subendocardium, endocardium, and myocardium • Stiffness and enlargement of tongue, decreased intestinal motility, malabsorption, bleeding, abdominal pain, constipation, and diarrhea • Appearance of peripheral neuropathy • Liver enlargement, usually with azotemia, anemia, albuminuria and, rarely, jaundice
Ankylosing spondylitis • No known cause; strongly associated with presence of human leukocyte antigen-B27 • Familial inheritance	Fibrous tissue of the joint capsule is infiltrated by inflammatory cells that erode the bone and fibrocartilage. Repair of the cartilaginous structures begins with the proliferation of fibroblasts, which synthesize and secrete collagen. The collagen forms fibrous scar tissue that eventually undergoes calcification and ossification, causing the joint to fuse or lose flexibility.	• Intermittent lower back pain that's most severe after inactivity or in the morning • Stiffness, limited lumbar spine motion • Pleuritic pain and limited expansion of chest • Peripheral arthritis in shoulders, hips, and knees • Kyphosis in advanced stages • Hip deformity and limited range of motion • Mild fatigue, low-grade fever, and anorexia or weight loss
Anthrax • Infection of the skin, lungs, or GI tract that results from contact with *Bacillus anthracis* spores	After infection, bacterium produces toxins that enter susceptible cells, leading to cell death; mechanism unknown.	Incubation is 12 hours to 5 days • Red-brown bump on skin enlarges and swells around edges; a black scab forms after the bump blisters and hardens • Swollen lymph nodes • Muscle ache and headache • Nausea, vomiting, fever **IN PULMONARY ANTHRAX:** • Respiratory problems that may progress to respiratory failure • Shock and coma **IN GI ANTHRAX (RARE):** • Extensive bleeding; tissue death • Fatal if enters the bloodstream

Disease and causes	Pathophysiology	Signs and symptoms
Aspergillosis • Fungal infection caused by *Aspergillus* species; transmitted by inhalation of fungal spores or invasion of spores through wounds or injured tissue	*Aspergillus* species produce extracellular enzymes, such as proteases and peptidases that contribute to tissue invasion, leading to hemorrhage and necrosis.	Incubation is a few days to weeks • May produce no symptoms or mimic tuberculosis, causing a productive cough and purulent or blood-tinged sputum, dyspnea, empyema, and lung abscesses **ALLERGIC ASPERGILLOSIS:** • Wheezing, dyspnea, pleural pain, and fever **ASPERGILLOSIS ENDOPHTHALMITIS:** • Appears 2 to 3 weeks after eye surgery • Cloudy vision, eye pain, and reddened conjunctiva • Purulent exudate in anterior and posterior chambers of the eye
Bell's palsy • Considered an idiopathic facial paralysis; infectious cause suggested	Blockage of the seventh cranial nerve due to inflammation around the nerve where it leaves bony tissue leads to unilateral or bilateral facial weakness or paralysis. The blockage may result from hemorrhage, tumor, meningitis, or local trauma.	• Unilateral facial weakness or paralysis, with aching at the jaw angle • Drooping mouth, causing salivation • Distorted taste • Impaired ability to fully close the eye on the affected side • Loss of taste and tinnitus
Botulism • Paralytic illness caused by an endotoxin produced by *Clostridium botulinum*; commonly caused by consumption of inadequately cooked, contaminated foods	The endotoxin acts at the neuromuscular junction of skeletal muscle, preventing acetylcholine release and blocking neural transmission, eventually resulting in paralysis.	Appears 12 to 36 hours after digesting food; severity depends on amount consumed **INITIAL SIGNS:** • Dry mouth, sore throat, weakness, dizziness, vomiting, and diarrhea **CARDINAL SIGNS:** • Acute symmetrical cranial nerve impairment, followed by weakness and muscle paralysis • Mental or sensory processes not typically affected; if they are affected, they're usually associated with fever
Bronchiectasis • Conditions associated with continued damage to bronchial walls and abnormal mucociliary clearance cause tissue breakdown to adjacent airways; such conditions include cystic fibrosis, immunologic disorders, and recurrent bacterial respiratory tract infections	Inflammation and destruction of the structural components of the bronchial wall lead to chronic abnormal dilation.	**IN EARLY STAGES:** • Asymptomatic with complaints of frequent pneumonia or hemoptysis • Chronic cough producing foul-smelling, mucopurulent secretions • Coarse crackles during inspiration • Wheezing, dyspnea, sinusitis, fever, and chills

Disease and causes	Pathophysiology	Signs and symptoms
Bronchiectasis (continued)		**IN ADVANCED STAGE:** • Chronic malnutrition and right-sided heart failure caused by hypoxic pulmonary vasoconstriction
Bronchiolitis • No known cause; may be associated with specific diseases or conditions, such as bone marrow, heart, or lung transplantation; rheumatoid arthritis; lupus erythematosus	Infection or other unknown factors cause necrosis of the bronchial epithelium and destruction of ciliated epithelial cells. As the submucosa becomes edematous, cellular debris and fibrin form plugs in the bronchioles.	**SUBACUTE SYMPTOMS:** • Fever, persistent nonproductive cough, dyspnea, malaise, and anorexia • Physical assessment reveals dry crackles **LESS COMMON:** • Productive cough, hemoptysis, chest pain, general aches, and night sweats
Celiac disease • Also called *gluten-sensitive enteropathy* or *celiac sprue*; results from a complex interaction involving dietary, genetic, and immunologic factors	Ingestion of gluten causes atrophy of the villi in the upper small intestine, leading to a decreased surface area and malabsorption of most nutrients. Inflammatory enteritis also results, leading to osmotic diarrhea and secretory diarrhea.	• Recurrent diarrhea, steatorrhea, abdominal distention, stomach cramps, weakness, or increased appetite without weight gain • Normochromic, hypochromic, or macrocytic anemia • Osteomalacia, osteoporosis, tetany, and bone pain in lower back, rib cage, and pelvis • Peripheral neuropathy, paresthesia, or seizures • Amenorrhea, hypometabolism • Mood changes and irritability
Cholera • Acute enterotoxin-mediated GI infection caused by gram-negative bacillus, which is transmitted through water and food that's contaminated with fecal material from carriers or people with active infections	After ingestion of a significant inoculum, colonization of the small intestine occurs. The secretion of a potent enterotoxin results in a massive outpouring of isotonic fluid from the mucosal surface of the small intestine. Profuse diarrhea, vomiting, fluid and electrolyte loss occurs and may lead to hypovolemic shock, metabolic acidosis, and death.	Incubation period is several hours to 5 days • Acute, painless, profuse watery diarrhea, and vomiting • Intense thirst, weakness, and loss of skin tone • Muscle cramps • Cyanosis • Oliguria • Tachycardia • Falling blood pressure, fever, and hypoactive bowel sounds
Creutzfeldt-Jakob disease • Rare form of dementia • Prion infection	Organism infects the central nervous system, leading to myelin destruction and neuronal loss.	• Myoclonic jerking, ataxia, aphasia, vision disturbances, paralysis, and early abnormal EEG

Disease and causes	Pathophysiology	Signs and symptoms
Endocarditis • Infection of the endocardium of the heart caused by bacteria, viruses, fungi, rickettsiae, or parasites	Endothelial damage allows microorganisms to adhere to the surface, where they proliferate and promote the propagation of endocardial vegetation.	• Weakness and fatigue • Weight loss, fever, night sweats, and anorexia • Arthralgia, splenomegaly, and new systolic murmur • Heart failure
Esophageal varices • Portal hypertension	Shunting of blood to the venae cavae caused by portal hypertension, leading to dilation of esophageal veins.	• Hemorrhage and subsequent hypotension • Compromised oxygen supply • Altered level of consciousness
Fanconi's syndrome • Inherited renal tubular transport disorder	Changes in the proximal renal tubules caused by atrophy of epithelial cells and loss of proximal tube volume result in a shortened connection to glomeruli by an unusually narrow segment. Malfunction of the proximal renal tubules leads to hyperkalemia, hypernatremia, glycosuria, phosphaturia, aminoaciduria, uricosuria, retarded growth, and rickets.	Mostly normal appearance at birth with slightly lower birth weights • After 6 months: weakness, failure to thrive, dehydration, cystine crystals in the corners of the eye, and retinal pigment degeneration • Yellow skin with little pigmentation • Slow linear growth
Hypersplenism • Increased activity of the spleen, where all types of blood cells are removed from circulation due to chronic myelogenous leukemia, lymphomas, Gaucher's disease, hairy cell leukemia, or sarcoidosis	Spleen growth may be stimulated by an increase in its workload, such as the trapping and destroying of abnormal red blood cells.	• Enlarged spleen • Cytopenia
Idiopathic pulmonary fibrosis • Chronic progressive lung disease associated with inflammation and fibrosis • No known cause	Interstitial inflammation made up of an alveolar septal infiltrate of lymphocytes, plasma cells, and histiocytes. Fibrotic areas are composed of dense acellular collagen. Areas of honeycombing that form are composed of cystic fibrotic air spaces, commonly lined with bronchiolar epithelium and filled with mucus. Smooth muscle hyperplasia may occur in areas of fibrosis and honeycombing.	• Dyspnea • Nonproductive cough • Chest heaviness • Wheezing • Anorexia • Weight loss

Disease and causes	Pathophysiology	Signs and symptoms
Kaposi's sarcoma • Acquired immunodeficiency syndrome–related cancer	A malignant cancer arising from vascular endothelial cells, Kaposi's sarcoma affects endothelial tissue, which compromises all blood vessels.	• Red-purple circular lesions, slightly raised on the face, arms, neck, and legs • Internal lesions, especially in GI tract and brain, identified by biopsy
Keratitis • Inflammation of cornea caused by bacteria or viruses	Infection leading to ulceration of the cornea.	• Decreased visual acuity • Pain and tearing • Photophobia
Kyphosis • An excessive anteroposterior curving of the spine caused by a congenital anomaly, malignant or compression fracture, arthritis, or spondylitis	Pathophysiology is related to causative factor.	• Abnormally rounded thoracic curve
Latex allergy • Hypersensitivity to products containing natural latex	Latex protein allergens trigger release of histamine and other mediators of the systemic allergic cascade in sensitized persons.	• Local dermatitis to anaphylactic reaction
Legionnaires' disease • Infection caused by gram-negative bacillus, *Legionella pneumophila*	Transmission of disease occurs with inhalation of organism carried in aerosols produced by air-conditioning units, water faucets, shower heads, humidifiers, and contaminated respiratory equipment.	• Dry cough • Myalgia • GI distress • Pneumonia • Cardiovascular collapse
Leprosy • Also know as *Hansen's disease*; infection caused by *Mycobacterium leprae*	Chronic, systemic infection with progressive cutaneous lesions that attacks the peripheral nervous system.	• Skin lesions • Anesthesia • Muscle weakness • Paralysis
Medullary sponge kidney • Genetic disorder	Collecting ducts in the renal pyramids dilate, forming cavities, clefts, and cysts that produce such complications as calcium oxylate calculi and infections.	• Renal calculi • Hematuria • Infection (fever, chills, and malaise)

Disease and causes	Pathophysiology	Signs and symptoms
Myocarditis • Inflammation of the myocardium caused by bacterial, fungal, viral, or protozoal infections; heat stroke; ionizing radiation; or rheumatic fever	Initial infection triggers an autoimmune, cellular and, possibly, humoral response resulting in myocardial inflammation and necrosis.	• Rapid, irregular, and weak pulse • Chest tenderness • First heart sound resembles second heart sound • Fatigue
Neurofibromatosis • Inherited disorder	Group of developmental disorders of the nervous system, muscles, bones, and skin that affects the cell growth of neural tissue.	• Café-au-lait spots • Multiple, pediculated, soft tumors • Hearing loss
Osgood-Schlatter disease • No known cause	Osteochondrosis of the tibia; disease of the growth or ossification centers in children.	• Frequent fractures • Pain at inferior aspect of patella
Pediculosis • Infestation by the lice parasite	Ectoparasite that attaches itself to the hair shaft with claws, and feeds on blood several times daily; resides close to the scalp to maintain its body temperature. Itching may be caused by an allergic reaction to louse saliva or irritability.	• Itching • Eczematous dermatitis • Inflammation • Irritability • Lice present in hair (head, axillary, and pubic)
Pheochromocytoma • Polyglandular multiple endocrine neoplasia	Tumor of the chromaffin cells of the adrenal medulla that causes an increased production of catecholamines.	• Hypertension • High blood glucose • High lipid levels • Headache • Palpitations • Sweating • Dizziness • Constipation • Anxiety
Pleurisy • Several causes, including lupus, rheumatoid arthritis, and tuberculosis	Inflammation of the pleura with exudation into the thoracic cavity and lung surface.	• Chilliness • Stabbing chest pain • Fever • Suppressed cough • Pallor • Dyspnea

Disease and causes	Pathophysiology	Signs and symptoms
Polycythemia vera • No known cause; possibly caused by a multipotential stem cell defect	Increased production of red blood cells, neutrophils, and platelets inhibits blood flow to microcirculation, resulting in intravascular thrombosis.	Usually no symptoms in early stages In later stages, related to expanded blood volume and system affected • Weakness, light-headedness, headache, vision disturbances, and fatigue • Hepatomegaly and splenomegaly
Pyloric stenosis • Congenital; no known cause	Pyloric sphincter muscle fibers thicken and become inelastic, leading to a narrowed opening. The extra peristaltic effort that's necessary leads to hypertrophied muscle layers of the stomach.	• Progressive nonbilious vomiting, leading to projectile vomiting at ages 2 to 4 weeks
Retinal detachment • Caused by trauma; can also occur after cataract surgery, severe uveitis, and primary or metastatic choroidal tumors	The neural retina separates from the underlying retinal pigment epithelium.	• Floaters, flashing lights, scotoma in peripheral visual field (painless) and, eventually, a curtain or veil occurs in the field of vision
Retinitis pigmentosa • Autosomal recessive disorder in 80% of affected children • Less commonly transmitted as an X-linked trait	Slow, degenerative changes in the rods cause the retina and pigment epithelium to atrophy. Irregular black deposits of clumped pigment are in equatorial region of retina and eventually in the macular and peripheral areas.	• Progressive night blindness, visual field constriction with ring scotoma, and loss of acuity progressing to blindness
Reye's syndrome • No known cause • Viral agents and drugs (especially salicylates) have been implicated	Mitochondrial dysfunction and fatty vacuolization of the liver and renal tubules leading to hepatic injury and central nervous system damage.	• Vomiting • Change in mental status progressing rapidly from lethargy to disorientation to coma
Rocky Mountain spotted fever • Infection caused by *Rickettsia rickettsii* carried by several tick species	*R. rickettsii* multiply within endothelial cells and spread through the bloodstream. Focal areas of infiltration lead to thrombosis and leakage of red blood cells into surrounding tissue.	• Fever, headache, mental confusion, and myalgia • Rash develops as small macules progress to maculopapules and petechiae (Initially, rash starts on wrists and ankles and spreads to trunk. A rash noted on palms and soles is especially diagnostic.)

Disease and causes	Pathophysiology	Signs and symptoms
Sarcoidosis • No known cause • Evidence suggests that the disease is the result of exaggerated cellular immune response to a limited class of antigens	Organ dysfunction results from an accumulation of T lymphocytes, mononuclear phagocytes, and nonsecreting epithelial granulomas, which distort normal tissue architecture.	• Mainly generalized, most commonly involving the lung, with resulting respiratory symptoms • Fever, fatigue, and malaise
Scabies • Human itch mite (*Sarcoptes scabiei* var. *hominis*)	Mite burrows superficially beneath stratum corneum, depositing eggs that hatch, mature, and reinvade the skin.	Occur from sensitization reaction against excreta that mites deposit • Intense itching, worsens at night; threadlike lesions on wrists, between fingers, and on elbows, axillae, belt line, buttocks, and male genitalia
Sjögren's syndrome • Autoimmune rheumatic disorder with no known cause; genetic and environmental factors may be involved	Lymphocytic infiltration of exocrine glands causes tissue damage that results in xerostomia and dry eyes.	IN XEROSTOMIA: • Dry mouth; difficulty swallowing and speaking; ulcers on the tongue, buccal mucosa and lips; severe dental caries IN OCULAR INVOLVEMENT: • Dry eyes; gritty, sandy feeling; decreased tearing; burning, itching, redness; and photosensitivity EXTRAGLANDULAR: • Arthralgias, Raynaud's phenomenon, lymphadenopathy, and lung involvement
Strabismus • Eye malalignment that's frequently inherited; controversy exists whether amblyopia is caused by or results from strabismus	In paralytic (nonconcomitant) strabismus, paralysis of one or more ocular muscles may be caused by an oculomotor nerve lesion. In nonparalytic (concomitant) strabismus, unequal ocular muscle tone is caused by supranuclear abnormality within the central nervous system.	• Eye malalignment noticeable by external eye examination, ophthalmoscopic observation of the corneal light reflex in center of pupils, diplopia, and other vision disturbances
Thrombocythemia • *Primary:* no known cause • *Secondary:* caused by chronic inflammatory disorders, iron deficiency, acute infection, neoplasm, hemorrhage, or postsplenectomy	A clonal abnormality of a multipotent hematopoietic stem cell results in increased platelet production, although platelet survival is usually normal. If combined with degenerative vascular disease, may lead to serious bleeding or thrombosis.	• Weakness, hemorrhage, nonspecific headache, paresthesia, dizziness, and easy bruising

Disease and causes	Pathophysiology	Signs and symptoms
Thrombophlebitis • Caused by endothelial damage, accelerated blood clotting, and reduced blood flow	Alteration in epithelial lining causes platelet aggregation and fibrin entrapment of red blood cells, white blood cells, and additional platelets; the thrombus initiates a chemical inflammatory process in the vessel epithelium that leads to fibrosis, which may occlude the vessel lumen or embolize.	• Varies with site and length of affected vein • Affected area usually extremely tender, swollen, red, and warm to the touch
Trigeminal neuralgia • No known cause; possibly a compression neuropathy • At surgery or autopsy, the intracranial arterial and venous loops are found to compress the trigeminal nerve root at the brain stem	Painful disorder along the distribution of one or more of the trigeminal nerve's sensory divisions, most commonly the maxillary.	• Searing or burning pain lasting seconds to 2 minutes at the trigeminal nerve distribution • Touching a trigger point typically elicits pain
Vitiligo • No known cause; usually acquired but may be familial (autosomal dominant) • Possible immunologic and neurochemical basis suggested	Destruction of melanocytes (humoral or cellular) and circulating antibodies against melanocytes results in hypopigmented areas.	• Progressive, symmetrical areas of complete pigment loss with sharp borders, generally appearing in periorificial areas, flexor wrists, and extensor distal extremities
Wilson's disease • Inherited copper toxicosis	Defective mobilization of copper from hepatocellular lysosomes for excretion by way of bile allows excessive copper retention in the liver, brain, kidneys, and corneas, leading to tissue necrosis and subsequent hepatic and neurologic disorders.	• *Kayser-Fleischer ring:* Rusty brown ring of pigment at periphery of corneas • Signs of hepatitis leading to cirrhosis • Tremors, unsteady gait, muscular rigidity, inappropriate behavior, and psychosis • Hematuria, proteinuria, and uricosuria

Glossary

acute illness: sudden onset of illness having severe symptoms and a short course

agranulocyte: leukocyte (white blood cell) not made up of granules or grains; includes lymphocytes, monocytes, and plasma cells

allele: one of two or more different genes that occupy a corresponding position (locus) on matched chromosomes; allows for different forms of the same inheritable characteristic

allergen: substance that induces an allergy or a hypersensitivity reaction

anaphylaxis: severe allergic reaction to a foreign substance

androgen: steroid hormone that stimulates male characteristic (The two main androgens are androsterone and testosterone.)

anemia: reduction in the number and volume of red blood cells, the amount of hemoglobin, or the volume of packed red cells

aneurysm: sac formed by the dilation of the wall of an artery, a vein, or the heart

angiography: radiographic visualization of blood vessels after injection of radiopaque contrast material

anoxia: absence of oxygen in the tissues

antibody: immunoglobulin molecule that reacts only with the specific antigen that induced its formation in the lymph system

antigen: foreign substance such as bacteria or toxins that induces antibody formation

antitoxin: antibody produced in response to a toxin that's capable of neutralizing the toxin's effects

atrophy: decrease in size of a cell, tissue, organ, or body part

autoimmune disorder: disorder in which the body launches an immunologic response against itself

autosome: any chromosome other than the sex chromosomes (Twenty-two of the human chromosome pairs are autosomes.)

bacterium: one-celled microorganism that breaks down dead tissue, has no true nucleus, and reproduces by cell division

baroreceptor: receptor that responds to changes in pressure

benign: not malignant or recurrent; favorable for recovery

bone marrow: soft organic material filling the cavities of bones

bursa: fluid-filled sac or cavity found in connecting tissue in the vicinity of joints; acts as a cushion

calculus: any abnormal concentration, usually made up of mineral salts, within the body; for example, gallstones and renal calculi

carcinogen: substance that causes cancer

carcinoma: malignant growth made up of epithelial cells that tends to infiltrate surrounding tissues and metastasize

cardiac output: volume of blood ejected from the heart per minute

cartilage: dense connective tissue made up of fibers embedded in a strong, gel-like substance; supports, cushions, and shapes body structures

cell: smallest living component of an organism; the body's basic building block

cholestasis: stopped or decreased bile flow

chondrocyte: cartilage cell

chromosome: linear thread in a cell's nucleus that contains deoxyribonucleic acid; occurs in pairs in humans

chronic illness: illness of long duration that includes remission and exacerbation

clearance: complete removal of a substance by the kidneys from a specific volume of blood per unit of time

coagulant: substance that promotes, accelerates, or permits blood clotting

collagen: main supportive protein of skin, tendon, bone, cartilage, and connective tissue

colonoscopy: examination of the upper portion of the rectum with an elongated speculum or colonoscope to visualize the colon, remove polyps, or biopsy suspicious growths

compensation: the counterbalancing of any defect in structure or function; measure of how long the heart takes to adapt to increased blood in ventricles

complement system: major mediator of inflammatory response; a functionally related system made up of 20 proteins circulating as functionally inactive molecules

cytoplasm: aqueous mass within a cell that contains organelles, is surrounded by the cell membrane, and excludes the nucleus

cytotoxic: destructive to cells

degeneration: nonlethal cell damage occurring in the cell's cytoplasm while the nucleus remains unaffected

demyelination: destruction of a nerve's myelin sheath, which interferes with normal nerve conduction

deoxyribonucleic acid (DNA): complex protein in the cell's nucleus that carries genetic material and is responsible for cellular reproduction

differentiation: process of cells maturing into specific types

disease: pathologic condition that occurs when the body can't maintain homeostasis

disjunction: separation of chromosomes that occurs during cell division

distal: farthest away

diverticulitis: inflammation of one or more diverticula in the muscular layer of the colon

dominant gene: gene that expresses itself even if it's carried on only one homologous (matched) chromosome

dyscrasia: a condition related to a disease, usually referring to an imbalance of component elements (A blood dyscrasia is a disorder of cellular elements of the blood.)

dysphagia: difficulty swallowing

dysplasia: abnormal development of tissue

embolism: sudden obstruction of a blood vessel by foreign substances or a blood clot

endemic: disease of low morbidity that occurs continuously in a particular patient population or geographic area

endochondral ossification: process in which cartilage hardens into bone

endocrine: pertaining to internal hormone secretion by glands (Endocrine glands, including the pineal gland, the islets of Langerhans in the pancreas, the gonads, the thymus, and the adrenal, pituitary, thyroid, and parathyroid glands secrete hormones directly into circulation.)

endogenous: occurring inside the body

erythrocyte: red blood cell; carries oxygen to the tissues and removes carbon dioxide from them

erythropoiesis: production of red blood cells or erythrocytes

estrogen: female sex hormone produced by the ovaries; produces female characteristics

etiology: cause of a disease

exacerbation: increase in the severity of a disease or any of its symptoms

exocrine: external or outward secretion of a gland (Exocrine glands discharge through ducts opening on an external or internal surface of the body; they include the liver, the pancreas, the prostate, and the salivary, sebaceous, sweat, gastric, intestinal, mammary, and lacrimal glands.)

exogenous: occurring outside the body

fasciculation: involuntary twitching or contraction of the muscle

fungus: nonphotosynthetic microorganism that reproduces asexually by cell division

gland: specialized cell cluster that produces a secretion used in some other body part

glomerulus: a network of twisted capillaries in the nephron, the basic unit of the kidney; brings blood and waste products carried by blood to the nephron

glucagon: hormone released during the fasting state that increases blood glucose concentration

granulocyte: any cell containing granules, especially a granular leukocyte (white blood cell)

hematopoiesis: production of red blood cells in the bone marrow

hemoglobin: iron-containing pigment in red blood cells that carries oxygen from the lungs to the tissues

hemolysis: red blood cell destruction

hemorrhage: escape of blood from a ruptured vessel

hemostasis: complex process whereby platelets, plasma, and coagulation factors interact to control bleeding

heterozygous genes: genes having different alleles at the same site (locus) (If each gene in a chromosome pair produces a different effect, the genes are heterozygous.)

homeostasis: dynamic, steady state of internal balance in the body

homologous genes: gene pairs sharing a corresponding structure and position

homozygous genes: genes that have identical alleles for a given trait (When each gene at a corresponding locus produces the same effect, the genes are homozygous.)

hormone: chemical substance produced in the body that has a specific regulatory effect on the activity of specific cells or organs

host defense system: elaborate network of safeguards that protects the body from infectious organisms and other harmful invaders

hyperplasia: excessive growth of normal cells that causes an increase in the volume of a tissue or organ

hypersensitivity disorder: state in which the body produces an exaggerated immune response to a foreign antigen

hypertension: abnormally high blood pressure

hypotension: abnormally low blood pressure

hypoxia: reduction of oxygen in body tissues to below normal levels

idiopathic: disease with no known cause

immunocompetence: ability of cells to distinguish antigens from substances that belong to the body and to launch an immune response

immunodeficiency disorder: disorder caused by a deficiency of the immune response due to hypoactivity or decreased numbers of lymphoid cells

immunoglobulin: serum protein synthesized by lymphocytes and plasma cells that has known antibody activity; main component of humoral immune response

immunosurveillance: defense mechanism in which the immune system continuously recognizes abnormal cells as foreign and destroys them (For example, an interruption in immunosurveillance can lead to overproduction of cancer cells.)

insulin: hormone secreted into the blood by the islets of Langerhans of the pancreas; promotes the storage of glucose, among other functions

ischemia: decreased blood supply to a body organ or tissue

joint: the site of the union of two or more bones; provides motion and flexibility

karyotype: chromosomal arrangement of the cell nucleus

leaflets: cusps in the heart valves that open and close in response to pressure gradients to let blood flow into the chambers

leukocyte: white blood cell that protects the body against microorganisms causing disease

leukocytosis: increase in the number of leukocytes in the blood; generally caused by infection

leukopenia: reduction in the number of leukocytes in the blood

ligament: band of fibrous tissue that connects bones or cartilage, strengthens joints, provides stability, and limits or facilitates movement

lymphedema: chronic swelling of a body part from accumulation of interstitial fluid secondary to obstruction of lymphatic vessels or lymph nodes

lymph node: structure that filters the lymphatic fluid that drains from body tissues and is later returned to the blood as plasma; removes noxious agents from the blood

lymphocyte: leukocyte produced by lymphoid tissue that participates in immunity

macrophage: highly phagocytic cells that are stimulated by inflammation

malabsorption: insufficient intestinal absorption of nutrients

malignant: condition that becomes progressively worse and results in death

megakaryocytes: giant bone marrow cells

meiosis: process of cell division by which reproductive cells (gametes) are formed

melanin: dark skin pigment that filters ultraviolet radiation and is produced and dispersed by specialized cells called *melanocytes*

metastasis: transfer of malignant cells via pathogenic microorganisms or vascular system from one organ or body part to another not directly connected with it

mitosis: ordinary process of cell division in which each chromosome with all its genes reproduces itself exactly

multifactorial disorder: disorder caused by genetic and environmental factors

myelin: a lipidlike substance surrounding the axon of myelinated nerve fibers that permits normal neurologic conduction

myelitis: inflammation of the spinal cord or bone marrow

necrosis: cell or tissue death

neoplasm: abnormal growth in which cell replication is uncontrolled and progressive

nephron: structural and functional unit of the kidney that forms urine

neuritic plaques: areas of nerve inflammation; found on autopsy examination of the brain tissue of people with Alzheimer's disease

neuron: highly specialized conductor cell that receives and transmits electrochemical nerve impulses

nevus: circumscribed, stable malformation of the skin and oral mucosa

nondisjunction: failure of chromosomes to separate properly during cell division; causes an unequal distribution of chromosomes between the two resulting cells

opportunistic infection: infection that strikes people with altered, weakened, immune systems; caused by a microorganism that doesn't usually cause disease but becomes pathogenic under certain conditions

organ: body part, made up of tissues, that performs a specific function

organelle: structure of a cell found in the cytoplasm that performs a specific function; for example, the nucleus, mitochondria, and lysosomes

osmolality: concentration of a solution expressed in terms of osmoles of solute per kilogram of solvent

osmoreceptors: specialized neurons located in the thalamus that are stimulated by increased extracellular fluid osmolality to cause release of antidiuretic hormone, thereby helping to control fluid balance

osteoblasts: bone-forming cells whose activity results in bone formation

osteoclasts: giant, multinuclear cells that reabsorb material from previously formed bones, tear down old or excess bone structure, and allow osteoblasts to rebuild new bone

pancytopenia: abnormal depression of all the cellular elements of blood

parasite: single-celled or multicelled organism that depends on a host for food and a protective environment

parenchyma: essential or functional elements of an organ as distinguished from its framework

pathogen: disease producing agent or microorganism

pathogenesis: origin and development of a disease

peristalsis: intestinal contractions, or waves, that propel food toward the stomach and into and through the intestine

phagocyte: cell that ingests microorganisms, other cells, and foreign particles

phagocytosis: engulfing of microorganisms, other cells, and foreign particles by a phagocyte

plasma: liquid part of the blood that carries antibodies and nutrients to tissues and carries wastes away from tissues

platelet: disk-shaped structure in blood that plays a crucial role in blood coagulation

polypeptide chains: chains of amino acids linked by a peptide bond; for example, hemoglobin

proximal: nearest to

pulmonary alveoli: grapelike clusters found at the ends of the respiratory passages in the lungs; sites for the exchange of carbon dioxide and oxygen

pulsus paradoxus: pulse marked by a drop in systemic blood pressure greater than 15 mm Hg during inspiration

pyrosis: heartburn

recessive gene: gene that doesn't express itself in the presence of its dominant allele (corresponding gene)

remission: abatement of a disease's symptoms

remyelination: healing of demyelinated nerves

renin: enzyme produced by the kidneys in response to an actual or perceived decline in extracellular fluid volume; an important part of blood pressure regulation

resistance: opposition to airflow in the lung tissue, chest wall, or airways

sepsis: pathologic state resulting from microorganisms or their poisonous products in the bloodstream

sigmoidoscopy: inspection of the rectum and sigmoid colon through a sigmoidoscope

stasis: stagnation of the normal flow of fluids, such as blood and urine, or within the intestinal mechanism

stenosis: constriction or narrowing of a passage or orifice

subchondral: below the cartilage

surfactant: lipid-type substance that coats the alveoli, allowing them to expand uniformly during inspiration and preventing them from collapsing during expiration

synovial fluid: viscous, lubricating substance secreted by the synovial membrane, which lines the cavity between the bones of free-moving joints

synovitis: inflammation of the synovial membrane

tendon: fibrous cord of connective tissue that attaches the muscle to bone or cartilage and enables bones to move when skeletal muscles contract

thenar: palm of the hand or sole of the foot

thrombolytic: clot dissolving

thrombosis: obstruction in blood vessels

tissue: large group of individual cells that perform a certain function

tophi: clusters of urate crystals surrounded by inflamed tissue; occur in gout

toxin: a poison, produced by animals, certain plants, or pathogenic bacteria

toxoid: toxin treated to destroy its toxicity without destroying its ability to stimulate antibody production

trabeculae: needlelike, bony structures that form a supportive meshwork of interconnecting spaces filled with bone marrow

transferrin: trace protein in blood that binds and transports iron

translocation: alteration of a chromosome by attachment of a fragment to another chromosome or a different portion of the same chromosome

trisomy 21: aberration in which chromosome 21 has three homologous chromosomes per cell instead of two; another name for Down syndrome

tubercle: a tiny, rounded nodule produced by the tuberculosis bacillus

tubules: small tubes; in the kidney, minute, reabsorptive canals that secrete, collect, and conduct urine

uremic frost: white, flaky deposits of urea on the skin of patients with advanced uremia

urate: salt of uric acid found in urine

urticaria: wheals associated with itching; another name for hives

vasopressor: drug that stimulates contraction of the muscular tissue of the capillaries and arteries

virus: microscopic, infectious parasite that contains genetic material and needs a host cell to replicate

$\dot{V}/\dot{Q}$ ratio: ratio of ventilation (amount of air in the alveoli) to perfusion (amount of blood in the pulmonary capillaries); expresses the effectiveness of gas exchange

X-linked inheritance: inheritance pattern in which single gene disorders are passed through sex chromosomes; varies according to whether a male or female carries the gene (Because the male has only one X chromosome, a trait determined by a gene on that chromosome is always expressed in a male.)

Selected references

Alipour, S., et al. "Effects of Environmental Tobacco Smoke on Respiratory Symptoms and Pulmonary Function," *Inhalation Toxicology* 18(8):569-73, July 2006.

Bennett, J.S. "Vasoocclusion in Sickle Cell Anemia: Are Platelets Really Involved?" *Arteriosclerosis, Thrombosis, and Vascular Biology* 26(7):1415-16, July 2006.

Bhoola, S., and Hoskins, W.J. "Diagnosis and Management of Epithelial Ovarian Cancer," *Obstetrics & Gynecology* 107:1399-1410, June 2006.

Bickley, L.S., and Szilagyi, P.G. *Bates' Guide to Physical Examination and History Taking*, 9th ed. Philadelphia: Lippincott Williams & Wilkins, 2006.

Canonica, G.W., and Passalacqua, G. "Sublingual Immunotherapy in the Treatment of Adult Allergic Rhinitis Patients," *Allergy* 61 Suppl 81:20-23, 2006.

Copstead-Kirkhorn, L.C., and Banasik, J.L. *Pathophysiology*, 3rd ed. Philadelphia: W.B. Saunders Co., 2005.

Daniels, R., et al. *Contemporary Medical-Surgical Nursing*, Clifton Park, N.Y.: Delmar Publishing, 2007.

Doughty, D., et al. "Issues and Challenges in Staging of Pressure Ulcers," *Journal of Wound, Ostomy & Continence Nursing* 33(2):125-30, March/April 2006.

Fox, F.I. *A Laboratory Guide to Human Physiology: Concepts and Clinical Applications*, 12th ed. New York: McGraw-Hill Book Co., 2007.

Gray, M., and Ratliff, C.R., "Is Hyperbaric Oxygen Therapy Effective for the Management of Chronic Wounds?" *Journal of Wound, Ostomy & Continence Nursing* 33(1):21-25, January/February 2006.

Hall, J.C. *Sauer's Manual of Skin Diseases*, 9th ed. Philadelphia: Lippincott Williams & Wilkins, 2006.

Hess, J.R., and Lawson, J.H. "The Coagulopathy of Trauma Versus Disseminated Intravascular Coagulation," *Journal of Trauma* 60(6 Suppl):S12-19, June 2006.

Ignatavicius, D.D., and Workman, M.L. *Medical-Surgical Nursing: Critical Thinking for Collaborative Care*, 5th ed. Philadelphia: W.B. Saunders Co., 2006.

Khandani, A.H., and Detterbeck, F.C. "Positron Emission Tomographic Scanning in the Diagnosis and Staging of Non-Small Cell Lung Cancer 2 cm in Size or Less," *Journal of Thoracic and Cardiovascular Surgery* 132(1):214-15, July 2006.

Lewis, S.L., et al. *Medical-Surgical Nursing, Assessment and Management of Clinical Problems*, 7th ed. St. Louis: Mosby–Year Book, Inc., 2007.

Martin, P.R., et al. "Noise as a Trigger for Headaches: Relationship between Exposure and Sensitivity," *Headache* 46(6):962-72, June 2006.

Porth, C.M. *Essentials of Pathophysiology: Concepts of Altered Health States*, 2nd ed. Philadelphia: Lippincott Williams & Wilkins, 2007.

Price, A.S., et al. "Impending Cardiac Tamponade: A Case Report Highlighting the Value of Bedside Echocardiography," *Journal of Emergency Medicine* 30(4):415-19, May 2006.

Rasmussen, K.G, et al. "Blood Glucose Before and After ECT Treatments in Type 2 Diabetic Patients," *The Journal of ECT* 22(2):124-26, June 2006.

Ruffolo, C., et al. "Urologic Complications in Crohn's Disease: Suspicion Criteria," *Hepatogastroenterology* 53(69):357-60, May-June 2006.

Smeltzer, S.C., et al. *Brunner and Suddarth's Textbook of Medical-Surgical Nursing*, 11th ed. Philadelphia: Lippincott Williams & Wilkins, 2006.

Stewart, E.A., and Morton, C.C. "The Genetics of Uterine Leiomyomata: What Clinicians Need to Know," *Obstetrics & Gynecology* 107:917-21, April 2006.

Tamura, T., and Picciano, M.F. "Folate and Human Reproduction," *American Journal of Clinical Nutrition* 83(5):993-1016, May 2006.

Williams, D.T,, and Liu, A.K. "Cerebral Venous Thrombosis: Hemorrhagic Stroke Requiring Acute Heparin Anticoagulation," *Journal of Emergency Medicine* 31(1):111-13, July 2006.

Credits

Chapter 3
Asbestosis, page 82. Photo 1 from Rubin, E., MD, and Farber, J.L., MD. *Pathology*, 3rd ed. Philadelphia: Lippincott Williams & Wilkins, 1999. Photo 2 from Cagle, P.T., MD. *Color Atlas and Text of Pulmonary Pathology*. Philadelphia: Lippincott Williams & Wilkins, 2005.

Chapter 5
Crohn's disease, page 185. From Rubin, E., et al. *Rubin's Pathology: Clinicopathologic Foundations of Medicine*, 4th ed. Philadelphia: Lippincott Williams & Wilkins, 2005.

Chapter 6
Muscle structure, page 215. From Premkumar, K. *The Massage Connection: Anatomy and Physiology*, 2nd ed. Philadelphia: Lippincott Williams & Wilkins, 2004.

Gout, page 226. Images provided by *Stedman's*.

Osteoporosis, page 235. From Smeltzer, S.C., and Bare, B.G. *Brunner and Suddarth's Textbook of Medical-Surgical Nursing*, 9th ed. Philadelphia: Lippincott Williams & Wilkins, 2000.

Chapter 11
Herpes zoster, page 374. From Goodheart, H.P., MD. *Goodheart's Photoguide of Common Skin Disorders*, 2nd ed. Philadelphia: Lippincott Williams & Wilkins, 2003.

Chapter 12
Breast quadrants, page 398. From Weber, J., and Kelley, J. *Health Assessment in Nursing*, 2nd ed. Philadelphia: Lippincott Williams & Wilkins, 2003.

We also gratefully acknowledge Anatomical Chart Company and LifeART for the use of selected images.

Index

A

Abdominal aortic aneurysm, 21-24
  dissecting, 22i
  types of, 21i
Absence seizure, 136
Acid-base balance, 282
Acid-base imbalances, 320-326
Acidosis, 282
  metabolic, 321t, 322, 323-324, 325-326
  respiratory, 320-321, 321t, 323, 324, 325
Acid perfusion test
  in gastroesophageal reflux disease, 191
  in hiatal hernia, 193
Acini, 173
Acquired immunodeficiency syndrome. *See
    also* Human immunodeficiency virus
    infection.
  opportunistic diseases associated with,
    350, 351-355t
  progression of human immunodeficiency
    virus infection to, 349
Acute coronary syndrome, 51
Acute demyelinating polyneuropathy. *See*
    Guillain-Barré syndrome.
Acute leukemia, 411-414, 413i
  risk factors for, 412
  types of, 411-412
Acute pancreatitis, 197-198, 198i, 200
Acute posterior ganglionitis as opportunistic
    disease, 354t
Acute poststreptococcal glomerulo-
    nephritis, 292
Acute renal failure, 303-307
  causes of, 304t
  classifying, 303
  phases of, 304-305
Acute respiratory distress syndrome, 75-78, 77i.
    See also Pulmonary edema.
Acute respiratory failure, 79-82

Acute tubular necrosis, 285-289
  pathophysiology of, 286, 287i
Acute tubulointerstitial nephritis. *See* Acute
    tubular necrosis.
Addisonian crisis, 250, 251i
Addison's disease, 249-250, 252-253
Adenovirus infection, 99t
Adrenal crisis, 250, 251i
Adrenal glands, 246-247
  disorders of, 249-250, 252-256
Adrenal hypofunction, 249-250, 252-253
Adrenal insufficiency, 249-250, 252-253
Adrenocorticotropic hormone, 244
  stimulation test for, 253
Akinesia, 155
Akinetic seizure, 136
Alcoholic cirrhosis, 179-180
Aldosterone, 247
  fluid balance and, 282
Aldosteronism as hypertension cause, 46
Alkalosis, 282
  metabolic, 321t, 322-323, 324, 325, 326
  respiratory, 321-322, 321t, 323, 324, 325
Allele, 436
Allergen, 343
Allergic rhinitis, 343-345
Allergic shiners, 344
Alveoli, 71, 72i
Alzheimer's disease, 125-130
  contributing factors for, 126, 128
  forms of, 126
  tissue changes in, 127i, 128
Amantadine, 156
Amyloidosis, 499t
Amyotrophic lateral sclerosis, 130-132
Anal canal, 168i, 171
Anaphylactic reaction. *See* Anaphylaxis.
Anaphylaxis, 345-348
  development of, 346, 347i
Androgens, 247

i refers to an illustration; t refers to a table.

Anemia, 318
  iron deficiency, 331-333
  sickle cell, 457-461
Aneurysm. *See* Abdominal aortic aneurysm.
Angina, 32
Angiography
  in coronary artery disease, 34
  in dilated cardiomyopathy, 37
  in pulmonary embolism, 110
  in stroke, 162
Anion gap, 325-326
Ankylosing spondylitis, 499t
Anterior cerebral artery as stroke site, 161t
Anthrax, 499t
Anticholinesterase drugs, 153
Antidiuretic hormone, 248
  fluid balance and, 281-282
Antigens, 341
Antihistamines, 345
Antiretroviral drugs, 357
Apneustic center, 74
Apoptosis, 359
Appendicitis, 174-175, 174i
Appendicular skeleton, 216i, 218
Arachnoid mater, 120
Arterial blood gas analysis
  in acute respiratory distress syndrome, 76
  in acute respiratory failure, 81
  in asbestosis, 83
  in asthma, 88
  in cardiogenic shock, 29
  in chronic bronchitis, 90
  in chronic renal failure, 309
  in cor pulmonale, 92
  in emphysema, 96
  in metabolic acidosis, 321t
  in metabolic alkalosis, 321t
  in pneumonia, 100
  in pneumothorax, 104
  in pulmonary edema, 106
  in pulmonary embolism, 110
  in respiratory acidosis, 321t
  in respiratory alkalosis, 321t
Arthrodesis, 231
Arthroplasty, 231

Asbestosis, 82-83, 82i
Aseptic viral meningitis, 142
Aspergillosis, 500t
Aspiration pneumonia, 97, 98
Asthma, 84-88. *See also* Chronic obstructive
     pulmonary disease.
  pathophysiology of, 84, 85i
Atherosclerosis, 30, 31
Atrophy, 5, 5i, 8
Autoimmune disorders, 343
Autoimmune thrombocytopenia, 329-331
Autoimmunity, 358
Autologous bone marrow transplantation, 430
Autonomic nervous system, 124-125
Autosomal dominant inheritance, 437, 438i
Autosomal recessive inheritance, 438-439, 439i
Autosomes, 436
Axial skeleton, 216i, 217i

B

Bacteremia, 384-386
Bacteria, 368
Bacterial meningitis, 141-142, 145
Bacterial pneumonia, 97-98, 99-100t. *See also*
     Pneumonia.
Barium studies
  in Crohn's disease, 186
  in diverticular disease, 188
  in gastroesophageal reflux disease, 191
  in hiatal hernia, 193
  in irritable bowel syndrome, 196
  in peptic ulcer, 203
  in ulcerative colitis, 206
Basal cell carcinoma, 396-397, 396i
Basal cell epithelioma, 396-397, 396i
Basophils, 315
B cells, 340, 341
Beck's triad, 25
Bell's palsy, 500t
Benign prostatic hyperplasia, 289-291, 290i
Bile, 173
Biliary cirrhosis, 180
Bladder, 279
Blasts, 318-319

Blood, 313-316, 317i, 318-319
    circulation of, 18-19
    clotting process and, 317i
    components of, 313-316
    functions of, 313
    pH of, 320
Blood disorders, 316, 318-335
    causes of, 316, 318-319
Blood dyscrasias, 316, 318-319. *See also* Blood
        disorders.
Blood pressure regulation, 284
Body movement, 220-221
Bone marrow, 340
    blood dyscrasias and, 316, 318
Bone marrow studies
    in acute leukemia, 413
    in idiopathic thrombocytopenic purpura, 330
    in iron deficiency anemia, 333
    in multiple myeloma, 425i, 426
    in thrombocytopenia, 335.
Bones, 215, 216i, 217-218, 217i
    classifying, 215
    density and strength of, 219
    formation of, 218-219
    functions of, 218
Bone scan
    in osteomyelitis, 234
    in osteoporosis, 238
Botulism, 500t
Bouchard's nodes, 230, 230i
Brain, structures and functions of, 120-122, 121i
Brain stem, 122
Breast cancer, 397-401
    risk factors for, 398
    susceptibility to, 398
    tumor sites in, 398, 398i
    types of, 398-399, 399i
Breathing, mechanics of, 73-74
Bronchiectasis, 500-501t
Bronchiolitis, 501t
Bronchodilators, 88
Bronchopneumonia, 96, 98i. *See also*
        Pneumonia.
Brudzinski's sign, 144i, 145
Bursae, 220

C

Calcium formation, 285
Cancer, 391-432. *See also specific type.*
    abnormal cell growth in, 392-393, 392i
    causes of, 393-395
    deaths related to, 391
    early detection of, 391
    metastasis in, 392, 393i
    warning signs of, 392
Candidiasis as opportunistic disease, 352t
Carcinogenesis, 393-394
Carcinomas, 392
Cardiac catheterization
    in cor pulmonale, 92
    in dilated cardiomyopathy, 37
    in hypertrophic cardiomyopathy, 51
    in rheumatic fever, 63
Cardiac cirrhosis, 180
Cardiac enzyme levels in cardiogenic shock, 29
Cardiac tamponade, 24-26, 25i
Cardiogenic shock, 27-29, 28i
Cardiomyopathy
    dilated, 34-37, 35i
    hypertrophic, 48-51, 49i
Cardiovascular disorders, 20-64
    risk factors for, 19-20
    susceptibility to, 20
Cardiovascular system, 17-19
Carditis, 61-62, 64
Carpal tunnel, 223i
Carpal tunnel syndrome, 222-224
Cartilage, 218, 219
Celiac disease, 501t
Cell
    adaptation of, 4-6, 5i
    aging of, 8
    components of, 1-2, 2i
    death of, 2, 4, 6, 8
    degeneration of, 7-8
    division and reproduction of, 2-4, 3i
    injury to, 6-7
Cell-mediated immunity, 341
Central nervous system, 120-124, 121i, 123i
Cerebellum, 122
Cerebrospinal fluid, 120
Cerebrovascular accident. *See* Stroke.

Cerebrum, 120-122, 121i
Cervical cancer, 401-403, 402i
Cervical neoplasm as opportunistic disease, 355t
Chemotaxis, 342
Chemotherapy
    for acute leukemia, 414
    for breast cancer, 400
    for chronic lymphocytic leukemia, 415
    for colorectal cancer, 406
    for endometrial cancer, 408
    for Hodgkin's disease, 409
    for lung cancer, 421
    for malignant melanoma, 422
    for multiple myeloma, 424
    for prostate cancer, 427
    for testicular cancer, 430
Chest X-ray. See also X-ray.
    in acute respiratory distress syndrome, 78
    in acute respiratory failure, 81
    in asbestosis, 83
    in asthma, 88
    in cardiac tamponade, 26
    in chronic bronchitis, 90
    in cor pulmonale, 92
    in dilated cardiomyopathy, 37
    in emphysema, 96
    in heart failure, 42
    in hiatal hernia, 193
    in hypertrophic cardiomyopathy, 51
    in lung cancer, 419
    in meningitis, 146
    in pancreatitis, 199
    in pneumonia, 100
    in pneumothorax, 104
    in pulmonary edema, 107
    in pulmonary embolism, 110
    in respiratory acidosis, 325
    in rheumatic fever, 63
    in severe acute respiratory syndrome, 111
    in systemic lupus erythematosus, 360
    in tuberculosis, 114
Chickenpox, 99t
Cholecystitis, 176-179
    gallstone formation in, 176, 177i
    predisposing factors for, 176

Cholera, 501t
Cholinergic crisis, 152
Cholinesterase inhibitors, 129
Christmas disease, 451-454
Chromosomal disorders, 442-444, 443i, 449-451, 450i
Chromosomes, 435
Chronic bronchitis, 88-90, 89i. See also Chronic obstructive pulmonary disease.
Chronic lymphocytic leukemia, 414-415, 415i
Chronic myeloid leukemia, 415-418, 416i
Chronic obstructive pulmonary disease, 84. See also Asthma, Chronic bronchitis, and Emphysema.
Chronic pancreatitis, 197, 200
Chronic renal disease as hypertension cause, 46
Chronic renal failure, 307-310
    stages of, 307
Chronic vasomotor rhinitis, 344
Chyme, 170, 171
Circulatory system, 18-19
Cirrhosis, 179-183
    nodular changes in liver in, 181i
    types of, 179-180
Clearance, 283
Cleft lip and cleft palate, 444-446, 445i
Closed pneumothorax, 101
Clotting cascade, 316, 317i
Coagulation factors, clotting and, 317i
Coccidioidomycosis as opportunistic disease, 352t
Coccidiosis as opportunistic disease, 353t
Colon, 168i, 171
Colonoscopy
    in Crohn's disease, 186
    in irritable bowel syndrome, 196
    in ulcerative colitis, 206
Colorectal cancer, 403-406
    risk factors for, 403-404
    types of, 405i
Common cold, 344
Complement, 359
Complement cascade, 342
Complement system, 342
Completed stroke, 157

i refers to an illustration; t refers to a table.

Complex partial seizure, 135i, 136
Compression test in carpal tunnel
        syndrome, 224
Computed tomography
    in abdominal aortic aneurysm, 24
    in Alzheimer's disease, 130
    in cirrhosis, 183
    in Cushing's syndrome, 255
    in epilepsy, 138
    in meningitis, 146
    in multiple sclerosis, 149
    in osteoporosis, 237
    in pancreatitis, 199
    in rhabdomyolysis, 240
    in stroke, 162
    in tuberculosis, 114
Congestive cardiomyopathy. *See* Dilated
        cardiomyopathy.
Consumption coagulopathy. *See* Disseminated
        intravascular coagulation.
Coronary artery bypass graft surgery, 33
Coronary artery disease, 29-34
    genes implicated in, 30
    risk factors for, 30-31
Cor pulmonale, 90-94
    pathophysiology of, 91, 92, 93i
Corticosteroids, 88, 253, 358
Corticotropin, 244
Cortisol, 247
Cranial motor neurons, 123
Creutzfeldt-Jakob disease, 501t
Crohn's disease, 183-186
    changes to the bowel in, 184, 185i
Crohn's disease of the colon, 183
Cryptococcosis as opportunistic disease, 352t
Cryptosporidiosis as opportunistic disease, 353t
Cushing's syndrome, 253-256
    as hypertension cause, 46
Cystic fibrosis, 446-448
    diagnostic criteria for, 448
Cytokinesis, 3
Cytomegalovirus infection, 99t
    as opportunistic disease, 354t

D

Da Nang lung, 75-78
Dead-space ventilation, 72i, 73
Decompensation, cycle of, 27, 28i
Deep brain stimulation, 156
Defibrination. *See* Disseminated intravascular
        coagulation.
Deficit injury to cell, 7
Dehydration test, 259
Demyelination, 147i
Deoxyribonucleic acid, 435
Dermatome, 373
Desmopressin acetate, 258
Dexamethasone suppression test, 255
Diabetes insipidus, 256-259
    pathophysiology of, 257, 257i
Diabetes mellitus, 259-265
    screening guidelines for, 262
    type 1, 260, 262, 264
    type 2, 260, 261i, 262, 264
Diabetic ketoacidosis, 263
Dialysis, 309
Diffusion, gas exchange and, 71
Digestion
    accessory glands and organs in, 171-173
    cephalic phase of, 169
    esophagus in, 169
    gastric phase of, 169-170
    mouth in, 169
    small intestine in, 170-171
    stomach in, 169-170
Dilated cardiomyopathy, 34-37, 35i
Discoid lupus erythematosus, 357
Disease
    cause of, 11
    development of, 11
    factors that influence outcome of, 10
    stages of, 11-12
    stress and, 12-13, 12i
    versus illness, 10
Disseminated intravascular coagulation,
        326-329
    pathologic processes in, 327
    pathophysiology of, 327, 328i
    precipitating causes of, 326-327

Diverticular disease, 187-189
  in colon, 187, 188i
  forms of, 187
Diverticulitis, 187, 188, 188i. *See also* Diverticu-
    lar disease.
Diverticulosis, 187. *See also* Diverticular
    disease.
Dowager's hump, 236, 237i
Down syndrome, 449-451, 450i
Duodenal ulcer, 202
Duodenum, 168i, 170, 172i
Dura mater, 120
Dysplasia, 5i, 6

E
Echocardiography
  in cardiac tamponade, 26
  in cardiogenic shock, 29
  in cor pulmonale, 92
  in dilated cardiomyopathy, 37
  in heart failure, 42
  in hypertrophic cardiomyopathy, 50-51
  in myocardial infarction, 57
  in pericarditis, 61
  in rheumatic fever, 63
Elastic cartilage, 219
Electrocardiography
  in acute respiratory failure, 81
  in acute tubular necrosis, 289
  in cardiac tamponade, 26
  in cardiogenic shock, 29
  in chronic bronchitis, 90
  in coronary artery disease, 32, 34
  in cor pulmonale, 92
  in dilated cardiomyopathy, 37
  in emphysema, 96
  in heart failure, 42
  in hypertrophic cardiomyopathy, 51
  in metabolic alkalosis, 326
  in myocardial infarction, 56
  in pericarditis, 60-61
  in pulmonary edema, 107
  in pulmonary embolism, 110
  in respiratory alkalosis, 325
  in rhabdomyolysis, 240
  in rheumatic fever, 63

Electroencephalography
  in Alzheimer's disease, 130
  in chronic renal failure, 310
  in epilepsy, 138
  in multiple sclerosis, 149
  in stroke, 163
Electromyography
  in amyotrophic lateral sclerosis, 131
  in carpal tunnel syndrome, 224
  in Guillain-Barré syndrome, 141
  in myasthenia gravis, 152
Embolism as cause of stroke, 158, 159i, 160
Emphysema, 94-96, 95i. *See also* Chronic
    obstructive pulmonary disease.
Endocarditis, 63, 502t
Endochondral ossification, 218
Endocrine disorders, 249-276
Endocrine system, 243-244, 245i, 246-249
Endoluminal stent grafting, 23
Endometrial cancer, 406-408
  predisposing factors for, 406
  progression of, 406, 407i
Endoscopic retrograde cholangiopancreatog-
    raphy, 179, 200
Enterocolitis, 384-386
Eosinophils, 315
Epidural space, 120
Epilepsy, 133-138, 135i. *See also* Status
    epilepticus.
Epinephrine, 247
  as emergency drug for anaphylaxis, 346
Epstein-Barr virus, glands affected by, 376i. *See
    also* Infectious mononucleosis.
Erythema chronicum migrans, 377, 378i
Erythema marginatum, 63
Erythrocytes. *See* Red blood cells.
Erythropoiesis, 314
Erythropoietin, 284-285, 314
Esophageal balloon tamponade, 182
Esophageal varices, 502t
Esophagogastroduodenoscopy, 183, 203
Esophagus, 168i, 169
Essential thrombocytopenia, 329-331
Estrogens, 247
Etiology, 11
Exacerbation, 11

i refers to an illustration; t refers to a table.

Excretory urography
  in benign prostatic hyperplasia, 291
  in chronic renal failure, 310
  in hydronephrosis, 296
  in hypertension, 47
  in renal calculi, 302
Extrapyramidal system, 153
Extrinsic causes of disease, 11
Extrinsic pathway, clotting and, 317i

F

Factor replacement, 453
Fanconi's syndrome, 502t
Feedback mechanisms, homeostasis and,
    9-10, 10i
Feedback system, regulation of endocrine
    system and, 244, 245i
Fibrinolytic therapy, 109
Fibrotic regeneration, 179
Fibrous cartilage, 219
Fight-or-flight response, 12i, 13, 247
Fissures, cerebral, 121i
Fluid balance, 281-282
Follicle-stimulating hormone, 244
Frank-Starling curve, 41
Frontal lobe, 121i
Functioning metastatic thyroid carcinoma, 268
Fungi, 368
Fusion inhibitors, 357

G

Gallbladder, 168i, 172-173, 172i
Gallstone formation, 176, 177i
  predisposing factors for, 176
Gas exchange, 67, 68, 71, 72, 73
Gastric lavage, 182
Gastric secretions, 169-170
Gastric ulcer, 202
Gastroesophageal reflux disease, 189-191
  factors that lead to, 189-190
  pathophysiology of, 190, 190i
Gastrointestinal disorders, 174-210
Gastrointestinal system, 167-173, 168i, 172i
Gastrointestinal tract, 167, 168i, 169-171
Generalized seizures, 135i, 136
Generalized tonic-clonic seizure, 136

Genes
  Alzheimer's disease and, 126
  amyotrophic lateral sclerosis and, 131
  asthma and, 86
  colorectal cancer and, 404
  coronary artery disease and, 30
  Crohn's disease and, 184
  lupus erythematosus and, 359
  malignant melanoma and, 423
  mutations in, 437
  rheumatoid arthritis and, 361
Gene therapy for cystic fibrosis, 448
Genetic disorders, 444-462
Genetic inheritance, 435
  autosomal dominant, 437, 438i
  autosomal recessive, 438-439, 439i
  sex-linked, 439-442, 440i, 441i
Genetics, 435-444
Genital herpes, 372
German measles. *See* Rubella.
Glands, 246-249
  inflammation and, 246
  tumors and, 246
Gliosis, 147
Glomerular filtration rate, 283
Glomerulonephritis, 292-294, 293i
Glucagon, 248
Glucocorticoids, 247
Gluconeogenesis, 247
Goiter, 265-268, 266i
  classifying, 265
Goodpasture's syndrome, 292-293
Gout, 225-228, 226i
  factors that may provoke attack of, 226
  stages of, 225
Granulocytes, 315
Granulomatous colitis, 183
Graves' disease, 268-272
Growth hormone, 248
Guillain-Barré syndrome, 138-141
  peripheral nerve demyelination in, 139, 139i
  phases of, 138
  risk factors for, 138

i refers to an illustration; t refers to a table.

H

Hay fever, 343-345
Heart attack. *See* Myocardial infarction.
Heartburn. *See* Gastroesophageal reflux disease.
Heart failure, 38-43
  adaptations in, 41-42
  classifying, 38, 41
  left-sided, 39i, 41
  predisposing conditions for, 38, 40
  right-sided, 40i, 41
Heberden's nodes, 230, 230i
Helper T cells, 341
  human immunodeficiency virus and, 349-350
Hematologic system, 313-316, 317i, 318-319. *See also* Blood disorders.
Hemophilia, 451-454
Hemorrhage as cause of stroke, 160
Hemostasis, 316
Heparin therapy, 328
Hepatitis. *See* Viral hepatitis.
Herpes simplex, 370-373
  as opportunistic disease, 354t
  types of, 370, 371
Herpes zoster, 373-375, 374i
  as opportunistic disease, 354t
Heterozygosity, 436
Hiatal hernia, 192-194, 193i
  types of, 192
Highly Active Antiretroviral Therapy, 357
Histoplasmosis as opportunistic disease, 352t
Hodgkin's disease, 409-411
  Ann Arbor staging system for, 410i
Homeostasis, 8-10, 10i
  feedback mechanisms and, 9-10, 10i
  structures responsible for maintaining, 9
Homozygosity, 436
Hormonal therapy, 400, 408, 427
Hormones
  abnormal concentrations of, 244, 246
  fluid balance and, 281
  hyporesponsiveness and, 246
  hypothalamic, 243-244
  negative feedback system and, 244, 245i
Host defense system, 339

Human immunodeficiency virus infection, 348-350, 356-357. *See also* Acquired immunodeficiency syndrome.
  antibody detection in, 356
  Centers for Disease Control and Prevention classification system for, 348, 349
  development of acquired immunodeficiency syndrome and, 349
  incubation period for, in children, 356
  testing recommendations for, 356
  transmission of, 350
Humoral immunity, 341-342
Hyaline cartilage, 219
Hydronephrosis, 294-296
  renal damage in, 295, 295i
Hyperosmolar hyperglycemic nonketotic syndrome, 263
Hyperplasia, 5, 5i, 8
Hypersensitivity reactions, classifying, 343
Hypersplenism, 502t
Hypertension, 43-48
  blood vessel damage in, 46-47, 47i
  classifying, 44
  development of, 44, 45i
  predisposing factors for, 47-48
Hyperthyroidism, 268-272. *See also* Thyroid storm.
  signs of, 270-271, 270i
  types of, 268
Hypertrophic cardiomyopathy, 48-51
  pathophysiology of, 48, 49i
Hypertrophic obstructive cardiomyopathy. *See* Hypertrophic cardiomyopathy.
Hypertrophy, 5, 5i, 8
Hyporesponsiveness, hormone receptors and, 246
Hypothalamus, 122, 243, 244, 245i
Hypothyroidism, 273-276
  signs of, 274-275, 275i
Hypoventilation, 79

I

Idiopathic diseases, 11
Idiopathic hypertrophic subaortic stenosis. *See* Hypertrophic cardiomyopathy.
Idiopathic pulmonary fibrosis, 502t

Idiopathic thrombocytopenic purpura, 329-331
Ileocecal valve, 168i, 171
Ileum, 168i, 170
Illness vs. disease, 10
Immune disorders, 342-364
Immune response, disorders of, 342
Immune system, 339-342
Immunity
    cell-mediated, 341
    humoral, 341-342
Immunocompetence, 340
Immunodeficiency disorders, 343
Immunoglobulins, classes of, 341-342
Immunosuppressant therapy, 331
Immunosurveillance, 395
Immunotherapy for malignant melanoma, 422
Infection, 367-370
    barriers to, 369
    development of, 369-370
    microorganisms that cause, 367-369
    opportunistic, 351-355t, 370
Infectious disorders, 370-388
Infectious injury to cell, 6-7
Infectious mononucleosis, 375-377, 376i
Infectious rhinitis, 344
Inflammation, hormone secretion and, 246
Inflammatory bowel disease. See Crohn's
        disease.
Inflammatory response, 342
Influenza, 99t
Insulin, 248
Insulin-dependent diabetes mellitus. See
        Diabetes mellitus, type 1.
Insulin replacement, 264
Insulitis, 260
Intra-aortic balloon pump, 29
Intrarenal failure, 303, 304t, 305
Intrinsic causes of disease, 11
Intrinsic pathway, clotting and, 317i
Intrinsic renal failure, 303, 304t
Iron deficiency anemia, 331-333, 333i
Iron preparations, administering, 332
Irritable bowel syndrome, 194-196, 196i
Irritant reflex, 68
Ischemic stroke, 159i. See also Stroke.
Islets of Langerhans, 173

J
Jacksonian seizure, 136
Jejunum, 168i, 170
Joints, 220
    types of, 220

K
Kaposi's sarcoma, 503t
    as opportunistic disease, 355t
Keratitis, 503t
Kernig's sign, 144i, 145
Kidneys
    anatomy of, 279, 280i
    functions of, 281-285
Kidney stones. See Renal calculi.
Kidney-ureter-bladder radiography
    in chronic renal failure, 310
    in glomerulonephritis, 294
    in renal calculi, 302
Killer T cells, 341
Klebsiella pneumonia, 99t
Kyphosis, 503t

L
Laënnec's cirrhosis, 179-180
Large intestine, 168i, 171
Laser angioplasty, 33
Latex allergy, 503t
Left-sided heart failure, 38, 39i, 41. See also
        Heart failure.
Left ventricular remodeling surgery, 43
Legionnaire's disease, 503t
Leprosy, 503t
Leukemia
    acute, 411-414, 413i
    chronic lymphocytic, 414-415, 415i
    chronic myeloid, 415-418, 416i
Leukocytes, 315
Levodopa, 156
Ligaments, 220
Lithotripsy, 179, 302
Liver, 168i, 171-172, 172i
Lobar pneumonia, 96, 98i. See also Pneumonia.
Locus, 436
Long bones, 217i
Lou Gehrig's disease, 130-132

i refers to an illustration; t refers to a table.

Lumpectomy, 400
Lung cancer, 418-421
    tumor infiltration in, 419i
    types of, 418, 420t
Lungs, 70-71
    airflow resistance and, 73-74
    compliance of, 73
    gas exchange and, 71, 72i, 73
    volume and capacity of, 73
Lupus erythematosus, 357-360
Luteinizing hormone, 244
Lyme disease, 377-379
    bull's-eye rash in, 377, 378i
    stages of, 377-378
Lymph nodes, 340
Lymphocytes, 315
Lymphocytopenia, 319
Lypressin, 258
Lysozymes, 369

M

Macrophages, 315
Magnetic resonance imaging
    in Alzheimer's disease, 130
    in cor pulmonale, 92
    in Cushing's syndrome, 255
    in epilepsy, 138
    in multiple sclerosis, 149
    in osteomyelitis, 234
    in rhabdomyolysis, 240
    in stroke, 162
    in tuberculosis, 114
Malignant lymphomas as opportunistic
        disease, 355t
Malignant melanoma, 421-423, 422i
    ABCDE's of, 423i
    risk factors for, 422
Marfan syndrome, 454-456
Mast cell stabilizers, 88
Mastectomy, 400
Meal planning, diabetes treatment and, 264
Measles, 99t
Mechanical ventilation, maximizing benefits
        of, 78
Medulla oblongata, 122
Medullary sponge kidney, 503t

Megakaryocytes, 335
Meiosis, 436
Memantine, 129
Meningeal irritation, signs of, 145
Meningitis, 141-146
    aseptic viral, 142
    meningeal inflammation in, 141, 143i
    risk factors for, 143
    signs of, 144i, 145
Meningococcal meningitis, 145. See also
        Meningitis.
Metabolic acidosis, 321t, 322, 323-324, 325-326
Metabolic alkalosis, 321t, 322-323, 324, 325, 326
Metaplasia, 5, 5i
Metastasis, 392, 393i
Midbrain, 122
Middle cerebral artery as stroke site, 161t
Mineralocorticoids, 247
Mitosis, 436
    phases of, 3-4, 3i
Monocytes, 315
Mononucleosis, infectious, 375-377, 376i
Monosomy, 442
Mosaicism, 442
Motor neuron diseases, 130
Mouth, 169
Mucociliary system, 70
Multifactorial disorders, 444-446, 445i
Multiple myeloma, 424-426
    bone marrow aspirate in, 425i
Multiple sclerosis, 146-149
    myelin breakdown in, 147, 147i
Muscles, 213, 214i, 215
    factors that cause variations in, 215
    structure of, 215i
    types of, 213, 215
Muscular aortic stenosis. See Hypertrophic
        cardiomyopathy.
Musculoskeletal disorders, 221-240
Musculoskeletal system, 213, 214i, 215, 215i,
        216i, 217-221, 217i
Myasthenia gravis, 150-153
    crisis in, 152, 153
    neuromuscular transmission in, 150, 151i
Myasthenic crisis, 152, 153

Mycobacterium avium complex as opportunistic disease, 351t
Mycotic infections, 368
Myocardial infarction, 51-57
  complications of, 54
  pain in, 56
  pathophysiology of, 52-53i
  predisposing factors for, 53-54
  sites of, 55-56
  warning signs of, 56
Myocardial ischemia in coronary artery disease, 30, 31, 32
Myocardial perfusion imaging
  in coronary artery disease, 34
  in myocardial infarction, 57
Myocarditis, 63, 504t
Myoclonic seizure, 136
Myxedema, 275. *See also* Hypothyroidism.
Myxedema coma, 273

N

Necrosis, 6
Nephron, 280i, 284
Nephrotomography in chronic renal failure, 310
Nerve conduction studies in myasthenia gravis, 153
Neurofibromatosis, 504t
Neurologic disorders, 125-163
Neurologic system, 119-125, 121i, 123i
Neuron, 119-120, 123i
Neutropenia, 319
Neutrophils, 315
Nondisjunction, 442, 443i
Non–insulin-dependent diabetes mellitus. *See* Diabetes mellitus, type 2.
Nonnucleoside reverse transcriptase inhibitors, 357
Nontoxic goiter. *See* Goiter.
Nuclear ventriculography in myocardial infarction, 57
Nucleoside reverse transcriptase inhibitors, 357
Nutritional cirrhosis, 179-180

O

Occipital lobe, 121i
Oliguria, 305
Open pneumothorax, 101
Opportunistic diseases associated with acquired immunodeficiency syndrome, 350, 351-355t
Osgood-Schlatter disease, 504t
Osteoarthritis, 229-231
  effects of, 230, 230i
Osteoblasts, 218, 219
Osteoclasts, 218-219
Osteomyelitis, 231-234
  common sites of, 232
  stages of, 232i
Osteoplasty, 231
Osteoporosis, 234-238
  contributing factors for, 234
  height loss in, 236, 237i
  pathophysiology of, 235i, 236
  types of, 234-235
Osteotomy, 231
Oxygen supply and demand, 17-18
Oxytocin, 248

PQ

Pain
  in abdominal aortic aneurysm, 23
  in appendicitis, 175
  in coronary artery disease, 32
  in gastroesophageal reflux disease, 191
  in herpes zoster infection, 373-374
  in irritable bowel syndrome, 195
  in myocardial infarction, 56
  in pancreatitis, 199
  in pericarditis, 58
  in renal calculi, 301
  in sickle cell anemia, 460
Pancreas, 168i, 172i, 173
  disorders of, 197-200, 259-265
  as endocrine gland, 247-248
Pancreatitis, 197-200
  forms of, 197-198
  necrotizing, 198, 198i
Paraesophageal hernia, 192
Parasites, 369

Parasympathetic nervous system, 125
Parathyroid glands, 249
Parathyroid hormone, 249
Parenchymal renal failure, 303, 304t
Parietal lobe, 121i
Parkinson's disease, 153-156
    neurotransmitter action in, 154, 154i
Partial seizures, 135i, 136
Pathogenesis, 11
Pediculosis, 504t
Peptic ulcer, 200-203
    common sites and types of, 200, 201i
    forms of, 201-202
    predisposing factors for, 202
Percutaneous myocardial revascularization, 33
Percutaneous transluminal coronary angio-
        plasty, 33
Perennial allergic rhinitis, 343-345
Pericardectomy, 60
Pericardial effusion, 58
Pericardial friction rub, 58
Pericardial window, 26
Pericardiocentesis, 26
Pericarditis, 57-61
    development of, 58, 59i
Peripheral nervous system, 124-125
Permissive hypercapnia, 78
Petrosal sinus sampling, 256
Peyer's patches, 184
Phagocytosis, 342
Phalen's wrist-flexion test, 224
Phenylketonuria, 456-457
Pheochromocytoma, 504t
    as hypertension cause, 46
Physical injury to cell, 7
Pia mater, 120
Pierre Robin malformation, 446
Pill-roll tremor, 155
Pituitary gland, 243-244, 248
    disorder of, 256-259
    neural stimulation of, 243-244
Plasma, 313, 314
Platelet count
    factors that decrease, 334
    in thrombocytopenia, 335

Platelets, 316
    disorders of, 319
Pleurisy, 504t
Pneumococcal meningitis, 145. *See also*
        Meningitis.
Pneumocystis carinii pneumonia as opportunis-
        tic disease, 353t
Pneumonia, 96-100
    classifying, 96-97
    location of, 96, 98i
    predisposing factors for, 97-98
    types of, 99-100t
Pneumotaxic center, 74
Pneumothorax, 100-104, 102i
    classifying, 101
Polycythemia, 318
Polycythemia vera, 505t
Pons, 122
Portal cirrhosis, 179-180
Portosystemic shunts, 182
Positron emission tomography
    in Alzheimer's disease, 130
    in stroke, 162
Postherpetic neuralgia, 373
Postmenopausal osteoporosis, 234
Postnecrotic cirrhosis, 180
Postrenal failure, 303, 304t
Postviral thrombocytopenia, 329-331
Potassium, factors that affect secretion of, 282
Pregnancy, dilated cardiomyopathy and, 36
Premenopausal osteoporosis, 235
Prerenal failure, 303, 304t, 305-306
Pressure-controlled inverse ratio ventilation, 78
Progressive multifocal leukoencephalopathy as
        opportunistic disease, 54t
Progressive stroke, 157
Prolactin, 248
Prostate cancer, 426-428, 428i, 429i
    risk factors for, 426-427
Prostatism, 290-291
Prostatitis, 296-299
    inflammation in, 297i
    types of, 296-298
Protease inhibitors, 357
Protein-A immunoadsorption therapy, 362

t refers to a table; i refers to an illustration.

Pulmonary artery pressure monitoring
  in acute respiratory distress syndrome, 76
  in acute respiratory failure, 82
  in cardiac tamponade, 26
  in cardiogenic shock, 28-29
  in cor pulmonale, 92
  in heart failure, 42-43
  in pulmonary edema, 107
Pulmonary edema, 104-107
  development of, 105i
  heart failure as cause of, 43
Pulmonary embolism, 107-110
  pathophysiology of, 108, 108i
  predisposing factors for, 107
Pulmonary function tests
  in asbestosis, 83
  in asthma, 87
  in chronic bronchitis, 90
  in cor pulmonale, 92
  in emphysema, 96
Pulse oximetry
  in acute respiratory distress syndrome, 78
  in acute respiratory failure, 81
  in asthma, 88
  in chronic bronchitis, 90
  in cor pulmonale, 92
  in emphysema, 96
  in pneumonia, 100
  in pneumothorax, 104
  in pulmonary edema, 107
Pump failure, 27-29, 28i
Pyloric stenosis, 505t
Pylorus, 170, 172i

R

Rabies, 379-381
  postexposure prophylaxis for, 380
Radiation therapy
  for cervical cancer, 403
  complications of, 403
  for endometrial cancer, 408
  for lung cancer, 421
  for malignant melanoma, 422
  for prostate cancer, 427
  for testicular cancer, 430
Radioactive iodine therapy, 272

Rapid corticotropin test, 253
Raynaud's phenomenon, 359
Rectum, 168i, 171
Red blood cells, 313, 314-315
  disorders of, 318
  erythropoietin and production of, 284-285
Regional enteritis, 183
Regurgitation in valvular disease, 18
Remission, 11
Remodeling, bones and, 219
Renal calculi, 299-303
  predisposing factors for, 299-300
  preventive measures for, 302
  types of, 300i
Renal disorders, 285-310
Renal failure
  acute, 303-307
  chronic, 307-310
Renal system, 279, 280i, 281-285
Renin-angiotensin system, blood pressure
      regulation and, 284
Resistance, airway, 73-74
Resorption, 218-219
Respiration, neurochemical control of, 74
Respiratory acidosis, 320-321, 321t, 323, 324, 325
Respiratory alkalosis, 321-322, 321t, 323,
    324, 325
Respiratory center, 74
Respiratory disorders, 75-115
Respiratory syncytial virus infection, 99t,
    381-382
Respiratory system, 67-74
  breathing mechanics and, 73-74
  function of, 67
  gas exchange in, 67, 68, 71, 72i, 73
  lower airway in, 68, 69i, 70, 70i
  lungs in, 70-71
  neurochemical control of ventilation and, 74
  upper airway in, 68, 69i
Reticular formation, 122
Reticuloendothelial cells, 315
Retinal detachment, 505t
Retinitis pigmentosa, 505t
Retrograde pyelography in hydronephrosis, 296
Revascularization therapy, 55
Reye's syndrome, 505t

Rhabdomyolysis, 238-240
Rheumatic fever, 61-64
Rheumatic heart disease, 61-64
    sequelae of, 61-63, 62i
Rheumatoid arthritis, 360-364
    effects of, on joints, 363i
    stages of joint inflammation in, 361-362
Rheumatoid factor, 361
Rhinitis, types of, 344
Rhinitis medicamentosa, 344
Ribavirin, 382
Robertsonian translocation, 449
Rocky Mountain spotted fever, 505t
Rotational ablation, 33
Rotational atherectomy, 33
Rubella, 382-384
    immunization against, 384
Rubeola, 99t

S

Salmonellosis, 384-386
    as opportunistic disease, 351t
Salvage therapy for multiple myeloma, 424
Sarcoidosis, 506t
Scabies, 506t
Sclerotherapy, 182
Secondarily generalized seizure, 136
Secretory immunity, 70
Seizures, 133-138. See also Status epilepticus.
    electrical impulses in, 135i
    types of, 136
Selye's General Adaptation Model, 12i, 13
Senile osteoporosis, 235
Sensory seizure, 136
Severe acute respiratory syndrome, 110-112
    pathophysiology of, 110, 111i
Sex-linked inheritance, 439-442, 440i, 441i
Shingles, 373-375, 374i
    as opportunistic disease, 354t
Shock lung, 75-78
Shunting, ineffective gas exchange and, 72i, 73
Sickle cell anemia, 457-461, 458i
Sickle cell crisis, 458-459, 459i
    types of, 460-461

Sigmoidoscopy
    in Crohn's disease, 186
    in irritable bowel syndrome, 196
    in ulcerative colitis, 206
Silent unit, ineffective gas exchange and, 72i, 73
Simple partial seizure, 135i, 136
Single-gene disorders, 437-442, 446-448,
        451-462
Sjögren's syndrome, 506t
Skin testing
    in asthma, 88
    in tuberculosis, 114
Sliding hiatal hernia, 192
Small intestine, 168i, 170-171
Somatic nervous system, 124, 125
Sphincter of Oddi, 170
Spinal cord, 122-124, 123i
Spinal nerves, 124
Spleen, 340
Splenectomy, 331, 335
Spontaneous pneumothorax, 101, 102-103
Sporadic Alzheimer's disease, 126. See also
        Alzheimer's disease.
Stalevo, 156
Staphylococcal pneumonia, 99t
Status epilepticus, 134
Stem cell, 314
Stenosis in valvular disease, 18
Stiff lung, 75-78
Stomach, 168i, 169-170
Stone dissolution therapy, 179
Strabismus, 506t
Streptococcal pneumonia, 99t
Stress
    disease and, 12-13, 12i
    homeostasis and, 8
Striations, 213
Stroke, 156-163
    classifying, 157
    completed, 157
    embolism as cause of, 158, 159i, 160
    hemorrhage as cause of, 160
    neurologic deficits in, 161t
    progressive, 157
    risk factors for, 158
    thrombosis as cause of, 158, 159i, 160
    transient ischemic attack and, 157

t refers to a table; i refers to an illustration.

Stroke-in-evolution, 157
Subacute thyroiditis, 268
Subarachnoid space, 120
Subclinical identification, 7-8
Subdural space, 120
Suppressor T cells, 341
Surfactant, 71
Sympathetic nervous system, 125
Synovial fluid, 220
Systemic lupus erythematosus, 357-360
    drugs that trigger, 359
    predisposing factors for, 359

T

Tay-Sachs disease, 461-462
T cells, 340, 341
Temporal lobe, 121i
Tendons, 220
Tensilon test, 152
Tension pneumothorax, 100, 101, 102i, 103
Testicular cancer, 429-432, 430i
    staging, 431i
Thalamus, 121-122
Thrombocytes. *See* Platelets.
Thrombocythemia, 506t
Thrombocytopathy, 319
Thrombocytopenia, 319, 334-335
Thrombocytosis, 319
Thrombolytic therapy, 163
Thrombophlebitis, 507t
Thrombosis as cause of stroke, 158, 159i, 160
Thrombus formation, 108
Thrombus-in-evolution, 157
Thrush as opportunistic disease, 352t
Thymus, 340
Thyroid gland, 248-249
    disorders of, 265-276
Thyroid hormone replacement, 267, 275
Thyroid-stimulating hormone, 244
Thyroid-stimulating hormone–secreting pitu-
        itary tumor, 268
Thyroid storm, 269, 272
Thyrotoxic crisis, 269, 272
Thyrotoxicosis. *See* Hyperthyroidism.
Thyrotoxicosis factitia, 268
Thyroxine, 248

Tinel's sign, 224
Tonsils, 340
Tophaceous gout, 225
Tophi, 225-226, 226i
Toxic adenoma, 268
Toxic injury to cell, 6
Toxoplasmosis, 386-388
    as opportunistic disease, 353t
Transient ischemic attack, 157
Transjugular intrahepatic portosystemic
        shunt, 182
Translocation, 443-444
Transmyocardial revascularization, 33
Traumatic pneumothorax, 101, 102-103
Trigeminal neuralgia, 507t
Triiodothyronine, 248
Trisomy, 442
Trisomy 21, 449-451, 450i
Tuberculosis, 112-115
    as opportunistic disease, 351t
    pathophysiology of, 113, 114i
Tumors, hormone secretion and, 246
Typhoid fever, 384-386

U

Ulcerative colitis, 203-206
    mucosal changes in, 204, 205i
Ultrasonography
    in abdominal aortic aneurysm, 24
    in cholecystitis, 178
    in Cushing's syndrome, 255
    in hydronephrosis, 296
    in pancreatitis, 199
    in renal calculi, 302
Uremia, 306
Ureters, 279, 280i
Urethra, 281
Urinary bladder, 279
Urine
    collection and excretion of, 279, 281
    components of, 279
Uterine cancer. *See* Endometrial cancer.

V

Vaginitis as opportunistic disease, 352t
Varicella pneumonia, 99t

i refers to an illustration; t refers to a table.

Vasopressin, aqueous, 258
Ventilation-perfusion ratio, 71, 72i, 73
Vesicle, 372, 372i
Viral hepatitis, 207-210
    stages of, 209
    types of, 207, 208t
Viral pneumonia, 97-98, 99t. *See also*
        Pneumonia.
Viruses, 368
Vitamin D regulation, 285
Vitiligo, 507t

W

Waste collection, kidneys and, 283
Werlhof's disease, 329-331
Wet lung, 75-78
White blood cells, 315
    disorders of, 318-319
White lung, 75-78
Wilson's disease, 507t

XY

X-linked inheritance, 439-442, 440i, 441i
X-ray. *See also* Chest X-ray.
    in abdominal aortic aneurysm, 24
    in cholecystitis, 178
    in chronic renal failure, 310
    in cirrhosis, 183
    in Crohn's disease, 185
    in diverticular disease, 188
    in gastroesophageal reflux disease, 191
    in gout, 228
    in meningitis, 146
    in osteoarthritis, 230
    in osteomyelitis, 234
    in osteoporosis, 237
    in pancreatitis, 199
    in peptic ulcer, 203
    in prostatitis, 299
    in rheumatoid arthritis, 364

Z

Zona as opportunistic disease, 354t
Zoster as opportunistic disease, 354t

t refers to a table; i refers to an illustration.

Notes

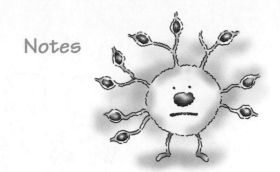

Notes

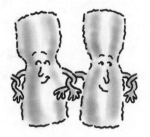

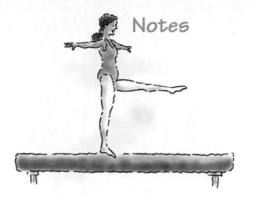

Notes

Notes